PAIN
MANAGEMENT
SECRETS

PAIN MANAGEMENT SECRETS

RONALD KANNER, MD

Chairman, Department of Neurology
Long Island Jewish Medical Center
New Hyde Park, New York
Associate Professor of Neurology
Albert Einstein College of Medicine
Bronx, New York

HANLEY & BELFUS, INC./ Philadelphia

Publisher: HANLEY & BELFUS, INC.
                    Medical Publishers
                    210 South 13th Street
                    Philadelphia, PA 19107
                    (215) 546-7293; 800-962-1892
                    FAX (215) 790-9330

United States sales and distribution:

                    MOSBY
                    11830 Westline Industrial Drive
                    St. Louis, MO 63146

Library of Congress Cataloging-in-Publication Data

Pain Management Secrets / [edited by] Ronald Kanner.
        p.   cm. – (The Secrets Series®)
    Includes bibliographical references and index.
    ISBN 1-56053-160-6 (alk. paper)
    1. Pain–Miscellanea.   2. Analgesia–Miscellanea.
  I. Kanner, Ronald, 1947-.   II. Series.
    [DNLM: 1. Pain–Therapy-examination questions.
WL 18.2 P144 1997]
RB127.P33239 1997
  616'.0472–dc21
  DNLM/DLC
  for Library of Congress   96-49764
                                                                     CIP

PAIN MANAGEMENT SECRETS   ISBN 1-56053-160-6

Last digit is the print number: 9 8 7 6 5 4 3 2 1

CONTENTS

IV. SYNDROMES IN WHICH PAIN IS A SIGNIFICANT COMPONENT

V. PSYCHOLOGICAL SYNDROMES

VI. SPECIAL PATIENT POPULATIONS

VII. PHARMACOLOGIC MANAGEMENT

VIII. NONPHARMACOLOGIC MANAGEMENT

CONTRIBUTORS

Zahid H. Bajwa, M.D.
Director of Education, Pain Management Center, Harvard Medical School; Beth Israel Hospital, Boston, Massachusetts

Allan Basbaum, Ph.D.
Professor, Department of Anatomy and W.M. Keck Center for Integrative Neuroscience, University of California, San Francisco, San Francisco, California

Susanne Bennett Clark, Ph.D.
Associate Professor, Research Medicine and Physiology, New York Medical College, Valhalla, New York

Martin R. Boorin, D.M.D.
Section Head, Dental Anesthesiology, Department of Dental Medicine, Long Island Jewish Medical Center, New Hyde Park, New York

James N. Campbell, M.D.
Professor, Department of Neurosurgery; Director, Blaustein Pain Treatment Center, Johns Hopkins University School of Medicine, Baltimore, Maryland

Mark David Canning, M.D.
Clinical and Research Fellow in Pain Management, Harvard Medical School; Beth Israel Hospital, Boston, Massachusetts

Meir Chernofsky, M.D.
Department of Anesthesiology, Long Island Jewish Medical Center, New Hyde Park, New York

W. Crawford Clark, Ph.D.
Professor of Psychology in Psychiatry, College of Physicians and Surgeons, Columbia University; Research Scientist VI, New York State Psychiatric Institute, New York, New York

Ellen Cooper, M.S.
Administrative Manager, Department of Neurology, Long Island Jewish Medical Center, New Hyde Park, New York

Robert A. Duarte, M.D.
Co-Medical Director, Pain and Headache Treatment Center, Long Island Jewish Medical Center, New Hyde Park, New York; Assistant Professor, Department of Neurology, Albert Einstein College of Medicine, Bronx, New York

Gilbert R. Gonzales, M.D.
Assistant Professor of Neurology, Mayo Medical School, Mayo Clinic Scottsdale, Scottsdale, Arizona

Helen Greco, M.D.
Assistant Professor, Department of Obstetrics and Gynecology, Albert Einstein College of Medicine, Bronx, New York

Ronald Greenberg, M.D.
Associate Professor of Clinical Medicine, Albert Einstein College of Medicine, Bronx, New York; Department of Medicine, Long Island Jewish Hospital, New Hyde Park, New York

Michael Hanania, M.D.
Assistant Professor of Anesthesiology, Albert Einstein College of Medicine, Bronx, New York; Department of Anesthesiology, Long Island Jewish Medical Center, New Hyde Park, New York

Nelson H. Hendler, M.D., M.S.
Clinical Director, Mensana Clinic, Stevenson, Maryland

Brian Kahan, D.O.
Clinical Instructor, Department of Rehabilitation Medicine, Montefiore Medical Center, Albert Einstein College of Medicine, Bronx, New York

Ronald Kanner, M.D.
Chairman, Department of Neurology, Long Island Jewish Medical Center, New Hyde Park, New York;
Associate Professor of Neurology, Albert Einstein College of Medicine, Bronx, New York

Abbas Kashani, M.D.
Long Island Jewish Medical Center, New Hyde Park, New York

Richard B. Lipton, M.D.
Professor of Neurology, Epidemiology, and Social Medicine, Albert Einstein College of Medicine; Co-
Director, Headache Unit, Montefiore Medical Center, Bronx, New York

Patricia A. McGrath, Ph.D.
Professor of Paediatrics, Child Health Research Institute, The University of Western Ontario; Director,
Pediatric Pain Program, Children's Hospital of Western Ontario, London, Ontario, Canada

Lawrence C. Newman, M.D.
Assistant Professor of Neurology, Albert Einstein College of Medicine, Bronx, New York; Director,
Headache Unit, Montefiore Medical Center, Bronx, New York

David S. Pisetsky, M.D., Ph.D.
Professor of Medicine, Duke University Medical Center, Durham, North Carolina; Chief of
Rheumatology, Allergy, and Clinical Immunology, Durham VA Hospital, Duke University Medical
Center, Durham, North Carolina

Russell K. Portenoy, M.D.
Co-Chief, Pain and Palliative Care Service, Memorial Sloan-Kettering Cancer Center; Associate
Professor of Neurology, Cornell University Medical College, New York, New York

Jill T. Silverman, M.A.
Pain and Headache Treatment Center, Long Island Jewish Medical Center, New Hyde Park, New York

Jason E. Silvers, M.D.
Johns Hopkins University School of Medicine, Baltimore, Maryland

Brian Thiessen, M.D.
Fellow, Department of Neurology, Memorial Sloan-Kettering Cancer, New York, New York

Mark A. Thomas, M.D.
Assistant Professor, Department of Rehabilitation Medicine, Albert Einstein College of Medicine,
Montefiore Medical Center, Bronx, New York

Dennis R. Thornton, Ph.D.
Assistant Professor of Psychology, Albert Einstein College of Medicine, Bronx, New York; Attending
Psychologist, Long Island Jewish Medical Center, New Hyde Park, New York

Carol A. Warfield, M.D.
Associate Professor of Anaesthesia, Harvard Medical School, Boston, Massachusetts; Chief, Division
of Pain Medicine, Beth Israel Hospital, Boston, Massachusetts

DEDICATION

To Ellen,
   Without whose support, wisdom, advice, and *nudzhing*, this volume would never have been completed.

PREFACE

The relief of pain and suffering is one of the most important tasks a physician can undertake. In many cases, the underlying cause of pain cannot be relieved (or even found), and management becomes the goal. Adequate pain management requires an understanding of pain mechanisms, appropriate assessment of pain syndromes, and a judicious selection of treatment modalities.

In *Pain Management Secrets*, clinicians and scientists from a number of disciplines, including the neurosciences, anesthesiology, psychiatry, psychology, neurosurgery, and rehabilitative medicine, have distilled decades of work into clear questions and answers. This book is not meant to be a comprehensive text on pain management or a handbook to guide practitioners through each step of management. Rather it is hoped that these questions and vignettes, representing the approach of experienced workers on specific topics, will stimulate the reader to look deeper into the problems of pain and suffering and to attack them with the same vigor that would be given to a life-threatening disease.

Ronald Kanner, M.D.
New Hyde Park, New York

I. Overview

1. DEFINITIONS

Ronald Kanner, M.D.

1. What is pain?

The International Association for the Study of Pain (IASP) defines pain as "an unpleasant sensory and emotional experience associated with actual or potential tissue damage, or described in terms of such damage." This definition may appear somewhat convoluted, but it states explicitly that pain always has a subjective component. It is both a physiologic sensation and an emotional reaction to that sensation. Another functional definition of pain is "whatever the patient says hurts."

2. What is the difference between pain and suffering?

Pain is a sensation plus a reaction to that sensation. Suffering is a more global concept. It is an overall negative feeling that impairs the sufferer's quality of life. Both physical and psychological issues are at play in suffering, and pain may be only a small component.

3. What is the difference between impairment and disability?

Impairment is a medical concept, and disability is a legal or societal concept. Impairment is any loss or abnormality of psychological, physiologic, or anatomic structure or function. According to the World Health Organization (WHO) definition, disability results from impairment; it is any restriction or lack of ability to perform an activity in the manner or within the range considered normal for a human. In governmental terms, disability is sometimes called a functional limitation. Another definition of disability is a disadvantage (resulting from an impairment or functional limitation) that limits or prevents the fulfillment of a role that is normal for an individual (depending on age, sex, social and cultural factors). This definition corresponds to the WHO classification of handicap.

4. What is meant by a pathophysiologic classification of pain?

Pathophysiologic classification implies that we understand the basic mechanisms underlying a pain syndrome. It has its functional utility in that it differentiates nociceptive and nonnociceptive syndromes (see Chapter 2). Pathophysiologic classification may be overly self-serving, because we can only infer, and rarely verify, the true mechanism.

5. What is nociception?

Nociception is the perception of a potentially tissue-damaging stimulus. It is the first step in the pain pathway.

6. What is a nociceptor?

A nociceptor is a neurologic receptor that is capable of differentiating between innocuous and noxious stimuli. In humans, nociceptors are the undifferentiated terminals of a-delta and c-fibers, which are the thinnest myelinated and unmyelinated fibers, respectively. A-delta fibers are also called high-threshold mechanoreceptors. They respond primarily to mechanical stimuli of noxious intensity.

7. What is the difference between pain threshold and pain tolerance?

Pain threshold refers to the lowest intensity at which a given stimulus is perceived as painful; it is relatively constant across subjects for a given stimulus. For example, most subjects will define a thermal stimulus as painful when it reaches about 50°C. Similarly, barring disease states, mechanical pressure produces pain at about the same amount of pressure across subjects. Pain tolerance, on the other hand, is the greatest level of pain that a subject is prepared to endure. Tolerance varies much more widely across subjects and depends on prescribed medications. Clinically, pain tolerance is of much more importance than pain threshold. More detailed discussions of threshold and tolerance are found in the chapter on Pain Measurement.

8. You touch an apparently normal area of skin and the patient jumps with pain. Why?

Allodynia is an abnormal circumstance in which a nonnoxious stimulus is perceived as painful. It is common in many neuropathic pain conditions, such as postherpetic neuralgia, chronic regional pain syndrome, and certain peripheral neuropathies. In cases of neuropathic pain, the underlying skin may appear normal. When skin is sensitized by a burn, a light touch may be painful, but the skin is obviously abnormal.

9. What is meant by analgesia?

Analgesia is the absence of pain in response to a normally noxious stimulus. It is conceptually the opposite of allodynia. Analgesia can be produced peripherally (at the site of tissue damage, receptor, or nerve) or centrally (in the spinal cord or brain). In general, the nonsteroidal antiinflammatory drugs and other minor analgesics act at the site of tissue damage, whereas opioids and adjuvant drugs act at the spinal cord or cerebral level.

10. What is meant by paresthesia?

A paresthesia is any abnormal sensation. It may be spontaneous or evoked. The most common paresthesia is the sense of "pins and needles" when a nerve in a limb is compressed. The limb "falls asleep." Paresthesias are not always painful.

11. What is a dysesthesia?

A dysesthesia is a painful paresthesia. By definition, the sensation is unpleasant. Examples include the burning feet that may be felt in alcoholic peripheral neuropathy or the spontaneous pain in the thigh felt in diabetic amyotrophy.

12. What is hypoesthesia?

Hypoesthesia is decreased sensitivity to stimulation. Essentially, it is an area of relative numbness and may be due to any kind of nerve injury. Areas of hypoesthesia obviously result therapeutically from local infiltrations of anesthetics.

13. What is anesthesia dolorosa? Give some examples.

Anesthesia dolorosa occurs when pain is felt in an area that is otherwise numb or desensitized. It commonly occurs after partial nerve lesions and is a relatively common complication of radiofrequency coagulation of the trigeminal nerve. Patients with intractable trigeminal neuralgia are sometimes treated by percutaneous radiofrequency lesioning of the nerve (see Chapter 17). In a certain percentage of patients, the original trigeminal neuralgia pain is replaced by spontaneous pain in a now denervated area.

14. What is meant by neuralgia?

Neuralgia is a clinically descriptive term, meaning pain in the distribution of a nerve or nerves. The condition described as sciatica is considered to be neuralgia of either the sciatic nerve or the S1 nerve root. Trigeminal neuralgia, one of the most common primary neuralgias, is characterized by a jabbing pain in one or more of the distributions of the trigeminal nerve. Neuralgic pain is fairly characteristic: it is an electrical, shocklike pain.

15. What is hyperpathia?

Hyperpathia literally implies too much pain. The term refers to an abnormally intense painful response to repetitive stimuli. Usually, the hyperpathic area of skin is not sensitive to a simple stimulus but overresponds to multiple stimuli. For example, a single pin prick may not be felt, but repetitive pin pricks produce intense pain. Hyperpathia is sometimes called summation dysesthesia.

16. What are algogenic substances?

Algogenic substances, when released from injured tissues or injected subcutaneously, activate or sensitize nociceptors. Histamines, substance P, potassium, and prostaglandins are thought to be algogenic substances.

17. What is meant by sensitization?

Sensitization is a state in which a peripheral receptor or a central neuron responds either to stimuli in a more intense fashion than it would under baseline conditions or to a stimulus to which it would normally be insensitive. Sensitization occurs both at the level of the nociceptor in the periphery and at the level of the second order neuron in the spinal cord (see the chapter on Basic Mechanisms). In the periphery, tissue injury may convert a high-threshold mechanoreceptor (which normally would respond only to noxious mechanical stimuli) into a receptor that responds to gentle stimuli as though they were noxious. Centrally, the second-order neurons (those on which the primary afferents synapse) also may become hyperexcitable. When spinal cord neurons are hyperexcitable, they may fire spontaneously, giving rise to spontaneous pain. This is typically the case after deafferentation.

18. What is deafferentation?

Deafferentation implies the loss of normal input from primary sensory neurons. It may occur after any type of peripheral nerve injury. Deafferentation is particularly common in postherpetic neuralgia and in traumatic nerve injuries. The central neuron on which the primary afferent was to synapse may become hyperexcitable.

19. What is the gate control theory of pain?

The basic premises of the gate control theory of pain are that activity in large (nonnociceptive) fibers can inhibit the perception of activity in small (nociceptive) fibers and that descending activity from the brain also can inhibit that perception. Given this construct, it is easy to understand why deafferentation may cause pain. If the large fibers are preferentially injured, the normal inhibition of pain perception does not occur.

20. What is meant by incident pain?

Incident pain is pain of sudden onset that may occur in a patient with chronic pain or in a patient who is otherwise pain-free. There are two major types. The first is expected incident pain, in which a patient has a bone metastasis or other lesion and knows that movement or weight-bearing will produce pain. The second type is unexpected and may arise from expansion of a hollow viscus or other medical complication.

21. What is tabetic pain?

Tabetic pain was first described in tabes dorsalis, a complication of syphilis. It is a sharp, lightning type of pain. Also called lancinating pain, it is one of the more common neuropathic pains.

22. What is central pain?

The term central pain is applied when the generator of the pain is believed to be in the spinal cord or the brain. The original insult may have been peripheral (nerve injury or postherpetic neuralgia), but the pain is sustained by central mechanisms. The basic process may be central sensitization. Central pain also may occur after central injuries, such as strokes or spinal cord injuries. Pain tends to be poorly localized and of a burning nature.

23. What is meant by referred pain?

Pain in an area removed from the site of tissue injury is called referred pain. The most common examples are pain in the shoulder from myocardial infarction, pain in the back from pancreatic disease, and pain in the right shoulder from gallbladder disease. The presumed mechanism is that afferent fibers from the site of tissue injury enter the spinal cord at a similar level to afferents from the point to which the pain is referred. This conjoint area in the spinal cord results in the mistaken perception that the pain arises from the referral site.

24. What is phantom pain?

Phantom pain is pain felt in a part of the body that has been surgically removed. It is common for patients to have phantom sensation postoperatively; that is, after limb amputation, the patient feels as though the limb were still present. This sensation occurs in nearly all patients undergoing amputation. It usually subsides over days to weeks. A small percentage of patients develop true phantom limb pain, which may be extraordinarily persistent and resistant to treatment.

25. What is meralgia paresthetica?

Meralgia paresthetica is a syndrome of tingling discomfort (dysesthesias) in an area of nerve injury, most commonly the lateral femoral cutaneous nerve. It is characterized by a patch of decreased sensation over the lateral thigh; this area is dysesthetic. Meralgia paresthetica may be due to more proximal nerve compression.

26. What is meant by fast and slow pain?

Fast pain is a relatively localized, well-defined pain that is carried in the neospinothalamic tract. Slow pain is more diffuse and poorly localized and presumed to be carried in the paleospinothalamic tract.

27. What is formication?

Formication is a form of paresthesia in which the patient feels as though bugs were crawling on the body. It is a common hallucinatory sensation in patients with delirium tremens.

28. What is the difference between primary and secondary pain syndromes?

In primary pain syndromes, the pain itself is the disease. Examples include migraine, trigeminal neuralgia, and cluster headache. A secondary pain syndrome is due to an underlying structural cause; for example, trigeminal neuralgia due to a tumor pressing on the cranial nerve. One of the major issues in any primary pain syndrome is to exclude an underlying destructive cause (tumor or infection).

BIBLIOGRAPHY

1. Merskey N, Bogduk N (eds): Classification of Chronic Pain. Task Force on Taxonomy, 2nd ed. Seattle, IASP Press, 1994.
2. Pain and Disability: Clinical, Behavioral and Public Policy Perspectives. Washington, DC, Institute of Medicine, National Academy Press, 1987.
3. Portenoy RK, Kanner RM: Definition and assessment of pain. In Portenoy RK, Kanner RM (eds): Pain Management: Theory and Practice. Philadelphia, F.A. Davis, 1996, pp 3–18.

2. CLASSIFICATION OF PAIN

Robert A. Duarte, M.D.

1. What are the most widely used classifications for pain?

The most recognized categories are based on inferred neurophysiologic mechanisms, temporal aspects, etiology, or region affected.

2. What is the neurophysiologic classification of pain?

This classification is based on the inferred mechanism for pain. There are essentially two types: nociceptive and nonnociceptive. Nociceptive pain can be subdivided into somatic or visceral and nonnociceptive into neuropathic and psychogenic.

3. What is nociceptive pain?

Nociceptive pain results from the activation of nociceptors (A delta and C fibers) by noxious stimuli that may be mechanical, thermal, or chemical. Nociceptors may be sensitized by endogenous chemical stimuli (algogenic substances) such as serotonin, substance P, bradykinin, prostaglandin, and histamine. The nervous system is intact and perceives noxious stimuli appropriately.

4. Under normal circumstances, where are algogenic substances found?

Serotonin, histamine, K^+, H^+, prostaglandins, and other members of the arachidonic acid cascade are in tissues; kinins are in plasma; and substance P is in nerve terminals of primary afferents. Histamine is found in the granules of mast cells, in basophils, and in platelets. Serotonin is present in mast cells and platelets.

Yaksh TL., Hammond DL: Peripheral and central substrates in the rostrar transmission of nociceptive information. Pain 13:1, 1982.

5. How do patients describe pain of somatic nociceptive origin?

Usually as a dull or achy sensation. It may be exacerbated by movement (incident pain) and relieved upon rest. It is well localized and consonant with the underlying lesion. Examples of somatic nociceptive pain include metastatic bone pain, postsurgical pain, musculoskeletal pain, and pain from arthritis.

6. How do patients describe pain of visceral nociceptive origin?

Pain arising from distention of a hollow organ is usually poorly localized, deep, squeezing, and crampy. It is often associated with autonomic sensations, including nausea, vomiting, and diaphoresis. There are often cutaneous referral sites (e.g., heart to the shoulder or jaw, gallbladder to the scapula, and pancreas to the back). Examples of visceral nociceptive pain include pancreatic cancer, intestinal obstruction, and intraperitoneal metastasis.

7. What is meant by neuropathic pain?

Neural injury or irritation is the source of pain. It persists long after the precipitating event and may be due to abnormal central sensitization (see Chapter 27).

8. How do patients describe pain of neuropathic origin?

The most common descriptors are burning or stabbing pains. Innocuous stimuli may be perceived as painful (allodynia). Patients often complain of paroxysms of electrical sensations (lancinating or lightning pains). Examples of neuropathic pain include trigeminal neuralgia, postherpetic neuralgia, and peripheral neuropathy.

9. What are examples of deafferentation pain?

Deafferentation pain is a subdivision of neuropathic pain that may complicate virtually any type of injury to the somatosensory system at any point along its course. Examples include well-defined syndromes precipitated by peripheral (phantom-limb) or central (thalamic pain) lesions. In all of these conditions, pain usually occurs in a region of clinical sensory loss. With phantom-limb pain, the pain is actually felt in an area that no longer exists. Patients with thalamic pain, also known as Dejerine-Roussy syndrome, report pain in all or part of the region of clinical sensory loss.

10. What is reflex sympathetic dystrophy (RSD)?

This term was originally coined to denote a diverse group of neuropathic disorders that shared several features: precipitation by trauma, persistent dysesthetic pains, local autonomic dysregulation (edema, vasomotor disturbances, sweating abnormalities), and local trophic changes. It was believed to be due to sympathetic hyperactivity, and many patients obtained transient relief from sympathetic blockade (see Chapter 36).

11. What is the difference between RSD and causalgia?

According to the International Association for the Study of Pain (IASP), reflex sympathetic dystrophy (more recently known as complex regional pain syndrome, or CRPS) is defined as "continuous pain in a portion of an extremity after trauma which may include fracture but does not involve a major nerve associated with sympathetic hyperactivity." The IASP considers causalgia, or CRPS 2, a separate entity defined as "burning pain, allodynia, and hyperpathia, usually in the foot or hand, after partial injury of a nerve or one of its major branches."

12. What is meant by psychogenic pain?

Psychogenic pain is presumed to exist when no nociceptive or neuropathic mechanism can be identified and there are sufficient psychologic symptoms to meet criteria for somatoform pain disorder, depression, or other DSM-IV diagnostic category commonly associated with complaints of pain.

13. What is the advantage of classifying pain?

It provides the clinician with invaluable information about the possible origin of the pain. More important, it directs the health care practitioner toward a proper pharmacologic treatment plan. For example, neuropathic pain syndromes generally respond to adjuvant medications such as tricyclic antidepressants and anticonvulsants. In nociceptive pain states, the implementation of NSAIDs alone or in combination with opioids is the mainstay.

14. What is the temporal classification of pain, and what are its shortcomings?

The temporal classification of pain is based on the time course of symptoms and is usually divided into acute, chronic, and recurrent. The major shortcoming is that the division between acute and chronic is arbitrary.

15. Define acute pain.

Acute pain is temporally related to injury and resolves during the appropriate healing period. It often responds to treatment with analgesic medications and treatment of the precipitating cause.

16. Define chronic pain.

Chronic pain is often defined as pain that persists for more than three months or that outlasts the usual healing process. Some authors choose six months as a cutoff. Chronic pain serves no useful biologic purpose. In some cases, psychologic factors play a significant role.

17. What is meant by an etiologic classification?

This classification pays more attention to the primary disease process in which pain occurs, rather than to the pathophysiology or temporal pattern. Examples include cancer pain, arthritis pain, and pain in sickle cell disease. Therapeutically, it is less useful than a pathophysiologic classification.

18. What is the basis of the regional classification of pain?

The regional classification is strictly topographic and does not infer pathophysiology or etiology. It is defined by the part of the body affected, then subdivided into acute and chronic.

BIBLIOGRAPHY

1. Bonica JJ: Definitions and taxonomy of pain. In Bonica JJ (ed): The Management of Pain. Philadelphia, Lea & Febiger, 1990.
2. International Classification of Diseases, 10th ed. Geneva, WHO, 1992.
3. Merskey H, Bogduk N (eds): Classification of Chronic Pain.Task Force on Taxonomy, 2nd ed. Seattle, IASP Press, 1994.

3. BASIC MECHANISMS: ANATOMY AND PHYSIOLOGY OF NOCICEPTION

Allan Basbaum, Ph.D.

1. What are nociceptors?

Nociceptors are neurons that respond to noxious thermal, mechanical, or chemical stimulation. They can distinguish noxious from innocuous stimuli. Some respond only to noxious stimuli, and others have graded responses, increasing their firing rate when stimuli reach noxious intensity. The term is used for both peripheral and central neurons. However, since the receptor is located in the periphery, the term is best associated with small myelinated (A delta) and unmyelinated (C) fiber primary afferent neurons. In the central nervous system (spinal cord), neurons that respond to noxious stimulation are considered nociresponsive.

2. What properties characterize A delta and C fibers?

A delta are small diameter (1 to 5 μm) myelinated primary afferent fibers; C fibers are very small in diameter (< 1 μm) unmyelinated primary afferent fibers. The A delta fibers conduct at velocities between 5 and 25 m/sec; C fibers conduct at 0.5 to 2 m/sec. A major component of the C fibers are polymodal nociceptors, which respond to thermal, mechanical, and chemical noxious stimulation. Other primary afferent nociceptors respond more selectively to noxious thermal or mechanical stimulation. It is unclear whether there are specific neurotransmitters associated with the modality subtypes of A delta and C fibers.

3. What physiologic characteristics differentiate thin fibers from large?

The thinner a fiber is, the more slowly it conducts. Thinner fibers are less sensitive to electrical stimuli. This may be part of the mechanism that underlies transcutaneous electrical nerve stimulation (TENS): through activation of inhibitory circuits in the spinal cord, activation of large-diameter fibers can inhibit the central transmission of messages generated by small-diameter nociceptive afferents, resulting in the reduction of pain. Small fibers are more sensitive to local anesthetics, so differential anesthetic blocks can be performed: sympathetic fibers are blocked before nociceptors, nociceptors before light mechanoreceptors, and light mechanoreceptors before motor nerves.

4. What are the characteristics of the dorsal root?

The dorsal root is the point of spinal cord entry of sensory afferents, the cell bodies of which reside in the dorsal root ganglion. The thinner fibers tend to be more lateral in the root, with the myelinated fibers located more medially. When rhizotomy (sectioning of the dorsal root) is performed for pain control, an attempt is made to section the lateral part of the root preferentially, thus destroying the nociceptors and sparing the fibers that subserve light touch.

5. What is sensitization, and how does it occur?

Sensitization refers to the phenomenon in which a receptor or cell responds to stimuli that would normally be below its threshold. In the periphery, release of substance P may lead to sensitization of nociceptors. In the spinal cord, dorsal horn neurons may become sensitized after prolonged pain or after peripheral nerve injury. This central sensitization is probably mediated through the N-methyl-D-aspartate (NMDA) receptor.

6. Distinguish between first and second pain.

First and second pain refers to the immediate and delayed pain responses to noxious stimulation. Other terms are "fast" and "slow" pain or sharp/pricking and dull/burning pain. The stimuli that generate first pain are transmitted by A delta fibers. Second pain results from activation of C fibers, which conduct impulses much more slowly, thus accounting for the timing difference.

7. Where do nociceptive fibers enter the spinal cord?

Nociceptive primary afferent fibers have their cell bodies in dorsal root ganglia. The central branches of these afferents enter the spinal cord via the tract of Lissauer. The central branches terminate predominantly in the superficial laminae of the dorsal horn, including lamina I (the marginal zone) and lamina II (the substantia gelatinosa). Some A delta primary afferent nociceptors also terminate more ventrally, in the region of lamina V and around the central canal. The fact that the level of analgesia observed following anterolateral cordotomy may be up to two segments below the segment at which the cordotomy was performed is presumed to reflect the anatomic course of axons in Lissauer's tract; some small diameter primary afferents ascend the spinal cord one to two segments in Lissauer's tract, ipsilaterally, before entering the spinal cord and synapsing on dorsal horn neurons, including cells at the origin of the spinothalamic and spinoreticular pathways.

8. What is the first synapse in the spinal cord?

There is a differential projection of small and large diameter primary afferent fibers to the spinal cord dorsal horn. The largest diameter Ia primary afferents arise from muscle spindles and make monosynaptic connection with motoneurons in the ventral horn. Large diameter, nonnociceptive primary afferents synapse on neurons in lamina IV that are at the origin of the spinocervical tract and on wide dynamic range neurons in lamina V. Small diameter nociceptive A delta and C fibers arborize most densely in the superficial dorsal horn. The C fibers predominantly synapse with neurons in lamina I; they also synapse on dorsally directed dendrites of neurons located more ventrally (e.g., in lamina V). In addition, there are connections with interneurons in the substantia gelatinosa.

9. What is meant by a second-order neuron?

Second-order neuron refers to all of the neurons that receive input from the primary afferent fibers. They are also the cells of origin of the ascending spinal sensory tracts. This includes interneurons and projection neurons. Second-order neurons are also located in the dorsal column nuclei; these receive input from large primary afferent fibers that ascend to the medulla via the dorsal/posterior columns. Many second-order neurons receive convergent input from small diameter nociceptive primary afferents and from large diameter nonnociceptive primary afferent fibers. It may be the balance of input that determines the quality of the sensation.

10. What is meant by a wide dynamic range neuron?

Wide dynamic range refers to neurons in the spinal cord that respond to a large range of intensity of stimulation; for example, neurons in lamina V that respond to nonnoxious brushing of the cell's receptive field as well as to intense mechanical stimulation and to noxious heat. Many wide dynamic range neurons also receive a visceral afferent input. By contrast, nociceptive-specific neurons respond exclusively to an intensity in the noxious range. Importantly, all primary afferent fibers are excitatory. Thus, any inhibitory effect that results from stimulation of large diameter fibers (e.g., by vibration) results from an indirect mechanism involving inhibitory interneurons that influence the firing of the wide dynamic range neuron. This inhibition is probably presynaptic.

11. Describe the two major ascending pathways that transmit nociceptive information.

The two major pathways are the spinothalamic tract and the spinoreticular tract. The cell origin of the spinothalamic tract is in the dorsal horn and intermediate gray matter of the spinal cord. Axons of these neurons cross to the anterolateral quadrant and ascend to the thalamus where they synapse on neurons in the lateral thalamus and in the intralaminar nuclei, located more medially. An additional ascending pathway, recently described, arises from neurons in the most superficial lamina of the dorsal horn, lamina I. These neurons project via pathways in the dorsal part of the lateral funiculus and terminate in the rostral brain stem, including the para-brachial nuclei. The output of these neurons would not be cut by the traditional spinothalamic tractotomy/anterolateral cordotomy, which in part may account for the failure of cordotomy and for the return of pain that often occurs.

Paralleling the spinothalamic tract is the spinoreticular pathway. Neurons at the origin of the spinoreticular pathway are abundant in the deeper parts of the dorsal horn and in the ventral horn (laminae VII and VIII). The output of the reticular neurons is predominantly to intralaminar thal-amic nuclei and to the hypothalamus. Thus, the origin of the term spinoreticulothalamic pathway.

12. What are the functional differences between the neospinothalamic and the paleo-spinothalamic tracts?

The neospinothalamic tract refers to the direct spinothalamic axons (a phylogenetically more recently evolved pathway). Many of these neurons, in normal conditions, have small receptive fields and are probably involved in the localization of acute noxious stimuli. By contrast, the paleospinothalamic tract (a phylogenetically older system) refers to the indirect pathway from spinal cord to thalamus (including the spinoreticulothalamic system). The receptive fields of the latter neurons are larger and are thought to contribute to the diffuse nature of clinical types of pain.

13. What are the major neurotransmitters involved in nociception?

Primary afferent nociceptors contain a variety of neurotransmitters, including the excitatory amino acid glutamate and a variety of neuropeptides, including substance P and calcitonin gene-related peptide (CGRP). Glutamate acts on several subtypes of receptors that mediate a rapid de-polarization of dorsal horn neurons, via influx of sodium and efflux of potassium. The NMDA receptor, which gates calcium (in addition to sodium and potassium), is involved in long-term changes in dorsal horn processing that are produced by noxious stimulation. Substance P acti-vates subpopulations of dorsal horn neurons and also contributes to some of the long-term changes produced by persistent injury.

14. What are the major neurotransmitters involved in antinociceptive functions?

Dorsal horn nociception can be regulated both by local inhibitory interneurons and by de-scending inhibitory pathways that arise in the brain stem. The majority of inhibitory interneurons use the neurotransmitters gamma-aminobutyric acid or glycine. These inhibit the firing of dorsal horn nociceptive neurons by both pre- and postsynaptic controls. Other interneurons contain one of the endorphin peptides, enkephalin or dynorphin. These increase potassium conductance, thereby hyperpolarizing neurons. In some cases, they presynaptically block the release of neuro-transmitters from primary afferent fibers by decreasing calcium conductance. The major de-scending inhibitory pathways use either serotonin or norepinephrine. Consistent with the presence of these diverse inhibitory neurotransmitter mechanisms, intrathecal injection of a vari-ety of compounds produces profound antinociceptive effects (e.g., opioids, clonidine). See Chapter 32.

15. What are the clinical and investigational roles of capsaicin?

Capsaicin, the algogenic substance in hot peppers, selectively stimulates primary afferent C fibers. Although selective antagonists to capsaicin have been developed, these do not block pain produced by substances other than capsaicin. Thus, the endogenous ligand for the capsaicin receptor has not been determined. When administered to neonatal animals, capsaicin destroys C fibers; when administered to adults, it produces a long-term desensitization of the C fibers, possibly by depletion of their peptide neurotransmitters, such as substance P. The desensitization is associated with a decreased response to noxious stimulation, which provides a rational basis for the therapeutic use of capsaicin in patients. To date, topical application of capsaicin has shown some promise in the treatment of the pain of postherpetic neuralgia and postmastectomy pain.

16. What is the laminar organization of the dorsal horn of the spinal cord?

The dorsal horn of the spinal cord can be divided into distinct laminae on cytoarchitectural grounds, using traditional cell (Nissl) stains. This anatomic organization is paralleled by a physiologic laminar organization. Neurons in laminae I and II, the substantia gelatinosa, respond exclusively either to noxious stimulation or to both noxious and nonnoxious stimuli. Neurons in laminae III and IV, the nucleus proprius, predominantly respond to nonnoxious stimuli. The majority of neurons in lamina V are of the wide dynamic range type, i.e., they respond to both nonnoxious and noxious stimuli and have visceral afferent inputs. Neurons in lamina VI respond predominantly to nonnoxious manipulation of joints.

17. How is the spinal cord influenced by peripheral nerve injury?

Peripheral nerve injury was originally thought only to functionally disconnect the periphery from the spinal cord. Since the dorsal root ganglion is not injured when the peripheral nerve is damaged, neither anatomic nor biochemical changes in the proximal limb of the dorsal root or in the dorsal horn were expected. Recent studies, however, indicate that there are significant changes in the dorsal root ganglia and in the spinal cord neurons with which they are connected. Among the changes are a significant decrease in the concentration of substance P message and substance P peptide in neurons of the dorsal root ganglia. There are also decreased substance P levels in the terminals of primary afferent fibers in the dorsal horn. Postsynaptic neurons are affected as well, with up-regulation of the opioid peptide, dynorphin, in dorsal horn neurons. The electrophysiologic consequences of peripheral nerve injury are also profound. The injury results in a massive release of glutamate, which acts on NMDA receptors to produce long-term changes in the physiologic properties of the dorsal horn neurons. Sensitization (i.e., hyperexcitability) of dorsal horn neurons in the setting of injury is particularly common and may contribute to postinjury pain states.

18. Provide a plausible explanation for the phenomenon of referred pain.

A very likely explanation relates to the convergence of visceral and somatic afferent input to wide dynamic range neurons of spinal cord lamina V. Thus, increased activity of visceral afferents secondary to injury to viscera is interpreted by the brain as having arisen from the source of the convergent somatic input. It is thus "referred" to the somatic site. Indeed, local anesthetic injection of the site of reference can reduce referred pain, even though the site of injury is clearly in the viscera.

19. What is neurogenic inflammation?

Neurogenic inflammation refers to the inflammation produced through the release of substances from the nervous system, in particular, from small diameter primary afferent fibers. Although most studies emphasize the contribution of the primary afferent C fibers, there is also evidence for a contribution of sympathetic postganglionic terminals. The primary afferents release peptides that act on postcapillary venules. These become leaky, resulting in plasmic extravasation and vasodilatation. Electrical stimulation of peripheral nerves that have been disconnected from the central nervous system can evoke neurogenic inflammation by antidromic activation of C fibers and the resultant release of neuropeptides in the periphery.

20. How is substance P implicated in the phenomenon of neurogenic inflammation?

Cell bodies in the dorsal root ganglion synthesize substance P and send it by axoplasmic transport both to the central (spinal) and peripheral terminals of the primary afferents. Substance P is stored in the periphery and can be released when the terminals are depolarized because of injury. The targets of substance P in the periphery include mast cells, blood vessels, and various immunocompetent cells. In concert with the concurring peptide, CGRP, which produces a profound vasodilatation, substance P significantly increases plasma extravasation from postcapillary venules. The extravasation of protein from vessels is accompanied by fluid, producing the characteristic swelling (tumor) of inflammation. The heat and redness (calor and rubor) of inflammation can be accounted for by neurogenic vasodilatation.

21. What is the contribution of the NMDA receptor to the production of pain?

Glutamate released from primary afferent fibers acts on two major receptor types in the dorsal horn: the AMPA and the NMDA receptors. Under normal conditions, the NMDA receptor is blocked by the presence of a magnesium ion in the channel. When neurons are depolarized, via the glutamate action at the AMPA receptor, the magnesium block is relieved and glutamate action at the NMDA receptor is effective. This results in entry of calcium into the postsynaptic neuron, which, in turn, activates various second-messenger systems that produce long-term biochemical and molecular changes in these neurons. The physiologic consequence of these changes is a hyperexcitability of the dorsal horn neuron manifested as an increase in the size of the receptive field of nociresponsive neurons and decreased threshold. The neuron may become spontaneously active. The allodynia (pain produced by nonnoxious stimuli) and hyperalgesia (exacerbated pain produced by noxious stimuli) associated with nerve injury may reflect NMDA-mediated long-term changes in dorsal horn neuronal processes.

22. Describe the regions of the thalamus that have been implicated in the processing of nociceptive information.

Two major regions of the thalamus have been implicated: the lateral thalamus, including the ventral posterolateral (VPL) and ventral posteromedial (VPM) nuclei; and the intralaminar nuclei of the medial thalamus. The VPL receives input via the spinothalamic tract. It subserves noxious stimuli from the torso and extremities. The VPM receives input via the nucleus caudalis and the principal trigeminal nucleus subserving the face. Stimulation of the lateral thalamus in patients who are not experiencing pain does not produce significant pain. By contrast, in patients who have ongoing pain, electrical stimulation can reproduce pain, suggesting a reorganization of the nociceptive input to thalamus under conditions of persistent injury. The output of the lateral thalamus is largely to the somatosensory cortex. However, connections with the limbic and insular cortex are probably necessary for the affective components of pain. The medial thalamus, including the intralaminar nuclei, receives direct spinothalamic and spinoreticular thalamic projections. Cells in this region have larger receptive fields and are thought to contribute to the diffuse character of pain perception (paleospinothalamic). The cortical connections of the more medial regions of the thalamus are presumed to be involved in the affective component of the pain perception.

23. Is there a cortical representation of pain?

Traditional teaching suggested that the cortex was not necessary for the experience of pain. This was based on clinical studies wherein stimulation rarely produces pain and in which large lesions do not completely disrupt the pain experience. Recent studies, however, using positron emission tomography (PET) have identified several cortical regions activated when humans experience pain (largely in an experimental setting). Among these are the somatosensory cortex, the anterior cingulate gyrus, and the insular cortex. This distributed processing in the cortex probably reflects the complex nature of the pain experience, which includes sensory discriminative, affective, and cognitive aspects. Lesions of any single region thus may not be sufficient to eliminate pain.

BIBLIOGRAPHY

1. Craig AD, Bushnell MC, Zhang ET, et al: A thalamic nucleus specific for pain and temperature sensation. Nature 372:770–773, 1994.
2. Dubner R, Basbaum AI: Spinal dorsal horn plasticity following tissue or nerve injury. In Wall PD, Melzack R (eds): The Textbook of Pain. London, Churchill-Livingstone, 1994, pp 225–241.
3. Hökfelt T, Zhang X, Wiesenfeld HZ: Messenger plasticity in primary sensory neurons following axotomy and its functional implications. Trends Neurosci 17:22–30, 1994.
4. Levine JD, Fields HL, Basbaum AI: Peptides and the primary afferent nociceptor. J Neurosci 13:2273–2286, 1993.
5. Talbot JD, Marrett S, Evans AC, et al: Multiple representations of pain in human cerebral cortex. Science 251:1355–1358, 1991.
6. Wilcox GL: Excitatory neurotransmitters and pain. In Bond MR, Charlton JE, Woolf CJ (eds): Proceedings of the VIth World Congress on Pain. New York, Elsevier Science Publishers, 1991, pp 97–111.

II. Clinical Approach

4. HISTORY-TAKING IN THE PATIENT WITH PAIN

Ronald Kanner, M.D.

1. What are the key elements in taking the clinical history of a patient presenting with a complaint of pain?

The first step is to evaluate the complaint of pain. The most important primary factors are location, intensity, characteristics, and temporal aspects. Secondary factors include exacerbating and relieving factors and circumstances surrounding the onset of pain.

2. If pain is a purely subjective phenomenon, how can its intensity be measured?

The only reliable measure of intensity is the patient's report. Measures of pain intensity are not meant to compare one person's pain with another's; rather, they compare the intensity of one patient's pain at any given time with its intensity at another given time. Thus, physicians and patients can judge whether pain intensity is increasing or decreasing with time and treatment. It is sometimes helpful to have the patient compare the intensity of the current pain experience with prior experiences.

3. How should pain intensity be recorded?

There are a number of different measurements for pain intensity (see Chapter 6), and it is not clear that any particular scale is universally better than any other. Some patients have greater ease with a verbal scale, some with a numerical, and some with a visual analog scale. It is, however, a good idea to use the same measure across time. Thus, verbal descriptors, such as "no pain, mild pain, moderate pain, severe pain, unbearable pain," or numerical scales, can be graded on each visit.

4. Can pain intensity be measured in children and the elderly?

Once children reach an age of verbal skills, pain intensity can usually be quantified on a verbal scale. However, a number of scales work even for preverbal children (see Chapter 29). Once children reach the pre-teen years, the same tools used in adults can be applied.

The elderly may face more difficult problems. If the patient is cognitively impaired, it is often difficult to assess pain intensity on a precise scale, and it becomes more valuable to judge the functional impairments due to pain. Furthermore, medications used to treat pain may increase cognitive impairment and make assessment even more difficult. Elderly patients tend to be stoic about pain and are reluctant to report high intensities.

5. What information can be gathered from the character of the pain?

The McGill Pain Questionnaire contains numerous descriptors for pain. Certain words that patients choose may help to infer a specific pathophysiology. For example, a burning, dysesthetic, or electric-shock–like pain usually implies neuropathic pain. An aching, cramping, waxing and waning pain in the abdomen usually indicates visceral, nociceptive pain.

6. Why are the temporal characteristics of pain important?

The onset of pain is extremely important. The approach to acute pain of relatively recent onset should follow more closely the medical model; that is, a search for underlying cause. Acute pain usually indicates a new pathologic process, correction of which will relieve the pain. Chronic pain of long duration is less likely to be amenable to a standard medical model and requires a biopsychosocial approach (see Chapter 39). Chronic pain often outlives the initial cause and develops a life of its own.

7. Why is the temporal course of the pain important?

Certain pain syndromes have classic temporal patterns. For example, cluster headaches may occur at the same time of the day, every day, during only certain months of the year. Rheumatoid arthritis is characteristically worse early in the morning on rising (morning stiffness), whereas osteoarthritis characteristically worsens later in the day (with prolonged weight-bearing). Similarly, chronic, daily abdominal pain that has persisted in an unchanging way for years is unlikely to have a clear medical cure, whereas episodic abdominal pain that allows long pain-free intervals punctuated by severe bouts of pain is more likely to be due to focal pathology. The intensity of pain over time is also of significance. An acute, severe pain in the back that gradually improves probably should be followed expectantly, assuming that there are no signs of tumor or infection. On the other hand, pain that increases over days to weeks is of more concern.

8. What is the best way to elicit the time course of a pain syndrome if the patient is having difficulty being specific?

For the onset, ask the patient what he or she was doing when the pain started. If the patient can give a specific act or time of day, it is likely that the pain was of acute onset. To judge whether the pain is worsening or improving, look for functional signs; that is, ask the patient what he or she cannot do now that he or she could do a few months ago. If functional ability is decreasing, the pain probably is increasing.

9. What is the importance of ascertaining exacerbating and relieving factors?

Specific pain syndromes have specific exacerbating and relieving factors. For example, tension headache is often relieved by alcohol, whereas cluster headache is characteristically exacerbated by alcohol intake. Back pain from a herniated disc is usually relieved by recumbency, whereas back pain from tumor or infection is either unrelieved or exacerbated by recumbency.

10. A patient complains of back and leg pain but has trouble describing the exact distribution. What can you do to clarify the matter?

Pain maps (body maps) are often useful for patients who have difficulty with verbal expression. A front and rear view of the body is presented on paper, and the patient simply pencils in the location of the pain. The patient may use different colors or different types of lines to describe different types of pain. This technique helps to define whether pain is in a nerve distribution or simply somatic.

11. A patient has a rather nondescript headache that is getting worse over days to weeks. What should you consider?

The temporal pattern of vague onset with rapid acceleration in symptoms should raise the question of a space-occupying lesion. Even in patients with back pain, one should consider tumor or infection as major possibilities.

12. An 80-year-old woman presents with severe pain in the chest wall after having a rash in that area. You made the diagnosis of postherpetic neuralgia and plan to use a tricyclic antidepressant. What questions should you ask in the history?

Before prescribing any medication, a careful history of prior medication use and prior medical illnesses is imperative. Particularly in an elderly person in whom we consider using a tricyclic antidepressant, these matters are of maximal importance. Tricyclic antidepressants have anticholinergic properties. Therefore, they can exacerbate glaucoma and increase confusion (two factors that are fairly common in the elderly). Orthostatic hypotension and other anticholinergic side effects are also more common in elderly than in young patients.

13. What specific questions should be asked about the medical history in patients with complaint of pain?

Questions should be directed at ascertaining three major factors. First, has the patient had other painful illnesses? The response to these illnesses helps to guide current therapy. Second, how has the patient responded to medications in the past? This may limit the drugs that can be prescribed. For example, in patients with a history of hypersensitivity to a given medication, any medication in the same group should be avoided. If the patient has an aspirin allergy, nonsteroidal antiinflammatory drugs (NSAIDs) cannot be used without great caution. If patients tend to develop orthostatic hypotension or confusion easily, the tricyclics probably should be avoided. Finally, medical conditions that may limit treatment should be investigated. For example, glaucoma, benign prostatic hypertrophy, and cognitive impairment are relative contraindications to the use of tricyclic antidepressants because their anticholinergic properties may precipitate crises. In patients with a history of opioid abuse, the opioids must be used only with great caution. In patients with peptic ulcer disease, aspirin and NSAIDs have limited utility. In patients with renal disease, acetaminophen and NSAIDs must be used with caution.

14. How does the family history affect a patient with pain?

Aside from the obvious issue of familial diseases, role models are often found in the family. A careful history should be taken to determine whether either parent or older siblings have suffered from a chronic pain syndrome. In addition, the family's reaction to the pain syndrome should be noted.

15. Is a history of disability benefits of any importance?

This issue has caused a great deal of argument in the literature, but there is no clear resolution. The general wisdom is that patients receiving significant compensation for illness are reinforced in their chronic pain. This has even been called compensation neurosis. However, the evidence is somewhat shaky, and such patients are probably best treated in the rehabilitative fashion.

16. On close questioning, a patient gives a history of alcohol abuse. Does this preclude the use of opioid analgesics?

In both hospital and ambulatory settings, it is not clear that substance abuse is any higher among patients with chronic pain than among patients with any other chronic illness. Although dependency on multiple substances is fairly common, there is no clear indication that a history of alcohol abuse predisposes to opioid abuse. The psychosocial history is addressed in Chapter 5.

BIBLIOGRAPHY

1. Fields HL (ed): Core Curriculum for Professional Education in Pain. Seattle, IASP Press, 1995.
2. Portenoy RK, Kanner RM: Definition and assessment of pain. In Portenoy RK, Kanner RM (eds): Pain Management: Theory and Practice. Philadelphia, F.A. Davis, 1996, pp 3–18.

5. PHYSICAL EXAMINATION OF THE PATIENT IN PAIN

Mark A. Thomas, M.D., and Brian Kahan, D.O.

1. What functional signs should be elicited in patients complaining of pain?

Some of the most useful information is found through observation. In general, try to observe the patient when he or she is not aware of your presence. Concentrate on how he or she walks, gets out of a chair, gets on to the examining table, or takes off garments. These observations point out areas of pain and restricted range of motion.

One should also examine how the patient gets dressed and leaves the office. Patients tend to be more relaxed after the doctor's visit is over. Observation at this time might detect subtle findings that weren't present during the initial evaluation because of guarding.

2. What are the fundamentals of the spinal exam?

The spine consists of cervical, thoracic, lumbar, and sacral areas. Each area should be examined individually and collectively.

The spinal column should be examined in at least two situations: (1) a dynamic situation: the spinal column is loaded (i.e., standing, sitting, or forward bending); and (2) a static situation: the spine is unloaded (i.e., supine, prone, or lateral recumbent). The examiner should look at the spine from the anterior, posterior, and lateral aspects. Check that normal curvature (cervical lordosis, thoracic kyphosis, lumbar lordosis) is maintained and note any asymmetry or unleveling (e.g., shoulder or sacral). From the lateral aspect, note whether there is any *increased* kyphosis or lordosis. This can be done by either hanging a plumb line from the office ceiling or drawing an imaginary line posterior to the external auditory meatus to the lateral malleolus. The line should bisect the humeral head and greater trochanter and travel slightly posterior to the knee to the lateral malleolus.

There are a number of provocative tests that, when they elicit pain, are indicative of specific disorders. Some of these have eponyms; others are simply descriptive. A table summarizing the tests appears at the end of the section. The next three questions relate to the cervical spine.

3. What is the axial compression test, and what are the implications of a positive test?

Axial compression involves compression of the cervical spine, directly caudad. When positive, pain is localized to the neck or radiates distally, indicating degenerative joint disease of the spine or nerve root impingement in the upper cervical spine.

4. What is Spurling's test, and what are the implications of a positive test?

Spurling's test involves compression of the cervical spine while it is slightly extended, rotated, and tilted toward one side (side bent). In a positive test, pain radiates distally, usually in a radicular distribution, indicating nerve root compression in the mid to lower cervical region. The nerve compression is ipsilateral to the side bent.

5. Under what circumstances is the chest expansion test used?

If ankylosing spondylitis is suspected, the chest expansion test may be used. In normal subjects, the difference between the totally deflated and totally inflated chest is usually more than 4 cm. In ankylosing spondylitis, it is almost invariably less than 4 cm. The patient is asked to exhale fully, and the chest is measured. He is then asked to inhale fully, and the chest is measured again. The difference between the two measurements is the chest expansion.

6. What is the straight leg raising test, and what are its implications?

Straight leg raising is used to check for lower lumbar radiculopathy. The patient lies supine, and the leg is passively elevated from the ankle. The knee is kept straight. Normal patients can reach nearly 90 degrees without pain. In lower lumbar nerve impingements, straight leg raising is relatively sensitive and produces pain in a radicular distribution. Somewhat less sensitive, but more specific, is contralateral straight leg raising. In this case, the nonpainful leg is elevated, and pain is felt on the affected side if there is nerve root involvement.

7. What is a sitting root test?

A sitting root test (SRT) is essentially the same as the straight leg raising test, but the patient is sitting rather than supine. The implications are the same.

In the Lasegue test, after the leg is extended from a sitting or supine position, the foot is dorsiflexed. This further stretches the root and causes pain.

8. What is the FABER test, and how is it different from Patrick's maneuver?

FABER is an acronym for flexion, abduction, and external rotation of both hips. When it produces low back pain on one side, it is indicative of sacroiliac joint dysfunction. When the same maneuver produces hip pain, it is called Patrick's maneuver and is indicative of hip joint pathology. Patrick's maneuver may be performed unilaterally, but the FABER test must be done bilaterally to avoid pelvic rotation.

9. How should painful extremities be examined?

Examination of the extremities should consist of having the patient perform active range of motion (ROM); then the examiner should perform passive range of motion for each joint to be tested. Limits of range and areas throughout the range that cause pain should be recorded. Active ROM should always be performed before passive ROM because voluntary guarding will avoid unintentional injury.

10. What is the impingement syndrome, and which clinical tests are used for its diagnosis?

The impingement syndrome is also called the painful arc syndrome. There is thought to be tendinitis of the rotator cuff. There may be mechanical impingement at the coracoacromial arc. The diagnostic test consists of stabilizing the scapula and elevating the patient's arm. Patients appear apprehensive, grimace, and experience pain. Pain relief from injection of lidocaine at the point of pain confirms the diagnosis.

11. What is Adson's test, and what does it signify?

Adson's test is used to support the diagnosis of a thoracic outlet syndrome. In this syndrome, the neurovascular bundle is compressed as it exits near the first rib and the scalenus anticus muscle. The examiner palpates the patient's radial pulse, as the patient extends the arm and the hand laterally while rotating the head. A positive result is the ablation of the radial pulse and may indicate vascular compromise. This is not, however, diagnostic of a neurologic thoracic outlet syndrome.

12. What signs are used in the diagnosis of carpal tunnel syndrome?

Carpal tunnel syndrome is compression of the medial nerve at the wrist. Phalen's test is performed by forced volar flexion of the wrist. After about one minute, the patient develops tingling in the first three fingers of the hand. Tinel's sign occurs when tapping over an injured nerve produces a jolt of pain in the distribution of that nerve. With carpal tunnel syndrome, the volar aspect of the wrist is percussed, and pain is felt in the first three fingers. This sign is not specific for carpal tunnel syndrome but can be seen anywhere a nerve injury occurs.

13. What is the piriformis syndrome, and which tests are used to detect it?

The piriformis syndrome is a type of sciatica. The sciatic nerve is believed to be compressed as it passes through the piriformis muscle. With the patient in the lateral decubitus position, the upper leg is held with the hip and knee flexed. If downward pressure produces pain over the buttock and into the leg, this is thought to indicate a piriformis syndrome.

14. A number of tests are indicative of pain amplification (embellishment) or malingering. Name and describe two tests that suggest that back pain is not due to organic disease.

For the axial loading test, the patient stands and pressure is applied over the skull. This would normally not produce low back pain. Similarly, for the rotation test the patient stands with feet together and shoulders and hips rotated in the same plane. Since neither of these tests stresses the low back, the elicitation of pain suggests that there is embellishment.

15. What is Hoover's test?

The patient lies supine and is asked to elevate the supposedly weak leg. The examiner keeps his or her hands under each of the heels. If there is true weakness, the patient presses down with the good leg to offer support for the bad leg. In Hoover's test, the downward pressure does not occur, indicating feigned weakness.

16. Which signs indicate feigned weakness in the arms?

Give-way weakness, or a ratchetlike sensation of weakness, is usually due to factitious weakness. If a patient is feigning weakness in one arm, he or she will have give-way weakness in that arm, and the other arm will be strong, when they are tested separately. However, when they are tested together, both may give way.

Provocative Tests for Eliciting Pain

AREA OF TESTING	TEST NAME	POSITIVE RESULT	IMPLICATIONS IF POSITIVE
Spine			
Cervical	Axial compression—compression of the cervical spine downward	Pain localized to neck or radiating distally	DJD or nerve root impingement in upper cervical area
	Spurling's—compression of cervical spine in slight extension, rotation, and side bent	Pain radiating distally	Nerve root impingement mid to lower cervical region
Thoracic	Chest expansion	< 4 cm	Rule out ankylosing spondylitis
Lumbar	Straight leg raising (SLR)	Pain radiating down leg from ROM 30–70°	Possible HNP L5–S1
	Sitting root (SRT)—patient in seated position and leg is extended	Pain radiating down leg when extended in sitting position from ROM 20–40°	In combination with SLR significant for lower lumbar HNP
	Lasegue	Same as SLR but pain is exacerbated with passive dorsiflexion of foot	Same as SLR/SRT
	FABER—flexion, abduction, and external rotation of the hip	Pain in low back with end ROM	SI joint dysfunction
	Gaenslen's—patient supine with one leg draped off the table asked to hip flex	Pain in low back	Pain in low back
	Shober's—mark made at level of S2 then 5 cm below and 10 cm above; measure distance between with spine erect and then flexed	Less than 5 cm increase in length	Ankylosing spondylitis

Continued on following page.

Provocative Tests for Eliciting Pain (Continued)

AREA OF TESTING	TEST NAME	POSITIVE RESULT	IMPLICATIONS IF POSITIVE
Extremities			
Shoulder	Painful arc—patient asked to move arm through flexed ROM. Performed actively and passively	Shoulder pain between 120–180°	Acromioclavicular disease
		Shoulder pain between 60–120°	Impingement syndromes
	Apprehension—arm flexed, abducted, and then passively externally rotated	Feeling of instability with abduction and external rotation	Joint laxity secondary to inferior glenohumeral ligament complex
	Drop arm—arm abducted passively	Patient unable to hold arm abducted	Rotator cuff tear
	Jerk—arm medially rotated forward flexed, then stress applied posteriorly into shoulder capsule	Clunk felt in posterior shoulder after stress applied	Posterior capsule instability
	Sulcus sign—arms at side, patient relaxed	Sulcus with inferior traction on arm	Inferior instability of the shoulder
	Yergason's—elbow flexed at 90°; examiner resists supination	Tenderness at bicipital groove	Bicipital tendinitis
	Impingement—patient's arm is forcibly elevated	Pain under acromion	Supraspinatus tendinitis, impingement syndrome
	Impingement sign—joint injected with xylocaine	Relief of pain	Impingement of supraspinatus under acromion
	Hawkin's—arm flexed at 90° and JR	Pain under acromion	Supraspinatus tendinitis
	Adson's—palpate radial pulse, head rotated ipsilaterally, head extended, and arm laterally rotated and extended	Disappearance of radial pulse	Thoracic outlet syndrome
Wrist	Phalen's	Numbness/tingling in first 3 digits	Carpal tunnel syndrome
	Tinel's sign	Electric shock in first 3 digits	Carpal tunnel syndrome
	Finkelstein's—thumb is actively opposed and finger flexed over thumb	Pain	DeQuervain's disease
	Watson's—wrist stabilized, scaphoid grasped and moved	Pain	Scaphoid instability or fracture
Hip	FABER	Pain before end ROM	Arthritis of hip joint
Thigh	Ober's—patient side-lying, hip flexed, examiner passively abducts and extends leg	Pain	Tightness of iliotibial band
	Piriformis—side-lying, hip flexed to 60°, knee flexed, pressure applied downward	Pain over buttock and radiating down leg	Compression of sciatic nerve secondary to spasm of piriformis
	Thomas—supine, flex one hip	Straight leg rises off table	Hip flexion contracture

Continued on following page.

Provocative Tests for Eliciting Pain (Continued)

AREA OF TESTING	TEST NAME	POSITIVE RESULT	IMPLICATIONS IF POSITIVE
Knee	Lachman's, anterior draw, pivot-shift—various forms of draw test	Pain and instability	Anterior cruciate ligament tear
	Varus stress	Pain, instability	Lateral collateral ligament damage
	Valgus stress	Pain, instability	Medial collateral ligament damage
	Apley's compression— patient supine, knee flexed, pressure applied through tibia to knee	Pain	Meniscal damage
	McMurray—patient supine, knee flexed, examiner medially rotates tibia as leg extended	Pain or locking of knee	Meniscal damage
	Bounce—patient supine, heel cupped and lifted off table	Pain or inability to reach full extension	Meniscal damage
	Childress' sign—patient performs duck walk	Pain or clicking	Posterior horn of meniscus damaged
Ankle	Anterior draw—patient supine, ankle in neutral, tibia stabilized, heel cupped and drawn anteriorly	Laxity	Tendon damage to deltoid ligaments or anterior talofibular ligaments
	Talar tilt—patient supine, foot relaxed, heel cupped and stressed internally	Laxity	Ligamentous instability
	Thompson—gastrocsoleus muscles grasped	Absence of plantar flexion	Rupture of Achilles tendon

BIBLIOGRAPHY

1. Greenman P: Principles of Manual Medicine. Baltimore, Williams & Wilkins, 1989.
2. Hoppenfeld S: Physical Examination of the Spine and Extremities. Norwalk, CT, Appleton-Century-Crofts, 1976.
3. Magee D: Orthopedic Physical Assessment. Philadelphia, W.B. Saunders, 1992.
4. Wadell G: Clinical assessment of lumbar impairment. Clin Orthop Rehabil Res 221:110, 1987.

6. PAIN MEASUREMENT

*W.Crawford Clark, Ph.D., Abbas Kashani, M.D.,
and Susanne Bennett Clark, Ph.D.*

1. Can children give reliable reports of pain?

At age two children can report that they feel pain, but they cannot rate its intensity. Preschool children require a degree of patience in eliciting reports of pain. Parents should be consulted on words the child is likely to recognize as pain-related, that is, words that are used within the family. When children are questioned by a stranger, they tend to deny pain. They believe they should be "brave." Furthermore, if they believe that admitting to pain will lead to a painful procedure, they are also likely to deny pain. By the age of four or five, children can use certain methods for quantifying the intensity of their pain. Children can use verbal rating scales and the other scales designed for adults by about age six or seven.

2. What standardized methods are available for quantifying children's pain?

Faces that vary in expression from smiling, to neutral, to severe misery are used in a variety of tests (see Chapter 29). This scale is suitable for the youngest children. Hester's Poker Chip Tool is suitable for children from age four to five. Four poker chips are placed in front of the child, and the chips are described to the child as "pieces of hurt," from "just a little hurt" to "a lot more hurt" to "more hurt" to "the most hurt you can have." The child is asked how many pieces of hurt he has.

3. Are there any physiologic measures that can be used as indicators of a patient's pain?

Heart rate initially increases with acute, sharp pain. It later decreases. Arterial oxygen tension decreases during painful procedures and stress-related hormones are released; however, fear alone produces similar changes in oxygen saturation, and blood hormone levels depend on age, diurnal rhythms, emotions, and baseline values. Evoked potentials recorded from the scalp have been shown to be linked with the intensity of the stimulus. However, no single parameter clearly distinguishes a painful from a nonpainful stimulus. In contrast to acute pain, there are few useful physiologic indicators of long-term, persistent pain.

4. How reliable are patients' reports of past pain?

In some studies, concordance between pain diaries and patients' later memories for the diaries' contents has been fairly good. However, other studies have shown that remembrance of past pain is influenced by present pain, anxiety, depression, and fear. Furthermore, it has been documented that when patients rated first their expectation of the pain they would experience during a procedure, then rated the pain they actually experienced immediately after a procedure, and finally, six months later rated the pain they remembered experiencing during a procedure, it was found that their memory of the pain reflected their original expectations, not the actual pain experienced.

5. What is a pain diary?

A continuous record of the patient's pain level, awake activity (sitting, walking, etc.), sleep pattern, and use of analgesics and other medications over a 24-hour period. The diary should record the intensity of pain and other symptoms (and their possible causes) at specified times during the day (upon awakening; at breakfast, lunch, and dinner; at bedtime, during the night, etc.). Some diaries record on an hourly basis (provided the patient is awake).[7,11]

6. What is the value of a pain diary?

Pain diaries are important for optimal pain management in hospitalized patients. Retrospective analysis of pain diaries can suggest improved strategies for analgesic dosage regimens.

They may also reveal exacerbating or relieving factors that the patient and practitioner would otherwise overlook.

7. What is pain assessment, and why is it important?

Pain assessment is a multidimensional approach to the evaluation of pain attributes. These attributes include the intensity, duration, and location of pain; its somatosensory qualities; and the accompanying emotions of the pain experience. Pain/suffering assessment is needed to tailor the patient's medication and dosage to her/his particular requirements and to allow the efficacy of different treatments to be compared reliably. Accurate pain assessment is necessary for all patients receiving analgesic medication or who are candidates for pain-relieving procedures. In particular, pain assessment is needed for patients whose pain report seems inappropriate to the physical findings.[7,9,11]

8. What is the most widely used pain questionnaire?

The McGill Pain Questionnaire, which has been translated into all major languages, was developed by Dr. Melzack of McGill University. It is a checklist of 87 descriptors of the sensory qualities of a patient's pain and related emotions, plus a line drawing of a body on which the patient sketches the location of the pain plus an overall intensity rating: the Present Pain Index.[8]

9. Which questionnaires are used to assess the general psychological status of pain patients?

The Derogatis Symptom Check List-90 (SCL-90), or its shorter version, the Brief Symptom Inventory (BSI), is often used. Using these written lists of symptoms, patients score how much they are bothered by a particular symptom.[7,11]

10. Which standardized questionnaires can be used to assess physical function?

Disability is assessed by the Health Assessment Questionnaire, the Sickness Impact Profile, and the Arthritis Impact Measurement Scale. Other scales measure productivity, ambulation, and self-care. The Karnofsky scale is a behavioral scale widely used in cancer patients to assess the stages of progression. Each scale assigns a numerical value to the patient's ability to perform a given task.[7,11]

11. Which questionnaires are used to assess the behavioral/cognitive aspects of pain and suffering?

Hypochondriasis, somatic concern, and denial behaviors are rated by the Illness Behavior Questionnaire developed by Pilowski. Other quantifiable measures of behavior include frequency of physician and/or hospital visits, number of surgeries for pain, changes in medication, sleep disturbances, and nonverbal pain behaviors such as limping, grimacing, or guarding.[7,11]

12. Which standardized questionnaires focus on emotional factors?

Depression is usually assessed by the Beck, Hamilton, or Zung Depression scales and anxiety by the Spielberger State Trait Anxiety Inventory. Hostility, paranoid ideation, and other psychological factors are often measured by the Derogatis Brief Symptom Inventory. The problem with some of these scales is that somatic symptoms (e.g., lack of appetite) are treated as indicators of depression; but a patient undergoing chemotherapy may very well suffer lack of appetite from physical, not emotional, causes.[7,11]

13. What is the Westhaven-Yale Multidimensional Pain Inventory (WHYMPI)?

A standardized questionnaire used in patients with chronic pain, WHYMPI is aimed at measuring the sensory, medical, neurologic, cognitive, and psychological aspects of pain as well as the patient's capacity for enduring pain.[6]

14. The Minnesota Multiphasic Personality Inventory (MMPI) classifies chronic pain patients into which four personality types?

1. Hypochondriacal   3. Somaticizers
2. Reactively depressed   4. Manipulators[11]

15. According to the taxonomy devised by the International Association for the Study of Pain, pain is established on which five axes?
1. Regions of the body
2. Systems affected
3. Temporal characteristics
4. Intensity and time since onset
5. Etiology[9]

16. Which major aspects (dimensions) of pain/suffering must be considered when assessing pain?
Melzack and Casey argue for three dimensions:
1. Sensory-discriminative
2. Affective-motivational
3. Cognitive-evaluative

The sensory-discriminative dimension comprises the sensory aspect of pain, including intensity, location, and temporal aspects. The affective-motivational dimension reflects the emotional and aversive aspects of pain and suffering. The cognitive-evaluative dimension reflects the patient's evaluation of the meaning and possible consequences of the pain and illness or injury, including impact on quality of life and even death itself. This three-dimensional model is widely accepted because it succeeds in integrating much of what is known about the physiology and psychology of pain and suffering.[11]

17. Name three accepted scales for measuring the intensity of pain.
1. A visual analogue scale
2. A numerical rating scale
3. A category rating scale

18. Which examples are applicable to pain assessment?
1. Visual analogue scales are 10-cm lines anchored at the ends by words that define the bounds of the pain/suffering dimension. The patient is asked to place a mark on the scale to indicate the level of intensity of her/his pain or anxiety.

For pain intensity:
No ———————————————————————————— Worst
Pain   Possible Pain

For anxiety:
No --- Worst
Anxiety   Possible Anxiety

2. Numerical rating scales are similar to analogue scales except that numbers (e.g., 0 to 5) are entered along the scale.

3. To use category scales, the patient is asked to circle the word that best describes her/his condition:

For pain intensity: None
                        Moderate
                        Severe
                        Unbearable[11]
For anxiety: None
                        Moderate
                        Severe
                        Unbearable
For depression: None
                        Moderate
                        Severe
                        Unbearable

19. What do the scores obtained from the above tests mean?
The overall score defines the relative importance of the sensory and emotional dimensions of pain/suffering to the individual patient.

20. What are the two essential characteristics of a questionnaire?
Reliability and validity.[11]

21. What is a *reliable* measure? Name three types of reliability tests.
A reliable measure has the property of yielding consistent results. The most common ways to assess reliability are:
1. By internal consistency, or split-half reliability
2. By test-retest reliability
3. By inter-rater reliability

For **split-half reliability**, similar items should receive similar scores. This requires questionnaires with two sets of similar items (Forms A and B) that are usually, but not necessarily, administered on different occasions. The advantage is that two independent assessments of the patient's symptoms can be made on separate occasions. The questions are designed so that patients cannot intentionally or unintentionally base their second responses on their memories of the previous test. **Test-retest reliability** indexes the consistency of the questionnaire. Patients should give the same answer to the same question if their status has not changed. For questionnaires that may be answered by an outside observer, **inter-rater reliability** is assessed by comparing the evaluations of the same patient by two or more raters.[11]

22. How is the reliability of a test quantified?
Reliability is usually expressed numerically as a correlation coefficient, with 0.0 signifying total unreliability and 1.0 indicating 100% reliability. Reliability coefficients above 0.85 are generally regarded as high and those between 0.65 and 0.85 as moderate.[11]

23. Is there an objective way to distinguish pain "amplifiers" from "deniers"?
For patients complaining of persistent pain, the response to calibrated noxious stimuli (e.g., a 3-second, 48°C thermal stimulus) can be a valuable tool in determining whether the patient is stoic or an "amplifier," i.e., whether she/he under- or over-reports pain. It has been shown that anxious individuals over-respond to calibrated noxious stimuli, while depressed and chronic pain patients under-respond to the same intensities of a stimulus, presumably because the calibrated stimulus is regarded as innocuous in comparison with their own suffering.[1,12]

24. Describe the magnitude estimation procedure. What are its major advantages and disadvantages?
In the magnitude estimation, or ratio scaling procedure, the subject is assigned a simple number, such as 10, to describe a calibrated stimulus (the modulus) of an intensity in the mildly painful range. The subject then assigns numbers to subsequently presented stimulus intensities that range both above and below that modulus value. Its advantage is that it is relatively simple to use and has a certain "face" validity. It has been shown that subjects are able to rate electrocutaneous stimuli separately with respect to sensory (pain) and affect (unpleasantness) dimensions. In one study, an anxiety-reducing drug (diazepam) reduced the intensity ratings of these stimuli on the affect, but not the sensory, dimension. Another study showed that an analgesic reduced sensory pain ratings of electrocutaneous stimuli while affect ratings remained unchanged. These results are in accord with the known tranquilizing and analgesic effects of these drugs and support the concept of separate sensory and emotional components of pain and suffering. A major disadvantage of the method is that the ratings are highly variable among subjects and typically are averaged over subjects. Thus, the method is of little value in understanding the responses of any individual patient to calibrated stimuli.[5]

25. Describe the method of limits (serial exploration) for measuring applied pain, and define threshold.

In the method of limits, the subject responds to each of a series of brief, physically calibrated stimuli (thermal, cold, pressure, pinch, or electrical) that are increased stepwise in intensity. Two thresholds are identified. The **pain sensitivity threshold** is the intensity at which the subject first reports pain, while the **pain tolerance threshold** is the intensity at which the subject withdraws from the stimulus. The method is useful for approximating the threshold in order to determine the intensities to be applied in more sophisticated and accurate procedures. Although the thresholds were once thought to be pure measures of sensory function, it is now clear that they lack validity because they are heavily influenced by nonsensory, psychological variables, such as the subject's expectations and attitudes.[8]

26. What is sensory decision theory?

The signal detection theory, or sensory decision theory (SDT), model requires the subject to make decisions about the presence or absence, or the strength (weak or strong), of calibrated stimuli. From the subject's responses, a 2×2 contingency table is created, and the hit and false alarm rates are computed.

	Response "Pain"	*Response "Not Painful"*
Higher intensity stimulus	Hits (sensitivity)	Misses
Lower intensity stimulus	False alarms	Correct rejections (specificity)

In the application of SDT to pain evaluation, a set of stimuli (about 10 at each of approximately five intensities) is presented randomly to the subject. The intensities range from blank (no stimulus administered) to the upper limits of the subject's tolerance.[1] The subject chooses a descriptor from a verbal category scale. For thermal stimuli, for example, the responses could be nothing, maybe something, warm, hot, faint pain, moderate pain, severe pain, withdrawal. The subject's ratings are translated into binary decisions for each pair of sequentially increasing physical intensities and are entered into a series of 2×2 tables for more details. This yields a quantitative evaluation of both the subject's actual pain experience and her/his attitude toward reporting pain (the report criterion).[8]

27. Why are sensory decision theory measures important for the understanding of pain?

A major problem in understanding pain and suffering is the seemingly inseparable mixture of sensory and psychological variables that determine a subject's oral report. This is as true for experimental pain as it is for clinical pain. Recent developments in psychophysical measurement (particularly in what is variously called medical decision making theory, signal detection theory, or sensory decision theory procedures, depending on its application) offer considerable promise for understanding the responses to calibrated noxious stimuli. These procedures separate the sensory component of the traditional method of limits threshold from its otherwise hidden psychological or attitudinal component. The method can be used with untrained subjects and has been applied not only to oral report but also to physiologic and motor indicators of pain.[1,8]

28. Which two indices of perceptual performance are obtained with sensory decision theory?

The discriminability index, d' or $P(A)$, is related to the functioning of the neurosensory system. High values suggest that neurosensory functioning is normal; low values suggest that the signal-related neurosensory activity has been attenuated as, for example, by damage to sensory pathways (e.g., diabetic neuropathy) or by an analgesic. Discriminability has been shown to be decreased by analgesics such as morphine and by nerve blocks, both of which attenuate neural activity and therefore the amount of information reaching higher centers. Unlike the traditional pain threshold obtained by the method of limits, d' or $P(A)$ has been shown to be essentially independent of changes in the subject's expectation, mood, and motivation.

The other measure of perceptual performance, the report criterion, Lx or B, measures response bias, which is the willingness (low or liberal criterion) or reluctance (high or stoical criterion) of a subject to use a particular response. The report criterion is related to the subject's attitude toward reporting painful experiences. Attitudes depend on cultural factors such as stoicism or on emotional factors such as anxiety and depression.[8,12]

29. What has sensory decision theory analysis of responses to calibrated noxious stimuli revealed about the effects of suggestion, attitude, emotional variables, age, and cultural differences on the pain report? Give examples.

Many studies have used sensory decision theory to demonstrate the effect of attitudinal and emotional variables on the pain report. For example, a placebo described and accepted by the subjects as a powerful analgesic raised the traditional threshold (equivalent to an apparently decreased pain sensitivity). Analysis of the same data by signal detection theory, however, demonstrated that only the report criterion had been raised (fewer pain reports); the discriminability, d', had not changed. Thus, the placebo-induced reduction in pain report was due not to an analgesic effect of the placebo but to a criterion shift in response to the social demand characteristics of the situation.

Other studies have shown elderly patients to be both more stoical (high report criterion) and to suffer some sensory loss (lower d'), compared with younger patients. People from non-Western cultures have been thought to be more tolerant of pain mainly because of physiologic differences. However, sensory decision theory has shown that the ability of Nepalese Sherpas to discriminate among noxious electrical stimuli (d') was the same as that of Westerners, which suggests that their nociceptive sensory systems were the same. However, the Sherpas gave much more stoical pain reports (higher report criteria), probably as a result of cultural/religious factors.[8,13]

30. What is known about pain assessment among different ethnocultural groups?

Higher pain thresholds to calibrated noxious stimuli have been reported among northern Europeans more than among Mediterranean people and African Americans; Irish Catholics and Yankee Protestants have been reported to have higher pain thresholds than Italians and Jews. However, as summarized in a recent review, there is little evidence for ethnocultural differences in the discrimination of noxious stimuli, but there are significant cultural differences in reporting pain. Probably all of the differences in pain thresholds that have been reported among various ethnocultural and religious groups are due entirely to cultural differences in the criterion for reporting pain and not at all to differences in the sensory experience of pain itself.[13]

31. Are there ethnocultural differences in how patients and practitioners view the source and estimate the intensity of a patient's pain?

There are striking differences in the particular body organ that a culture focuses upon as a source of pain. Germans are much more apt to complain of heart pain (and German cardiologists are more likely to read an electrocardiogram as abnormal). The French focus on the liver and even refer to a migraine headache as the "liver crisis." The English are most concerned about the gastrointestinal tract. Other studies have found that foreigners and minority groups in the United States tend to be undermedicated.[10]

32. What is the best method to evaluate clinical pain in an individual patient?

The Multidimensional Affect and Pain Survey (MAPS) is a useful tool. The patient is shown a set of 101 words that encompass three major superclusters. The first, **somatosensory qualities**, includes the full range of noxious and nonnoxious somatosensory experiences such as stabbing, burning, localized, cramping. The second, **suffering**, includes negative emotional states such as anxiety, depression, guilt, hostility, and fear. The third, **well-being**, includes positive states such as energetic, relaxed, and other indicators of good health. These 101 words, which fall into 30 subclusters, are presented to the patient in the form of questions. The patient rates the closeness of each descriptor to his or her pain and suffering on a numerical scale. Thus, the sensory and affect dimensions important to the individual patient are revealed in a quantitative form.[3]

33. Which test is most commonly used to measure the emotional aspects of pain and suffering?

The SCL-90, or preferably its shorter version, the Brief Symptom Inventory (Derogatis). It has nine subscales: somatization, obsessive compulsive, interpersonal sensitivity, depression, anxiety, hostility, phobic anxiety, paranoid ideation, and psychoticism.[7,11]

34. Why must responses to the psychological scales be interpreted with caution when given to patients who are suffering pain?

An item (e.g., loss of appetite) that reflects depression in psychiatric patients may, in a medical patient, be due to a physical condition or treatment (e.g., chemotherapy).

35. What is meant by validity?

Validity means that the test measures what it is supposed to measure. To determine this, the scores on the measure are compared with various kinds of external standards and validity coefficients (comparable to reliability coefficients) are calculated.[11]

36. What is content, or face, validity?

This informal approach simply asks a group of experts to confirm the suitability, clarity, and organization of the questionnaire items.[11]

37. What is concurrent validity?

Responses to the new pain measure being investigated (predictor variable) are correlated with results from a previous well-established (criterion variable) test.[11]

38. What is predictive validity?

Predictive validity is examined through longitudinal or prospective studies. The predictor variable may be the score on a pain questionnaire or a physiologic measure, e.g., hypertension. The criterion variable is an independently measured physical event, e.g., pre- and postsurgery pain or various stages of cancer, before and after administration of an analgesic.[11]

39. What is discriminant validity?

A statistical technique that validates a pain measure by evaluating a test item's ability to group patients according to an underlying shared characteristic, for example, how well a test item discriminates among patients with cluster, tension, and migraine headaches.[11]

40. Is it possible to assess pain indirectly?

Yes. For example, by determining the extent to which pain interferes with cognitive functioning using a range of choices from "mostly unaware of it" to "concentration on a mental task is impossible."

41. Are there structured interviews with a computerized format?

Yes. The Interactive Microcomputer Patient Assessment Tool for Health (IMPATH) and the Behavioral Assessment of Pain (BAP) questionnaires, among others.

42. Which three instruments are commonly used to measure the psychological status of chronic pain patients?

1. The MMPI (Minnesota Multiphasic Personality Inventory) is a 566-item self-report questionnaire that includes 10 scales designed to assess psychological disturbance and three validity scales. A revision, MMPI-2, is also available. However, it is very long, and many of its questions have very little to do with pain.

2. The Millon Behavioral Health Inventory (MBHI) is a 150-item self-report questionnaire designed to evaluate the psychological functioning of *medical* patients; thus, it has the advantages of being shorter and more specific than the MMPI.

3. The Illness Behavior Questionnaire (IBQ) is a 62-item questionnaire designed to measure symptom complaints in the absence of somatic pathology.[7,11]

43. Name a questionnaire that measures disability and suffering.

The Sickness Impact Profile (SIP) provides a profile of patient disability that includes ambulation, body care, social interaction, alertness, sleep, work, and recreation.[7,11]

44. Which questionnaires evaluate the impact of chronic pain syndromes on the patient's psychosocial life?

The Multidimensional Pain Inventory (MPI) and the Quality of Life Enjoyment and Satisfaction Questionnaire (Q-les-Q). Their particular advantage is that they distinguish overall severity of illness and severity of depression.[4,11]

45. Is it possible to measure the relative physiologic and psychological contributions to treatment outcome—that is, to separate specific and nonspecific treatment effects?

Specific effects of physiologically based procedures combine with nonspecific psychophysiologic effects to determine treatment outcome. As portrayed in the table, there are two treatment conditions and two belief states. The specific treatment is assumed to produce a real, i.e., physiologically based, therapeutic effect, and the sham treatment is assumed to be physiologically ineffective. In addition, the patient's belief as to whether she or he was in the real treatment or the sham treatment group is determined at the end of the study. The cell entries are the number of patients rated as improved according to some objective criterion. This approach yields the four-cell table into which patients with positive outcomes are placed on the basis of (1) physical treatment and (2) subjective opinion about which treatment they had received. A comparison of results according to (a) the treatment the patients **believed** they had received, compared with (b) what they **actually** received, permits comparison of how much of the group improvement was due to the specific effect of an alternative-medicine treatment and how much of the improvement was due to nonspecific psychophysiologic effects.[2]

Successful Outcome Contingent on Treatment and Belief

	PATIENT'S BELIEF IN TREATMENT RECEIVED	
	REAL TREATMENT	SHAM TREATMENT
Specific treatment*	A	B
Sham treatment†	C	D

* Accepted-site acupuncture, TENS, etc.
† Off-site acupuncture, drug placebo, sham TENS, etc. The cells: A, B, C, and D represent the four possible objective and subjective treatment conditions.

BIBLIOGRAPHY

1. Clark WC: Quantitative models for the assessment of clinical pain: Individual differences scaling and sensory decision theory. In Burrows GD, Elton D, Stanley GV (eds): Handbook of Chronic Pain Management. Amsterdam, Elsevier, 1987, 57–67.
2. Clark WC: Pin and pang: Research methodology for acupuncture and other "alternative medicine" therapies. Am Pain Soc J Forum 3:84–88, 1994.
3. Clark WC, Janal MN, Carroll JD: Multidimensional pain requires multidimensional scaling. In Loeser JD, Chapman CR (eds): The Measurement of Pain. New York, Raven, 1989.
4. Endicott J, Nee J, Harrison W, Blumenthal R: Quality of life enjoyment and satisfaction questionnaire: A new measure. Psychopharmacol Bull 29:321–326, 1993.
5. Gracely RH, McGrath P, Dubner R: Validity and sensitivity of ratio scales of sensory and affective verbal pain descriptors: Manipulation of affect by diazepam. Pain 5:5–18, 1986.
6. Kern RD, Turk DC, Rudy TF: The Westhaven-Yale Multidimensional Pain Inventory (WHYMPI). Pain 23:345–356, 1985.
7. Mersky H (ed): Classification of chronic pain: Descriptors of chronic pain syndromes and definitions of pain terms. Pain 3(Suppl):226, 1983.
8. Kornblith AB, Holland JC: Handbook of measures for psychological, social and physical function in cancer. New York, Memorial Sloan-Kettering Center Center, 1994.
9. Melzack R (ed): Pain Measurement and Assessment. New York, Raven Press, 1983, 15–25.

10. Payer L: Medicine and Culture. New York, Holt, 1988.
11. Turk DC, Melzack R (eds): Handbook of Pain Assessment. London, Guilford Press, 1992.
12. Yang JC, Richlin D, Brand L, Wagner JM, Clark WC: Thermal sensory decision theory indices and pain threshold in chronic pain patients and healthy volunteers. Psychosom Med 47:461–468, 1985.
13. Zatzick DF, Dimsdale JE: Cultural variations in response to painful stimuli. Psychosom Med 52:544–557, 1990.

7. PSYCHOLOGICAL ASSESSMENT OF CHRONIC PAIN PATIENTS

Dennis Thornton, Ph.D., and Jill Silverman, M.A.

1. Why is a good psychological assessment essential?

The purpose of a psychological evaluation is to frame the pain experience in the context of a patient's life. Specifically, it evaluates the impact of pain on patients' functioning and the role that patients' psychological makeup has in the experience of pain. It is not designed to differentiate between organic and psychogenic pain. It should, however, assess the impact of anxiety, depression, and prior life experiences on pain.

2. What are the essential elements of a good pain evaluation?

First, belief that pain is real. Whether an organic framework can be defined is somewhat less important in chronic pain than it is in acute pain. However, both physical and psychological issues must be addressed on the first visit.

3. What methods can be used for the psychological assessment of patients with chronic pain?

The psychological interview can be supported by a number of "pencil and paper" tests. The interview should establish a conceptual framework, and the pencil and paper tests can be used to quantify such issues as pain intensity, severity of mood disorder, and level of function.

4. What factors commonly interfere with the accurate assessment of chronic pain?

Pain is an entirely subjective experience. Therefore, personal factors impact the process and accuracy of pain assessment. Cultural, ethnic, and linguistic patterns may influence both how the pain is expressed and how it is interpreted. Furthermore, clinicians are classically trained in the biomedical model, in which pain is believed to be due to a clearly identifiable point of tissue injury. In chronic pain, this may no longer be the case. A shift must occur to a biopsychosocial model, in which the complaint of pain is viewed in a more global framework.

5. What is the most common conceptual mistake that the examining clinician makes?

Physicians often try to conceptualize pain as either organic or psychological. This dichotomy is rarely absolute. True delusional pain is extraordinarily rare. Most commonly, psychological factors impact on the expression of pain, and pain has its impact on a patient's psychological well-being.

6. How important are behavioral signs in assessing pain intensity in chronic pain?

The autonomic "flight-or-fight response" that we commonly associate with acute pain is often lacking in chronic pain. Therefore, tachycardia, diaphoresis, and agitation are often absent. Over time, patients adapt to chronic pain. This adaptation may be appropriate or inappropriate, given the circumstances.

7. Is there a specific format for interviewing patients with pain?

Interviews must be tailored to fit the situation. However, there is some organization to the structure. A biopsychosocial format is the most appropriate. It starts with the patient's complaint, which is clearly foremost in his or her mind. Aside from the usual questions regarding intensity, location, and character, the psychosocial variables to be addressed include the circumstances under which the pain began, its duration, the success or failure of various interventions, the patient's responses to these treatments and results, the impact of the pain on the patient's life, and the patient's expectations of goals or treatment.

8. Why is determining the time of onset important?

The circumstances under which the pain arose may give some insight into the psychological phenomenon surrounding the pain syndrome. For example, traumatic injuries, such as motor vehicle accidents or major surgeries, may give rise to a posttraumatic stress disorder. Diseases with an insidious onset and an exacerbating-remitting course may provoke anxiety with each exacerbation of pain. If the pain syndrome was the result of a coworker's negligence, poorly directed anger may be a significant component. Similarly, litigation and compensation surrounding an injury may be an important factor.

9. What psychological insights can be gained from reviewing treatments that have failed?

Patterns of response and nonresponse may imply certain specific psychological syndromes. For example, patients who claim dramatic relief from certain treatments, only to fail a short while after, may be engaging in idealization/demythification. This is typical of the hysterical personality disorder and may put the clinician at great risk for defeat. Similarly, patients who are unable to tolerate any medications, describing bad reactions to all, may be sabotaging treatment. Thus, a careful history of all prior treatments, successful or otherwise, can be a guide to expectations of future interventions. The same is true of the patient's perception of the prior treating clinicians. Much the same as a treatment can be rapidly valued and devalued, the same holds for a treating clinician.

10. Is emotional distress a normal consequence of illness and pain? What does the absence of such a response imply?

Serious illness, especially when accompanied by pain, raises numerous anxieties. Patients may fear very significant illness, death, or incapacitation. If they emphatically deny any anxiety or emotional impact, it is likely that these emotions are threatening to the patient and require further psychological evaluation.

11. What devices can be used to elicit the psychological impact of pain if a patient is unable to express it?

The first step is to put the patient at ease, suggesting that psychological reactions to pain are quite normal. Certain specific examples should be cited. These may include posttraumatic stress disorder after war injuries, and so on. Should this fail, interviewing family members and significant others may be helpful. They can describe pain behaviors, drug use patterns, altered functional roles, and mood changes. In addition, observing the interaction between the patient and significant others may provide useful insights into family dynamics and level of frustration.

12. What specific areas of function should be addressed?

The patient should be questioned about his or her ability to work (either outside the house or the usual household duties), and the impact on social life, mood, sleep, sexual activity, and relationships with others.

13. What specific work-related issues should be addressed?

Determine what the patient's prior work status was and the feasibility of his or her returning to that type of work. Specifically, questions should be asked regarding the amount of skill required for the job, physical qualifications, and job satisfaction. The financial impact of working vs. collecting disability payments should also be addressed. The patient's work history should also be questioned with regard to relative job satisfaction, progress on the job, and time lost because of pain or illness.

14. How can chronic pain affect social function?

First, it can impede a patient's ability to seek gainful employment. If the patient was originally the breadwinner, this role as head of household and power figure may diminish. Along with that, self-esteem may diminish, and the patient's interactions may necessarily change. Pain may limit a patient's social sphere. In certain instances, this may actually serve a subconscious psychological function. Most commonly, patients complain that the pain strips them of their desire to interact with other people and that they feel "too tired to do anything."

15. What are the normal affective reactions to chronic pain?

It is probably more useful to define adaptive and maladaptive rather than normal and abnormal. While frustration and irritability are very common affective reactions, channeling them into job rehabilitation may be an adaptive use of those emotions. If they lead to insomnia and social isolation, they are maladaptive.

16. What influence can be exerted by family members?

In classic behavioral theory, certain behaviors are reinforced and others are discouraged. While some degree of solicitousness on the part of a spouse or caretaker is appropriate for a patient in pain, excessive attention to the complaint may lead to infantilization and to less adaptive behavior by the patient. Families should be questioned very directly about how they react to the patient's pain complaints or behaviors.

17. Why should family dynamics be assessed?

In certain circumstances, family interactions can serve to perpetuate pain. For example, if a couple has been at odds, they may unite to combat a common enemy (the pain). When this happens, they have an investment in maintaining the complaint of pain to shift focus away from their own problems.

18. Why are questions about sexual activity important?

Chronic pain is a common symptom employed to avoid sexual contact. Passive acquiescence to the waning of sexual contact may reflect premorbid marital difficulties that can be conveniently overshadowed by the physical discomfort. Furthermore, decreased sexuality may be another manifestation of chronic depression.

19. What are the recommended approaches for eliciting a family history?

It is often advisable to have the spouse or other family members present at the initial interview. This will serve to substantiate the patient's complaints and to give some insight into family interactions. The clinician can judge whether the family is supportive and whether they have a shared objective. Issues of interpersonal dependence can be brought out.

20. How can the family issues be elicited?

Observe how the family interacts in the office. Patients and family members should be asked to describe their daily routines. The significant other should be asked how he or she knows that the spouse is in pain, and what their response is.

21. Name some adaptive coping mechanisms exhibited by patients with chronic pain.

These include seeking information, demonstrating interdependence (appropriate reliance on family members), setting realistic goals, and successfully reallocating tasks and roles. Maladaptive coping responses include overdependence on the partner, unwillingness to undertake activities that promote independence, personal and social isolation, and anger.

22. What is meant by pain behaviors, and how should they be assessed?

Pain behaviors are the outward signs of pain and suffering. These may be simple verbal expressions of pain or physical manifestations such as grimacing, posturing, or limping. More complex behaviors include functional limitations, changes in social interaction, or seeking health care.

23. What is meant by secondary gain?

The patient is reaping tangible benefits from having pain. This may be something as obvious as compensation payments or as subtle as getting more attention from a family member.

24. What is the purpose of using "pencil and paper" tests?

These tests are aimed at quantifying what would normally be subjective findings. The measures most commonly used address either the intensity of pain or its emotional component.

25. What is the WHYMPI scale, and what does it measure?

WHYMPI is the West Haven Yale Multidimensional Pain Inventory. It addresses a number of components of pain, including the sensory, neurologic, and cognitive aspects. It contains 52 items comprising 12 scales and is divided into three parts. The first section assesses the perceived impact of pain on vocational and social functions. The second section measures the patient's perception of how others respond to his or her pain. Section 3 evaluates the patient's perception of his or her own involvement in activities of daily life.

26. Which psychological measure is most widely used to assess patients with pain?

The MMPI (Minnesota Multiphasic Personality Inventory) is the most broadly used and validated scale. It is a self-report instrument that asks patients to answer questions as true or false. It attempts to classify patients according to personality types. Unfortunately, this tool was first used in psychiatric patients who did not have chronic pain. Many of the questions answered by chronic pain patients would lead to their classification in the hypochondriacal scale. The MMPI has 567 true/false questions. Analysis of response patterns yields a psychological profile.

27. How has the MMPI been used in the setting of compensation?

Various scales on the MMPI have been touted as predicting the probability of a patient's returning to work. However, no single scale is capable of doing this. The scales that were associated with hysteria and with job dissatisfaction tended to predict the patients who would not return to work.

28. What is the neurotic triad?

This refers to scales 1, 2, and 3 of the MMPI: respectively, hypochondriasis, depression, and hysteria. However, this cannot be taken to mean that the pain does not have an organic basis. Elevations on the neurotic triad were found among arthritis patients who were clinically assessed as not very distressed. The conclusion is that the presence of a physical disorder automatically elevates scores on these scales simply as an accurate reflection of the underlying disease process, rather than neurotic tendencies.

29. What is the SCL-90R?

Symptom Checklist 90, revised. It was designed to quantify the degree of psychological distress. It assesses nine clinical dimensions: obsessive-compulsive disorder, depression, anxiety, paranoid ideation, somatization, interpersonal sensitivity, hostility, psychoticism, and phobic anxiety. Patients are asked to rate how much they are distressed by each of 90 described situations. Ratings are quantified on a six-point scale, ranging from zero (not at all) to 5 (extremely).

30. What indices are commonly used for assessing depression?

Three of the most commonly used tests are the Beck Depression Inventory (BDI), the Hamilton, and the Zung. The BDI is a questionnaire consisting of 21 sets of statements. Each set of statements is ranked in terms of severity and scored from 0 to 3. Each set contains statements that express feelings commonly seen in depression. These are issues of guilt, self-worth, and suicidal ideation. It has 10 positive and 10 negative statements, and patients sometimes find it confusing. The Hamilton Depression Scale is actually scored by the observer, rather than the patient.

31. What rating scales are used to estimate a patient's perceived level of disability?

The Sickness Impact Profile (SIP) consists of 136 items divided into 12 categories. These categories include sleep and rest, eating, work, home management, recreation and pastimes, ambulation, mobility, body care and movement, social interaction, alertness behavior, emotional behavior, and communication. The patient is asked to respond true or false to statements that reflect their impairments in the various areas. The advantage is that this test can be readministered, yielding a pattern of improvement or deterioration.

32. What is meant by locus of control, and how does it affect chronic pain?

Locus of control refers to a patient's perception of what it is that governs experiences. There are three categories: internal (the patient feels in charge), powerful others (caregivers or family members are in charge), and chance. These last two are referred to as external locus of control and the first is internal locus of control. Patients with an external locus of control tend to adopt passive coping mechanisms, expecting others to provide remedies for their pain, and see these remedies as ineffective.

33. What are some of the medical consequences of a history of abuse?

A history of physical or sexual abuse is commonly elicited in patients with chronic pain. Abused patients are more likely to report chronic upper and lower abdominal pain, fatigue, headache, back pain, shortness of breath, unexplained bleeding, chest pain, more lifetime surgeries, greater use of the health care system, functional bowel disorders, drug and alcohol abuse, and attempted suicides.

34. Name the pain complaint most often associated with a history of abuse.

Patients with pelvic pain commonly report a history of sexual abuse. On the basis of interviews and self-report, compared with either normal controls or other pelvic pain sufferers without histories of abuse, the abused group scored higher on indices of psychological distress and somatization, tended to view themselves as disabled, perceived themselves as lacking control, experienced social and vocational impairment, amplified reports of pain, and used dissociation as a coping strategy. Those who have suffered severe abuse appear to be more vulnerable.

35. What other symptoms are common sequelae of abuse?

Individuals with histories of childhood sexual abuse, compared to nonabused or less severely abused, were also found to have higher lifetime histories of depression, drug abuse, panic disorder, phobias, somatization disorders, and medically unexplained symptoms. The number of somatization symptoms along with drug dependence and long-standing panic disorder was predictive of a history of severe sexual abuse in childhood.

36. How can prior experiences of abuse impact the current rehabilitation process?

Among the long-term sequelae of any form of abuse are depressive symptoms, low self-esteem, and a sense of powerlessness. The process of rehabilitation requires that patients be motivated to recover, assert themselves to engage in those activities that will decrease symptoms while increasing functioning, and view themselves as worthy to be helped and recover. Abused patients may view their pain as just another way they will continue to suffer. Lacking a sense of empowerment, these patients may be less likely to engage in rehabilitative efforts in their own behalf.

37. Does abuse at work impact health and the reporting of symptoms?

A few studies have been conducted in the medical community and strongly indicate that medical personnel experience abuse both at home and at work. Seventy-two percent of medical students surveyed stated that they experienced at least one abusive experience during their medical training. When similar experiences among emergency department medical and support personnel were assessed, 67% perceived abuse in their workplace. Abuse not only included sexual or physical abuse but also verbal abuse, intimidation, and behaviors that were an affront to self-esteem. Abuse in one venue, work or home, was seen as contributing to abuse in the other. In addition to poor staff morale, lower productivity, underlying fear, and increased tensions among coworkers, a high turnover rate was noted along with increased absenteeism. Virtually all felt that abuse in any setting contributed to health problems. When groups of nurses, ED staff, government employees, manufacturing employees, and MBA students were compared, 50% of the respondents perceived abusive or neglectful behaviors occurring at least monthly both at home and at work.

38. What is alexithymia?

The literal meaning of alexithymia is "no words for mood." The term is applied to those individuals who have difficulty describing their emotions. This phenomenon is commonly observed among individuals suffering from chronic somatic problems, including chronic pain. The construct is derived from principles of Western philosophy, which places an emphasis (positive value judgment) on the verbal expression of emotions. Possessing the ability to perceive and verbally express one's emotions is regarded as a reflection of mental health and maturity. In contrast, Eastern philosophy views somatization and intellectualized description of inner experiences as normative.

39. List some of the cardinal features of the alexithymic individual.

• Complains about countless physical symptoms.
• Displays an absence of fantasy production and rarely dreams.
• The content of speech lacks relevant facts and is replaced by repetitive details.
• Interpersonal relationships are either dependent or estranged in nature.
• Clinicians often feel bored interacting with such individuals.

40. What does the term compensation neurosis denote?

Compensation neurosis has traditionally carried a negative connotation. The construct presumes that the patient's complaints of pain and disability are motivated by the prospect of financial rewards, are encouraged by lawyers, and have little or no organic basis, and that the patient's condition would improve dramatically and quickly upon receipt of a favorable settlement.

41. Are individuals receiving compensation for pain complaints less likely than those not receiving rewards to respond positively to treatment?

This has been and remains one of the more debated topics in the field of pain management. The general clinical impression is that receipt of compensation or the prospect of a litigious windfall acts as a disincentive to participate actively and derive maximum benefit from rehabilitative efforts. Despite this popular belief, research data have failed to substantiate this assumption.

42. If the patient is applying for compensation and there are no organic findings, should you conclude that the pain problem is psychogenic in origin?

In one word, no. There are a number of pain syndromes, e.g., headaches or back pain, where the neuromedical examination may be negative. If gross inconsistencies between pain complaints and medical findings exist, questions should be raised but conclusions should not be drawn hastily.

43. What personality characteristics make an individual more prone to claiming disability?

Dependent individuals who have low self-esteem with poor tolerance for, and lack the ability to deal with, stress appear more apt to become a victim of an accident. These individuals are often dissatisfied with a stressful job and may also experience family and interpersonal tensions and feel at an impasse for coping with them effectively. Under these circumstances, a sanctioned disability provides a face-saving way to absolve the individual of personal responsibility, place the onus for recovery on the physician and quietly avoid the undesirable situation. When reinforced by social acceptance (because the injury or illness is not their fault), financial factors (disability payment may be equal to that received for work), and attention (sympathy from family and friends along with being the focus of inquiry by health care professionals), dysfunction can rapidly become an entrenched way of life.

44. What single factor is most predictive for return to work in the patient with back injuries?

While both physicians and patients alike tend to view organic findings, e.g., herniated disc, as the critical factor in predicting a return to functioning, the literature does not support this notion. In a series of clinical studies, the patient's fear of reinjury consistently accounted for the greatest proportion of the variance for predicting successful rehabilitation.

45. Are there specific personality types associated with headache?

In the 1960s, investigators were publishing reports that certain personality characteristics were associated with the occurrence of headaches. Conclusions were based mostly on clinical impressions, and the population of migraineurs was described as anxious, depressed, hostile, angry, obsessive, and rigid, with a tendency toward hypochondriasis. The classic portrait of migraine sufferers persisted despite the potential for bias in data collection.

46. Has further research clarified questions regarding headaches and personality?

Additional community-based epidemiologic studies have supported the notion that headache sufferers, particularly those with more frequent headaches, scored higher on an index of neuroticism, as assessed by the Eysenck Personality Questionnaire. Neuroticism was defined as a tendency to be emotionally labile, to overreact, and to be at risk for developing neurotic disorders under stress. A recent study supported this basic premise, showing that migraine with and without aura was associated with neuroticism.

47. Are migraine sufferers at greater risk for depression?

Community-based studies have pointed to an association between depression and migraine. Estimated risk for first onset of major depression among migraineurs was 3.2-fold higher than in controls. The risk for migraine was 3.1-fold higher among those with histories of depression. Findings applied equally to both males and females, although women had a higher incidence of both disorders. The study concluded that there is a bidirectional influence between the two disorders.

BIBLIOGRAPHY

1. Alston RJ, Lenhoff K: Chronic pain and childhood sexual abuse: Implications for rehabilitation education. Rehabilitation Education 9(1):37–49, 1995.
2. Bradley LA, McDonald HJ, Jaworski TM: Assessment of psychological status using interviews and self-report instruments. In Turk DC, Melzack R (eds): Handbook of Pain Assessment. New York, The Guilford Press, 1992.
3. Breslau N, Andreski P: Migraine, personality, and psychiatric comorbidity. Headache 382–386, July/August 1995.
4. Breslau N, et al: Migraine and major depression: A longitudinal study. Headache 34(7):387–393, 1994.
5. Crisson JE, Keefe FJ: The relationship of locus of control to pain coping strategies and psychological distress in chronic pain patients. Pain 35:147–154, 1988.
6. Derogatis L: The SCL-90R Manual-II: Administration, Scoring and Procedures. Baltimore, Clinical Psychometric Research, 1983.
7. Drossman DA, Leserman J, Nachman G, et al: Sexual and physical abuse in women with functional or organic gastrointestinal disorders. Ann Intern Med 113(11):828–833, 1990.
8. Fordyce WE, Bigos SJ, Batti'e MC, Fisher LD: MMPI scale 3 as a predictor of back injury report: What does it tell us? Clin J Pain 8:222–226, 1992.
9. Pilowsky I: Pain and illness behavior: Assessment and management. In Wall PD, Melzack R (eds): Textbook of Pain. New York, Churchill Livingstone, 1994.
10. Pincus T, Callahan LF, Bradley LA, Vaughn WK, Wolfe F: Elevated MMPI scores for hypochondriasis, depression and hysteria in patients with rheumatoid arthritis reflect disease rather than psychological status. Arthritis Rheum 29:1456–1466, 1986.
11. Randall T: Abuse at work drains people, money, and medical workplace not immune. Medical News & Perspectives. JAMA 267:1439–1440, 1992.
12. Walker EA, Katon WJ, Neraas K, et al: Dissociation in women with chronic pelvic pain. Am J Psychiatry 149(4):534–537, 1992.
13. Walker EA, Katon WJ, Hansom J, et al: Medical and psychiatric symptoms in women with childhood sexual abuse. Psychosom Med 54(6):658–664, 1992.
14. Wolff HG: Headache and Other Head Pains, 2nd ed. New York, Oxford University Press, 1963.
15. Wurtele SK, Kaplan GM, Keairnes M: Childhood sexual abuse among chronic pain patients. Clin J Pain 6:110–113, 1990.

III. Clinical Syndromes Defined by Pain

8. TENSION-TYPE HEADACHE

Richard B. Lipton, M.D., and Lawrence C. Newman, M.D.

1. Are tension-type headaches the headaches of everyday life?

Yes. Most of us experience tension-type headache at one time or another, and almost 80% of the population has had a tension-type headache within the past year. While there is a slight preponderance of females, the gender ratio is very close to 1:1. Tension-type headache is a disorder of middle life, affecting people during their peak productive years. It is seven times more common than migraine and may be disabling. Because it is so frequent, tension-type headache actually causes more work loss than migraine.

2. What is the approach to diagnosing tension-type headache?

The steps in the diagnosis of tension-type headache resemble the steps in the diagnosis of migraine. Secondary headache disorders are excluded based on a directed history and a careful general medical and neurologic examination. If no alarms are present by history or exam, try to apply the diagnostic criteria for the primary headache disorders. If the patient fits neatly into a standard diagnostic category, a diagnosis is assigned and treatment is initiated. If alarms are present or if the headache features are atypical, a directed diagnostic search is necessary to exclude secondary headache.

3. How is tension-type headache defined?

Tension-type headaches are characterized by recurrent attacks of head pain without specific associated features. To diagnose tension-type headache, the International Headache Society requires a lifetime history of 10 typical attacks. Obviously, at some point in their natural history, patients will have not yet experienced that number of attacks. To diagnose tension-type headache, two out of four of the following pain features should be present: pain on both sides of the head (bilateral pain), pain that is a steady ache or a pressure pain, pain that is mild or moderate in severity, and pain that is not exacerbated by routine physical activity. The pain of tension type headache is often bifrontal, bioccipital, or binuchal. On occasion, the pain is associated with tenderness of the paracranial muscles to palpation and may be described as a squeezing sensation akin to wearing a hat that is too tight, as a headband of pain, or as a pressure sensation at the vertex of the head.

4. What is the differential diagnosis of tension-type headache?

Tension-type headache must be distinguished from other primary and secondary headache disorders. Its bilateral location, mild to moderate pain intensity, and the absence of autonomic features make differentiating it from cluster headache relatively easy. Its distinction from migraine is discussed in question 5.

Unfortunately, early in their course, brain tumors and other intracranial mass lesions tend to produce bilateral dull headaches, which may be difficult to distinguish from tension-type headache. Headaches due to brain tumors tend to progress in frequency and severity and focal neurologic symptoms and signs or evidence of increased intracranial pressure usually develop (see Chapter 13).

5. How are tension-type headache and migraine differentiated?

The diagnostic features of tension-type headache and migraine contrast rather sharply. Migraine pain tends to be unilateral; tension-type headache pain tends to be bilateral. Migraine pain tends to be throbbing or pulsatile; tension-type headache pain tends to be a steady ache or a squeezing or pressure sensation. Migraine pain tends to be moderate to severe, tension-type headache pain tends to be mild or moderate. Migraine pain is aggravated by routine physical activity like climbing stairs; tension-type headache pain is not. In addition, tension-type headache is characterized by the absence of the migraine-defining associated symptoms. Specifically, tension-type headache is not accompanied by nausea, photophobia, or phonophobia. On the rare occasion that these features are present, they are mild.

6. Are there other forms of tension-type headache?

It's traditional to divide tension-type headache into two broad groups: episodic tension-type headache and chronic tension-type headache. By definition, episodic tension-type headache attacks occur less than 15 days per month and less than 180 days per year while chronic tension-type headache occurs 15 or more days per month or greater than 180 days per year. Otherwise, the clinical features of the attacks are quite similar. Chronic tension-type headache affects about 3% of the population.

The term chronic tension-type headache is sometimes used as a synonym for transformed migraine. While both chronic tension-type headache and transformed migraine are characterized by frequent attacks of mild to moderate headache, these disorders should be differentiated. As its name would indicate, transformed migraine evolves out of episodic migraine, as headaches increase in frequency and decrease in severity and the specific migraine features remit. Chronic tension-type headache does not evolve from migraine; it may arise de novo or in individuals with episodic tension-type headache.

7. What are the mechanisms of tension-type headache?

The mechanism of pain in tension-type headache remains uncertain. This disorder was once called muscle contraction headache, based on the assumption that excessive contraction of skeletal muscle produced pain. The term tension headache was sometimes used to suggest that stress or psychologic tension was the fundamental cause of the disorder. The term tension-type headache is intended to imply that we don't know what, if anything, is "tense." While there are excess levels of muscle contraction in tension-type headache, these levels don't exceed those found in patients with migraine. While stress is a trigger for some people with tension-type headache, the disorder can occur in the absence of stress, and high levels of stress can occur without tension-type headache.

The prevailing ideas suggest that tension-type headache may be a brain disease like migraine. Pathophysiologic changes in the brain may produce secondary changes in pain-sensitive blood vessels or nerve endings, giving rise to headache pain. However, the fundamental mechanism of tension headache remains uncertain.

8. Is tension-type headache a genetic disorder?

There is essentially no evidence that tension-type headache runs within families. In contrast, family and twin studies suggest an important role for genetic factors in migraine. Because it is so common, tension-type headache occurs within families by chance alone.

9. How is tension-type headache treated?

The treatment of tension-type headache, like the treatment of migraine, can be divided into two major categories: nonpharmacologic and pharmacologic therapies. The nonpharmacologic therapies are divided into acute (abortive) and preventive (prophylactic).

10. What are the nonpharmacologic treatment options for episodic tension-type headache?

As with migraine, it's important to begin by identifying factors that exacerbate or trigger headaches. It is important to distinguish trigger factors from causes. Trigger factors precipitate headache in a biologically vulnerable individual; they are not the fundamental cause of headache. Psychologic stress may be an important exacerbating factor. Stress may be related to a job or family situation. Resolving the stressful situation sometimes helps improve headache control. When this is not possible, stress management methods, including relaxation techniques or biofeedback, may be helpful. Sometimes, cognitive/behavioral therapy is useful (see Chapter 39).

Some patients find that postural factors (such as working long hours with an awkward head position) contribute to headache. For these patients, ergonomic changes in the workplace or simply getting up to stretch may be helpful. The traditional triggers of migraine (see Chapter 9), including dietary factors, missed meals, disrupted sleep, changes in the weather, and hormonal factors, occasionally contribute to tension-type headache as well. Regular meals, consistent sleep patterns, and exercise can help eliminate headache.

When tension-type headache is associated with spasm or tenderness of the pericranial or cervical musculature, physical modalities are sometimes useful. Local application of heat or ice packs and the use of a cervical pillow may be useful. Diathermy, massage, and trigger point injections are sometimes used. Transcutaneous electrical nerve stimulation (TENS) has been reported to alleviate tension-type headache as well.

For most patients, it is worthwhile to explore headache triggers and recommend a regular pattern of sleeping and eating along with a program of regular exercise and stress management.

11. What are the acute treatment options for episodic tension-type headache?

Tension-type headache can be treated with simple over-the-counter (OTC) analgesics such as aspirin, acetaminophen (Tylenol), ibuprofen (Advil, Nuprin), naproxen sodium (Aleve), and ketoprofen (Actron, Orudis KT). When simple analgesics fail or provide incomplete relief, OTC combination-of-ingredient products provide a useful alternative. Clinical trials demonstrate that the addition of caffeine to a simple analgesic significantly increases pain relief. This effect, referred to as the analgesic adjuvancy action of caffeine, is the basis for combination-of-ingredient products such as Excedrin and Anacin.

When OTC medications do not provide adequate relief, prescription drugs should be use. Nonsteroidal anti-inflammatory agents such as naproxen sodium (Anaprox), 550 mg, or diflunisal (Dolobid), 500 mg, may succeed where OTC nonsteroidal anti-inflammatory agents are inadequate. The isometheptene-containing combination-of-ingredient capsules (Midrin) are useful and produce few side effects. The butalbital and caffeine-containing combination-of-ingredient products (Fiorinal, Fioricet, Esgic) are very effective. Minor narcotics, including codeine combinations (acetaminophen with codeine) and butalbital and codeine combinations (e.g., Fioricet with codeine), are highly effective, but doses must be limited. Transnasal narcotics (Stadol NS) are useful for severe tension-type headaches refractory to other treatments. In general, caffeine, butalbital, or narcotic-containing products should not be used more than two or three days per week to avoid tolerance and dependence as well as rebound headache.

12. Isn't caffeine a cause of headache? Why is caffeine found in so many headache remedies?

Caffeine (more specifically, caffeine withdrawal) can be a headache trigger. If a patient drinks several cups of caffeinated beverages or takes caffeine-containing medications on a daily basis, the absence of caffeine can trigger headache. Some patients awaken on weekend mornings with a headache because they slept through their regular cup of coffee; caffeine withdrawal headaches are quite common even in moderate caffeine users.

When caffeine is taken at the time of a headache, it increases the efficacy of analgesics. For this reason, patients often learn to drink a cup of coffee when they take a pain killer or use combination drugs that contain caffeine. The best advise is to limit caffeine intake on nonheadache days (to one cup of coffee or tea a day) and to save caffeine for its medicinal effects on headache days.

13. What are the limits on the use of acute treatment for tension-type headache?

All acute headache treatments should be limited to avoid side effects and overuse of medication. Virtually all of the drugs used to treat headache can become a cause of headache if overused.

As a habitually used analgesic wears off, that process can, in itself, trigger a headache; these headaches are generally termed rebound headache. Aspirin and nonsteroidal anti-inflammatory agents are less likely to cause rebound than are products that contain caffeine, isometheptene, butalbital, or narcotics. As a rule, acute treatments should not be used more than three days a week.

14. Does prevention have a role in the treatment of tension-type headache?

Preventive treatment is used for only a small minority of patients who suffer from tension-type headache. Preventive medication should be considered in patients who have disability because of headaches three or more days each month. In addition, preventive medication may play a role in patients at risk for rebound headache because of a frequent need for analgesics. If symptomatic medication is ineffective or contraindicated, preventive therapy is a treatment option. Finally, if the patient has a comorbid condition (such as depression) that requires treatment, it is appropriate to treat both the headache disorder and the comorbid condition with a single drug, when possible.

15. What are the preventive treatments of choice for tension-type headache?

The most widely used drugs are the antidepressants. The tricyclic antidepressants are a standard choice. We prefer nortriptyline (Pamelor) and doxepin (Sinequan) because they have fewer anticholinergic side effects than amitriptyline (Elavil). The usual regimen starts with a low bedtime dose (10 or 25 mg), and the dose is gradually increased as needed and as tolerated. The selective serotonin reuptake inhibitors (SSRIs) are sometimes used for prevention of tension-type headache. Fluoxetine (Prozac) has been shown to be effective in a small controlled study of chronic daily headache. The other SSRIs have not been studied but are widely used.

If antidepressants are unsuccessful or contraindicated, many of the drugs used for the prevention of migraine may also be used for tension-type headache. Calcium-channel blockers and divalproex sodium are generally more successful than beta blockers. Daily administration of nonsteroidal anti-inflammatory agents is also sometimes used for prevention.

16. Is the management approach the same or different for chronic tension-type headache?

Behavioral interventions to reduce the frequency of attack are especially important for chronic tension-type headache. Although the acute treatment options are similar, because of the frequency of attacks, patients with chronic tension-type headache are at increased risk for rebound headache. Use of acute treatments that cause rebound headache should be avoided or severely limited. It is usually desirable to treat these patients with preventive medications.

BIBLIOGRAPHY

1. Couch, JR: Medical management of recurrent tension-type headache. In Tollison CD, Kunkel RS (eds): Headache Diagnosis and Treatment. Baltimore, Williams & Wilkins, 1993, pp 151–162.
2. Headache Classification Committee of the International Headache Society. Classification and diagnostic criteria for headache disorders, cranial neuralgias, and facial pain. Cephalalgia 8 (Suppl 7):1–96, 1988.
3. Rasmussen BK, Jensen R, Schroll M, Olesen J: Epidemiology of headache in a general population—A prevalence study. J Clin Epidemiol 44:1147–1157, 1991.
4. Solomon S, Lipton RB, Newman LC: Clinical symptomatology and differential diagnosis of tension-type headache. In Tollison CD, Kunkel RS (eds): Headache Diagnosis and Treatment. Baltimore, Williams & Wilkins, 1993, pp 123–127.

9. MIGRAINE

Richard B. Lipton, M.D., and Lawrence C. Newman, M.D.

1. Is migraine an important health problem?

Yes, by virtually any standard. Migraine is a highly prevalent disorder that affects 11% of the U.S. population and produces enormous suffering for individual sufferers and their families. Recent estimates indicate that 23 million Americans suffer from migraine headaches and that more than 11 million experience significant levels of headache-related disability. Economic estimates show that the cost of migraine in the United States may be as high as $17 billion a year. The principal factor of the cost of illness is missed work and disability at work (indirect costs). In addition, headaches are the seventh leading reason for outpatient visits in the United States and account for 2 to 4% of all emergency room visits.

2. What are the phases of the migraine attack?

1. The prodrome
2. The aura
3. The headache phase
4. The resolution phase

The prodrome typically occurs hours or days before the headache. The aura occurs immediately before or during the headache. The headache phase is characterized by pain and associated symptoms as discussed below. In the resolution phase, spontaneous pain subsides, but other symptoms are present. Most patients do not experience all four phases.

3. What is the difference between a prodrome and an aura?

Prodromal features vary enormously from person to person but typically include changes in mood or behavior hours or days before the headache. Patients may feel depressed, euphoric, irritable, or restless, and occasionally may report fatigue or hyperactivity. Constitutional symptoms may include changes in appetite, fluid balance, and bowel function. Some patients report food cravings while others describe a poorly characterized feeling that an attack is coming.

In contrast, the aura consists specifically of focal neurologic symptoms that usually precede, but that may accompany, the attack. Only 20 to 30% of migraine sufferers ever experience auras, and most people who have attacks with aura also have attacks without aura. The aura symptoms typically develop over 5 to 20 minutes and usually last less than 60 minutes. Auras are most commonly characterized by changes in vision, although changes in motor and sensory function may also occur. The classic visual aura of migraine is characterized by both positive symptom features such as flashes of light (scintillations) or zig-zag lines and negative symptom features such as visual loss (scotoma). The visual aura may begin in a small portion of the visual field and gradually expand to encompass an entire visual hemifield.

Sensory auras are also characterized by a mix of positive features (tingling) and negative features (numbness). These sensory features may begin on one side of the face or hand and slowly expand to encompass an entire side of the body. Hemiparesis may occur, and if the dominant hemisphere is involved, dysphasia or aphasia develops on rare occasions.

4. How do you differentiate migraine aura from other kinds of focal episodes of neurologic dysfunction?

Transient neurologic deficits may have several causes. These include seizures, stroke, metabolic derangements, and psychiatric disease. Seizure is most typically characterized by positive phenomena such as tonic or tonic/clonic movements. Stroke is most often characterized by negative phenomena such as weakness. Both seizures and stroke tend to come on relatively suddenly.

The gradual evolution of symptom features and the mix of positive and negative features as well as the temporal association with headache help identify migraine aura. The patient's age and risk-factor profile may also point the clinician in one diagnostic direction or another.

5. What are the characteristics of the headache phase?

The headache phase of migraine is characterized by a combination of pain features and associated symptoms. The pain is typically unilateral and pulsatile. It is generally moderate to severe in intensity and aggravated by routine physical activities. Not every patient has all four of the characteristic pain features. Pain may be bilateral at onset or may begin on one side and then become generalized. Eighty-five percent of patients with migraine describe their pain as throbbing or pulsatile, although this description is not specific for migraine. The pain is commonly aggravated by routine physical activity, like climbing stairs, or by head movement.

By definition, the pain of migraine must be accompanied by other features. Nausea occurs in up to 90% of patients and vomiting in up to 33% of migraineurs. Many patients experience sensory hyperexcitability in the form of photophobia, phonophobia, and osmophobia. Other accompanying features include anorexia or food cravings, blurry vision, nasal stuffiness, abdominal cramps, polyuria, and pallor. Although impaired concentration is common, measurable memory impairment has rarely been documented.

6. What is the postdrome?

The postdrome, or termination phase, of the migraine attack begins as the pain wanes. Following the headache, the patient may feel irritable, listless, tired, or washed-out. Many patients report residual scalp tenderness in the distribution of the remitted spontaneous pain. Some patients will feel unusually refreshed or euphoric after a migraine attack.

7. What feature or features are absolutely required to diagnose migraine?

It is important to recognize that there is no single headache feature and no single associated symptom that is pathognomonic for migraine. For example, 20 to 30% of migraineurs have auras, and 90% have nausea or vomiting. Therefore, the physician who relies exclusively on any one single feature to establish or exclude the diagnosis will invariably make mistakes.

In 1988, the International Headache Society (IHS) provided a classification system for headache disorders. That system defined seven different types of migraine. The two most important types are migraine without aura and migraine with aura.

Diagnostic Criteria for Migraine without Aura

A. At least five attacks fulfilling B–D.

B. Headache attacks lasting 4–72 hours (untreated or unsuccessfully treated).

C. Headache has at least two of the following characteristics:
   1. Unilateral location.
   2. Pulsating quality.
   3. Moderate or severe intensity (inhibits or prohibits daily activities).
   4. Aggravation by walking stairs or similar routine physical activity.

D. During headache at least one of the following:
   1. Nausea and/or vomiting.
   2. Photophobia and phonophobia.

E. At least one of the following:
   1. History, physical, and neurologic examinations do not suggest one of the disorders listed in groups 5–11.
   2. History and/or physical and/or neurologic examinations do suggest such disorder, but it is ruled out by appropriate investigations.
   3. Such disorder is present, but migraine attacks do not occur for the first time in close temporal relation to the disorder.

Diagnostic Criteria for Migraine with Aura

A. At least two attacks fulfilling B.

B. At least three of the following four characteristics:
   1. One or more fully reversible aura symptoms indicating focal cerebral cortical and/or brain stem dysfunction.
   2. At least one aura symptom develops gradually over more than 4 minutes, or two or more symptoms occur in succession.
   3. No aura symptom lasts more than 60 minutes. If more than one aura symptom is present, accepted duration is proportionally increased.
   4. Headache follows aura with a free interval of less than 60 minutes. (It may also begin before or simultaneously with the aura.)

C. At least one of the following:
   1. History, physical, and neurologic examinations do not suggest one of the disorders listed in groups 5–11.
   2. History and/or physical and/or neurologic examinations do suggest such disorder, but it is ruled out by appropriate investigations.
   3. Such disorder is present, but migraine attacks do not occur for the first time in close temporal relation to the disorder.

8. What diagnostic tests are required to establish the diagnosis of migraine?

Diagnostic testing in migraine serves primarily to exclude secondary causes of headache. In our practice, when we confront the patient complaining of headache, the first step is to identify headache alarms that suggest the possibility of secondary headache. These clinical alarms are discussed in Chapter 13. If the patient has no history of clinical alarms, the general medical and neurologic examinations sometimes provide evidence that raises the possibility of secondary headache. If there is a possibility of secondary headache, an appropriate diagnostic workup is required. In the absence of alarms, the next step is to try to diagnose a specific primary headache disorder. If the patient has typical migraine or tension-type headache, it is appropriate to proceed with treatment. If the headache features are atypical, even in the absence of alarms, it is important to consider diagnostic testing to exclude secondary causes. If treatment is initiated and the expected response to therapy is not obtained, it is appropriate to revisit the issue of secondary headache. Because migraine and tension-type headache are so common, however, it is not appropriate or cost-effective to obtain neuroimaging on every patient.

9. Why is migraine considered a neurologic disease?

Migraine is viewed as a disease of the brain. Changes in the brain give rise to inflammatory changes in cranial blood vessels which, in turn, produce pain. The prodrome itself, with its characteristic changes in mood, behavior, and autonomic function, is best understood on the basis of central nervous system dysfunction. Neuroimaging procedures, including PET scanning, electro-nencephalogram, and magneto-encephalography, demonstrate abnormalities of the brain during or between attacks in patients with migraine. Finally, the drugs used to treat migraine often act either on the brain itself or on the cranial blood vessels.

10. What is the mechanism of the aura?

The phenomenon of "spreading cortical depression" may underlie the aura of migraine. Spreading depression is characterized by a wave of excitation (depolarization) followed by a wave of inhibition that spreads over the cortical surface of experimental animals after mechanical stimulation or the application of potassium salts. Neuronal activity decreases during a wave of inhibition, producing decreased cerebral blood flow through the mechanism of cerebral autoregulation. As a consequence, the wave of inhibition is accompanied by a wave of spreading oligemia (decreased blood flow). In migraine with aura, cerebral blood flow studies demonstrate a wave of oligemia that accompanies the aura, as predicted by the model of spreading depression. This wave of oligemia progresses at a rate of 2 to 3 mm/minute, the same rate reported for spreading depression in experimental animals.

In addition, the rate of spreading oligemia and spreading depression corresponds with the evolution of the scintillating scotoma that marches across the visual field of the typical migraine aura.

11. What is the substrate of migraine pain?

The work of Michael Moskowitz and coworkers suggests that the trigeminovascular system may be involved as a final common pathway for migraine pain. The trigeminovascular system includes the trigeminal nerve and the cranial blood vessels that it innervates. The trigeminal nerve endings contain a wide range of neurotransmitters, including substance P, calcitonin gene-related peptide (CGRP), and neurokinin A. Release of these transmitters causes a sterile inflammatory response within the cranial blood vessels accompanied by extravasation of plasma proteins. The fibers of the trigeminal nerve provide an interface between the blood circulation and the brain. The pain of migraine may result from the activation of trigeminal sensory afferents and the development of a neurogenically mediated inflammatory response.

12. What is the role of serotonin in migraine?

Serotonin plays a pivotal role in the pathophysiology of migraine. Blood levels of serotonin decrease during the migraine attack. Urinary concentrations of serotonin's metabolites increase during a migraine attack. A serotonin-releasing factor is present in the plasma of migraine patients during migraine attacks but not at other times. In addition, activation of the serotonergic dorsal raphe nucleus causes migraine-like headaches. Finally, evidence from positron emission tomography demonstrates increased metabolism in the brain stem in the region of the serotonergic dorsal raphe nucleus during migraine attacks.

13. What are the subtypes of serotonin receptors, and what role may they play in migraine?

The neuropharmacology of serotonin has become increasingly complex in recent years. There are four major numbered classes of serotonin receptors in the brain, including 5-HT1, 5-HT2, 5-HT3, and 5-HT4 classes. There are many subclasses as well. The 5-HT1 class of receptors may play a role in acute migraine therapy on at least two levels. There is one subtype of 5-HT1 receptor found on cranial blood vessels. A distinct subtype of 5-HT1 receptor is found on trigeminal nerve endings. Activation of the 5-HT1 receptor on the trigeminal nerve terminal blocks the release of the mediators of neorogenic inflammation. This class of 5-HT1 agonist drugs effectively treats the acute migraine attack. Activation of another subclass of 5-HT1 receptors produces a vasoconstrictor response that may also play a role in relieving the pain of migraine. Many of the acute treatments for migraine, including ergotamine, dihydroergotamine, and sumatriptan, are 5-HT1 agonists. Sumatriptan is a highly selective agonist at this class of receptors.

Many of the medications used as preventive treatments for migraine act on 5-HT2 receptors. Methysergide is a 5-HT2 receptor antagonist. Tricyclic antidepressants may act by down-regulating the 5-HT2 receptor.

14. What is the role of genetics in the pathophysiology of migraine?

We have long known that migraine is a familial disorder. Twin studies demonstrate that identical twins are more likely to be concordant for migraine than fraternal twins. More recently, specific genetic linkage has been identified for the rare subtype of migraine known as familial hemiplegic migraine (FHM). A locus on chromosome 19 has been identified for familial hemiplegic migraine. That locus plays a role in some, but not all, families with FHM. Given that FHM is genetically heterogeneous, it seems virtually certain that there are multiple genetic forms for the other types of migraine and also quite likely that there may be nongenetic forms of the syndrome.

15. What are the strategies for treating migraine?

1. Make a specific diagnosis
2. Identify factors that trigger the patient's headache
3. Introduce other behavioral interventions
4. Provide medications to either treat acute attacks or prevent their recurrence.

Obtaining a thorough headache history and understanding the impact of migraine on the patient's life are critical preludes to treatment. Patients and their relatives should be educated about the nature of migraine and the approach to therapy. When possible, headache triggers should be identified, and patients should be taught to avoid them. Patients should understand that triggers do not generally operate through allergic mechanisms. Many dietary triggers contain biologically active chemicals that act on blood vessels or the brain to initiate an attack.

16. How do you help patients identify their headache triggers?

The first step in identifying headache triggers is simply to take a history. Many patients are aware of alcohol, chocolate, or medications that trigger their headaches. In addition, patients should be encouraged to keep headache diaries. This will provide accurate information about headache features, including the frequency and severity of attacks and potential triggers. Patients should record possible triggers so that patterns can be reviewed over time. Trigger factors may be difficult to identify because they cause a headache on one day but not on another. For example, a small glass of wine may not lead to a headache, while a half bottle of wine will initiate an attack. Chocolate may cause headache during menses or at a time of stress but not at other times of the month. Patients should understand that important triggers do not necessarily initiate an attack with every exposure. In addition, vulnerability to trigger factors varies widely from person to person.

Selected Migraine Trigger Factors

Alcohol	Hunger
Aspartame	Light (bright or flashing)
Barometric pressure changes	Medication overuse
Cheese	Menstruation
Cigarette smoke	Monosodium glutamate
Estrogens	Odors (perfume, gasoline, solvents)
Excessive or insufficient sleep	Oral contraceptives
Head trauma	Stress and worry

17. What other nonpharmacologic options are available?

In discussing nonpharmacologic treatment with patients, it is very important to distinguish exacerbating factors from the fundamental cause of migraine. Stress may make many illnesses worse, including asthma, heart disease, or ulcers. Just as stress can precipitate headaches, relaxation methods, including biofeedback, may diminish their severity or frequency. Behavioral interventions are often effective treatments and help give the patient a feeling of control.

Nonpharmacologic prevention strategies include changing the diet, teaching relaxation methods, using biofeedback, and applying cognitive behavioral therapy. Biofeedback is essentially a relaxation method that gives patients information about a measured physiologic parameter such as electromyography (EMG) or skin temperature. Biofeedback training may help decrease the frequency of attacks by decreasing reactivity to stress. It can also be used to treat acute attacks for patients who have learned the methods well.

18. Is migraine associated with psychiatric disease?

Migraine is associated with depression and anxiety disorders, as well as manic-depressive illness. This comorbidity does not imply that migraine has psychogenic mechanisms. More likely, it suggests that perturbations in particular neural transmitter systems predispose patients both to migraine and to certain forms of psychiatric illness. When comorbid psychiatric disease is present, it is important to address it in treatment.

19. What is an appropriate strategy for migraine pharmacotherapy?

The drugs used to treat migraine are generally classified as acute agents and preventive agents. Acute therapy is administered at the time of the attack to relieve or prevent pain, disability, and the associated symptoms of migraine. Preventive therapy is taken on a daily basis, whether or not headache is present, to reduce the frequency and severity of attacks. Almost everyone with migraine needs acute treatments. A minority of migraine sufferers require preventive treatments.

There are a number of acute treatment options for migraine. When migraine is mild or moderate, simple analgesics such as aspirin, acetaminophen, or nonsteroidal antiinflammatory agents may be sufficient for treatment. Caffeine enhances the effectiveness of simple analgesics and may have special benefits in migraine (e.g., Excedrin, Anacin). The addition of codeine or a barbiturate also increases treatment effects (e.g., Fiorinal, Fioricent, Esgic). These compounds may be associated with an increased risk of sedation, rebound headache, tolerance, or dependence so they should not be used more than two or three times a week. Isometheptene is a simple, safe vasoactive compound that can be used in combination with analgesics to relieve headache. When nausea or vomiting is present, adding an anti-emetic/prokinetic agent, such as metoclopramide, may enhance the effectiveness of the simple analgesics.

In addition, there is a category of migraine-specific acute treatments, also called "abortive agents."

20. What are the migraine-specific acute treatments, and how do they work?

The migraine-specific acute treatments include ergotamine, dihydroergotamine, and sumatriptan. All three agents are believed to activate presynaptic 5-HT1 receptors on trigeminal nerve endings. Activation of the 5-HT1 receptor blocks the release of substance P, calcitonin gene-related peptide, and neurokinin A and ameliorates the development of neurogenic inflammation. Ergotamine and dihydroergotamine activate a broad range of receptors while sumatriptan is highly selective for the 5-HT1 class of receptors. Other 5-HT1 agonist drugs are currently in development for the acute treatment of migraine.

21. How do you choose from among the acute treatment options?

Acute treatments need to be matched to the overall severity of the patient's illness, to the severity of the patient's attack, to the profile of associated symptoms, and to the patient's treatment preferences. Simple analgesics and combination analgesics may be adequate for the treatment of mild to moderate migraine attacks. More severe attacks often require specific migraine therapy. In addition, when nausea or vomiting is prominent, the associated gastric paresis may limit the effectiveness of oral agents. Nonoral agents for migraine currently include injections, suppositories, and nasal sprays. Patients often have strong treatment preferences for one route versus another. Some patients consider suppositories anathema, while others would prefer to avoid injections. Many patients favor nasal sprays as the nonoral route of administration.

For the patient who awakens with severe, full-blown attacks, with prominent nausea and vomiting, nonoral therapy may be the only appropriate choice. For patients who have attacks that begin gradually or who are unsure if the attack will be mild or severe, it is best to begin with oral agents and escalate therapy if the attack increases in severity. Treatment requirements also vary with the context of an attack. If an attack begins before a major business meeting, a rapid parenteral treatment may be needed. If the attack begins on a Saturday morning, the patient may prefer to use a slower oral treatment.

Optimal therapy often requires that patients receive more than one treatment. For a patient with both moderate and severe attacks, treatment may begin with a nonsteroidal anti-inflammatory agent (plus metoclopramide), and sumatriptan can be used either as an escape medication or for the more severe attacks.

22. What is the role of sumatriptan in migraine therapy?

Sumatriptan is the most specific of the available acute treatments for migraine. Currently available as an oral tablet or a subcutaneous injection, sumatriptan rapidly relieves the pain and associated features of migraine. Response rates to the 6 mg subcutaneous injection range from 70 to over 90%, depending on the study. Response to sumatriptan tablets develops more slowly, with overall response rates of about 60%. Sumatriptan is best used for moderate to severe attacks. The choice between oral and injectable sumatriptan should be based on the need for rapid relief and the effectiveness of the alternative routes of administration. If the headaches begin slowly and gradually progress in severity, oral sumatriptan is most appropriate. For patients who awaken with disabling headache, for patients who require very rapid relief, or patients who have prominent gastrointestinal disturbances, subcutaneous sumatriptan offers important advantages. Subcutaneous sumatriptan should not be given during the aura; it is best to wait until pain develops before treating.

23. What are the contraindications for sumatriptan?

All of the 5-HT1 agonists are contraindicated in patients with a history of myocardial infarction, ischemic heart disease, migraine with prolonged or complicated aura, and other forms of vascular compromise. Patients with risk factors for heart disease need to be evaluated carefully before sumatriptan is prescribed. Serious side effects are extremely rare, but mild side effects are common. These side effects include pain at the injection site, tingling, flushing, burning, warmth, or hot sensations. In addition, noncardiac chest pressure occurs in approximately 4% of migraine sufferers.

24. How do you treat the nausea and vomiting of migraine?

The associated symptoms of migraine, including nausea and vomiting, may be as disabling as the head pain. Gastric stasis and delayed gastric emptying can decrease the effectiveness of all medications. Antiemetics such as metoclopramide, promethazine, or prochlorperazine may be used both to treat the nausea and the pain of migraine. Sumatriptan relieves the nausea as well as the pain of migraine. Ondansetron, a selective 5-HT3 receptor antagonist, can also be used as an antiemetic in treating migraine.

25. What is the role of opiates in the treatment of migraine?

Oral narcotics, usually in the form of aspirin or acetaminophen and codeine (with or without caffeine and butalbital), are widely prescribed. If these agents relieve pain and restore the ability to function, they provide an appropriate therapeutic option. Because of the risk of tolerance, dependence, and rebound headache, they are best reserved for compliant patients with relatively infrequent attacks.

Injectable narcotics and antiemetics are still widely used in urgent care settings. In double-blind studies, these drugs have proved to be moderately effective at relieving pain. Pain relief may be accompanied by sedation, limiting the ability of these agents to restore normal function.

26. What is the role of transnasal butorphanol (Stadol NS)?

Transnasal butorphanol (Stadol NS) is a mixed opiate agonist-antagonist now available in the form of nasal spray. This convenient route of administration leads to rapid absorption and rapid pain relief even in patients with prominent nausea and vomiting. It produces sedation or orthostatic hypotension in about half of patients. It provides an important therapeutic option for the relief of migraine pain. It is especially useful in patients with nocturnal headaches or prominent gastrointestinal symptoms as well as those with contraindications, side effects, or lack of response to the specific antimigraine agents. Use should be limited to two headache days per week. Patients should be instructed to lie down after administration of the drug to minimize side effects.

27. Who should get preventive therapy?

While acute treatment is necessary for virtually everyone with migraine, preventive medication should be used only under special circumstances. Preventive therapy should be considered when patients have two or more attacks per month that produce disability lasting three or more days. In addition, if symptomatic medication is contraindicated or ineffective, patients with less frequent pain and disability may be treated. When abortive medication is required more than twice a week or when headache attacks produce profound, prolonged disruption, preventive therapy may also be appropriate.

28. What are the preventive treatment choices?

The major groups of medication used for migraine prophylaxis include the beta blockers, the calcium-channel blockers, antidepressants, serotonin antagonists, and anticonvulsants. Many of these agents may work either by blocking 5-HT2 receptor sites or by down-regulating them.

29. How do you choose from among the agents of first choice?

If preventive medication is indicated, treatments are selected primarily based on their side-effect profiles and comorbid conditions. For example, in a patient with migraine and hypertension, beta blockers or calcium-channel blockers may be used to treat both conditions simultaneously. Similarly, in a patient with migraine and depression, antidepressants may be especially useful. In the patient with migraine and epilepsy or migraine and manic-depressive illness, divalproex sodium provides an opportunity to treat two conditions with a single drug. Comorbid illnesses may also impose therapeutic restrictions. For example, in the patient with migraine and low blood pressure, beta blockers or calcium-channel blockers are difficult to use. Similarly, in the patient with migraine and epilepsy, caution may be advisable as antidepressants may lower seizure threshold. The patient with migraine and asthma or Raynaud's syndrome probably should not be treated with beta blockers. Finally, in patients concerned about sedation or increased appetite, tricyclic antidepressants may be an inappropriate choice. The table summarizes the categories of drugs used to treat migraine, the evidence for their efficacy, their side effect profiles and the comorbid conditions which provide relative indications as well as relative contraindications.

Preventive Agents for Migraine

CATEGORY	DRUG NAME	TOTAL DAILY DOSE	DAILY FREQUENCY	SIDE EFFECTS
Beta-Blockers	Propranolol	80–320 mg	2–4 times	Fatigue, depression, lightheadedness, impotence. Should not be used or should be used with caution if patient suffers from asthma, emphysema, heart failure, or diabetes.
	Nadolol	40–160 mg	Once	
	Atenolol	50–100 mg	Once	
	Timolol	10–60 mg	1–3 times	
Calcium-Channel Blockers	Verapamil	240–480 mg	1–4 times*	Lightheadedness, constipation.
Tricyclic Anti-depressants	Amitriptyline	50–150 mg	Divided or at bedtime	Drowsiness, dry mouth, weight gain, blurred vision, constipation, difficulty urinating. Should not be used if patient suffers from glaucoma, prostate disorders, or arrhythmias.
	Nortriptyline	50–150 mg		
	Doxepin	50–150 mg		
Other	Methysergide	4–8 mg	3–4 times with meals	Nausea, hallucinations, tingling of extremities, retroperitoneal fibrosis. Must have a 1-month drug-free period after 6 months of treatment. Use other ergot preparations with caution.
	Cyproheptadine	12–32 mg	3–4 times	Drowsiness, increased appetite, weight gain.
	Divalproex	500–2000 mg daily	2–4 times	Tremor, sedation, weight gain, hair loss, hepatic dysfunction.

* Ordinary verapamil must be administered in divided doses. There is a sustained release preparation that can be used daily.

30. What are the principles of using preventive drugs?

In general, drugs should be started at a relatively low dose to avoid side effects. The dose should then be gradually increased until therapeutic effects develop, side effects develop, or the ceiling dose for the agent in question is reached. Because of the need to gradually increase the dose of most of these drugs, a therapeutic trial may take several months. Patients should be advised that treatment effects develop slowly, so that therapy is not discontinued prematurely.

If one agent fails an adequate therapeutic trial, it is best to choose an agent from a different therapeutic category. In the presence of strong relative indications or contraindications, it may be appropriate to choose a second agent within a therapeutic category.

31. What is transformed migraine?

Transformed migraine is the single most common condition seen in headache specialty centers in the United States. The patient with transformed migraine typically begins with ordinary attacks of episodic migraine. Over time, attacks increase in frequency but decrease in average severity. The patient is left with a condition characterized by daily or near-daily attacks that resemble tension-type headache, often with superimposed interval headaches with all of the features of full-blown migraine. Transformed migraine must be defined based on a longitudinal history of headache, not simply the headache features at the time of consultation.

32. How can transformed migraine be treated?

Transformed migraine presents a formidable therapeutic challenge. Eighty percent of the patients with transformed migraine overuse analgesics, combination-of-ingredient tablets, or ergot alkaloids. These medications sustain the cycle of ongoing daily headache through the mechanism of medication withdrawal. The key to treatment is eliminating the overused medications. Preventive therapies generally do not become fully effective until the pattern of medication overuse is broken.

The best approach to treating transformed migraine is prevention. Rebound headaches can be prevented by restricting the use of ergotamine and caffeine or narcotic- or barbiturate-containing analgesics to two or three days per week. Nonsteroidal anti-inflammatory agents can be used more frequently with minimal risk of rebound headache. In the outpatient setting, the treatment of rebound headache generally involves substituting a nonsteroidal anti-inflammatory drug for the overused medication. As overused medications are tapered, caution is advisable to avoid barbiturate and opiate withdrawal. At times, rebound headaches require inpatient therapy.

The key to inpatient treatment of transformed migraine is the use of parenteral drugs such as intravenous dihydroergotamine in combination with metoclopramide. These agents are often given every 8 hours over a period of several days to taper the pattern of medication overuse. At the same time, an effective program of migraine prevention is initiated, and various behavioral modalities of pain control are introduced.

33. Who needs inpatient treatment and why?

The overwhelming majority of migraine sufferers do not require inpatient treatment. Inpatient treatment is indicated when patients experience frequent disabling attacks that do not respond to optimal outpatient therapy. Patients with significant medical or psychiatric comorbidities, patients who are emotionally exhausted by ongoing pain, and patients who are fearful of headache pain sometimes require inpatient therapy. For these patients, early inpatient treatment may be optimally cost-effective.

BIBLIOGRAPHY

1. International Headache Society: Classification and diagnostic criteria for headache disorders, cranial neuralgias and facial pain. Cephalalgia 8 (Supp. 7):1–96, 1988.
2. Lipton RB, Silberstein SD, Stewart WF: An update on migraine epidemiology. Headache 34:319–328, 1994.
3. Olesen J, Tfelt-Hansen P, Welch KMA: The Headaches. Raven Press, 1993, 165–436.
4. Silberstein SD, Lipton RB: Overview of diagnosis and treatment of migraine. Neurology 44 (Suppl. 7):6–16, 1994.

10. CLUSTER HEADACHE

Lawrence C. Newman, M.D., and Richard B. Lipton, M.D.

1. Is cluster headache just a more severe form of migraine?

Like migraine, cluster is a primary headache disorder, but it represents a distinct entity. Cluster headaches are characterized by attacks of excruciatingly severe unilateral head pain. Attacks last 15–180 minutes and recur from once every other day up to 8 times daily. These painful episodes are associated with autonomic features on the side of the pain. Autonomic features include ptosis, miosis, conjunctival injection, lacrimation, and rhinorrhea. For episodic cluster, attacks occur in "clusters" lasting weeks to months separated by periods of pain-free "remissions" lasting months to years. Times of frequent headache are called cluster periods. The clinical criteria for cluster headache as defined by the International Headache Society are found in the table below. As discussed below, migraine and cluster are differentiated by their symptom profiles and patterns of treatment response.

IHS Diagnostic Criteria for Cluster

(A)	At least 5 attacks fulfilling B–D
(B)	Severe unilateral, orbital, supraorbital, and/or temporal pain lasting 15–180 minutes
(C)	Headache is associated with at least one of the following signs, which have to be present on the pain side:
	(1) Conjunctival injection
	(2) Lacrimation
	(3) Nasal congestion
	(4) Rhinorrhea
	(5) Forehead and facial sweating
	(6) Miosis
	(7) Ptosis
	(8) Eyelid edema
(D)	Frequency of attacks: from one every other day to eight per day
(E)	At least one of the following:
	(1) History, physical and neurologic examinations do not suggest one of the disorders listed in groups 5–11
	(2) History and/or physical and/or neurologic examinations do not suggest such disorder, but it is ruled out by appopriate investigations
	(3) Such disorder is present, but cluster does not occur for the first time in close temporal relation to the disorder.

2. Are cluster headaches common? Who is affected?

Fortunately, cluster headache is relatively rare, affecting approximately 0.05–0.1% of the U.S. population. Men are affected six times more often than women. In contrast, migraine occurs in women three times more often than in men. Most patients report headache onset between the ages of 20 and 50 (mean 30). The age of onset ranges from early childhood through age 80. Women with cluster have a later average age of onset than men. Unlike migraine, there is no link between menses and cluster headaches; like migraine in women, clusters may disappear during pregnancy and may be triggered by the use of oral contraceptives.

3. What are the characteristics of the headaches?

The pain of cluster begins abruptly, usually without warning, and reaches maximum intensity within one to 15 minutes. The pain is excruciating, deep, and boring and is often described as a "red-hot poker" in or behind the affected eye. The pain is usually most severe in the orbital and retro-orbital regions and may radiate into the ipsilateral temple, upper teeth and gums, and neck. Unlike migraine, where attacks may alternate sides, the pain of cluster is strictly unilateral; only 10–15% of sufferers report side-shift in subsequent bouts.

4. When do bouts occur?

The majority of cluster sufferers note a phenomenon called periodicity; attacks recur around the same time each day during the entire cluster cycle. Approximately 75% of attacks occur between 9:00 p.m. and 10:00 a.m. About half of all cluster sufferers report nocturnal attacks that awaken them from sleep. Attacks typically occur within two hours of falling asleep and are often associated with REM sleep. Manzoni et al. studied the attack characteristics in 180 cluster sufferers and noted a higher incidence of individual attacks occurring between 1:00–2:00 a.m., 1:00–3:00 p.m., and at 9:00 p.m. Thus, cluster patients cycle in and out of cluster periods; during cluster periods, the individual headaches occur with regular patterns. For these reasons, cluster is considered a chronobiologic disorder.

5. Are cluster headaches triggered by the same things as migraine?

A very small minority of cluster sufferers report that typical migraine triggers induce their headaches. These include stress, relaxation after stress, exposure to heat or cold, and certain foods such as chocolate, dairy, or eggs. Alcohol is a common precipitant of cluster headache, affecting over half of all sufferers. Alcohol tends to trigger attacks within 5–45 minutes after ingestion. Interestingly, this trigger is present only during the active "cluster" phase of the disorder; imbibing alcohol-containing beverages during the "remission" phase will not trigger an attack. Sublingual nitroglycerine can also induce attacks.

6. Are there different types of cluster?

Yes. Typical cluster may be divided into three forms: episodic, chronic, and chronic-evolved from episodic. About 90% of cluster sufferers experience the episodic form, in which discrete attacks recur in cycles, usually lasting 1–3 months, separated by pain-free remissions lasting from one month to several years. Many patients with episodic cluster headaches experience one or two bouts yearly (typically in the spring or fall). In chronic cluster, attacks recur on a daily or near-daily basis for more than one year without remission or with remissions lasting less than two weeks. In approximately 10% of cluster sufferers, an initial episodic cluster cycle evolves into a chronic unremitting form in which attacks recur for 4–5 years or longer, without remission. This evolved pattern may occur more frequently in patients who experience a later onset of the episodic form.

The International Headache Society (IHS) also considers chronic paroxysmal hemicrania a form of cluster headache. This disorder is discussed in Chapter 11.

7. How are cluster headaches diagnosed?

The diagnosis of cluster headaches rests primarily on the history. Despite the distinctive features of the headache, cluster sufferers consult an average of five physicians prior to receiving the correct diagnosis. Their severe headaches are often misdiagnosed as migraine (see Chapter 9). If pain radiates into the upper teeth and gums, it is mistakenly related to dental pathology. Frontal pain, nasal congestion, and/or rhinorrhea may be attributed to sinus disease.

The distinction between cluster and the paroxysmal hemicranias and hemicrania continua is discussed in detail in Chapter 11. Briefly, cluster is distinguished from the paroxysmal hemicranias by the overwhelming male predominance; by the lack of mechanical trigger mechanisms; and by a lesser number of daily attacks, the longer duration of each attack, and the patterns of treatment response.

Cluster is differentiated from migraine by a number of important features. Migraine tends to be more prevalent in females, begins at an earlier age, demonstrates side-shift from attack to attack and is associated with nausea, vomiting, photophobia, phonophobia, and osmophobia. In migraine, attacks last longer, do not occur multiple times daily, and are usually not associated with autonomic features ipsilateral to the pain. There is no aura in cluster. During cluster, patients pace, sit upright in a chair, or bang their heads against a wall, whereas migraineurs lie quietly in a dark room and attempt to sleep; recumbency actually increases the pain of cluster. There are headaches with features of both migraine and cluster that cannot be adequately categorized in either group; these patients often have an intermediate disorder referred to as cluster-migraine variant.

Hemicrania continua is a rare, benign disorder characterized by a continuous baseline low-level discomfort. Superimposed on the baseline pain, sufferers report exacerbations of more severe pain lasting from five minutes to a few days. These exacerbations are often associated with the ipsilateral autonomic features of cluster, although when present, they tend to be less pronounced than those of cluster. The disorder is mistaken for cluster if the clinician or patient focuses on the exacerbations and misses the continuous less severe pain. Hemicrania continua is uniquely responsive to treatment with indomethacin and fails to remit with standard anti-cluster therapy.

Differential Diagnosis of Cluster Headaches

	CLUSTER	HEMICRANIA CONTINUA	MIGRAINE	PAROXYSMAL HEMICRANIAS
Sex F:M	1:6	1.8:1	3:1	2.13:1
Age of onset	20–40	11–58	Teens–20s	6–81
Pain quality	Stabbing, boring	Baseline dull ache, superimposed throbbing/stabbing	Throbbing, pulsatile	Stabbing, pulsatile, throbbing
Site of maximal pain	Orbit/temple	Orbit/temple	Temple/forehead	Orbit/temple
Attacks per day	0–8	Varies	0–1	1–40
Duration of untreated attacks	15–180 min (average 20–45)	Minutes → days	4–72 hr	2–120 min (average 2–25)
Autonomic features	+	+ (but less pronounced than cluster)	–	+
Aura	–	–	+ in 15–20%	–
Patient's behavior during attack	Pacing/rocking	Pacing or rest	Rest/sleep	Pacing/rocking
Oxygen may abort acute attacks	+ in 80%	–	+ in 20%	–

8. Is it possible to prevent cluster attacks?

Nearly all patients with cluster headache require preventive treatment. The short duration, high frequency, and remarkable severity of attacks make acute treatment unsatisfactory. A variety of anti-cluster agents may be used (see table). Most headache specialists begin treatment with verapamil and a prednisone taper. Prednisone usually induces a rapid remission but has too many side effects for long-term use. Verapamil is generally safe and well tolerated, but its benefits develop over one to two weeks. Accordingly, prednisone is started at 60 to 80 mg daily for one week. In the second week, prednisone is tapered by 10 mg per day. Verapamil is started at a dose of 240 mg daily and often increased to 480 mg per day if tolerated. Sometimes, additional dose escalations are required. Prednisone is intended to induce a rapid remission; verapamil is intended to prevent attacks until the cluster cycle is over. If verapamil fails, lithium carbonate and methysergide are the major alternatives. Lithium tends to be more efficacious in the chronic form. Valproic acid has been proven useful in both forms.

Treatment of Cluster Headaches

DRUG	DOSE (MG/DAY)	COMMENTS
Medications used preventively		
Verapamil	240–960	Useful in all forms; sometimes doses above the 480 mg maximum on the label are required
Valproic acid	500–3000	Useful in all forms
Lithium carbonate	300–1500	Best for chronic cluster
Methysergide	4–10	Best for episodic form; must discontinue every six months for one month drug-free holiday
Medications used abortively		
Oxygen	8–10 mg L/min via face mask for 10–15 min	
Sumatriptan	6 mg SQ	Maximum of two injections daily
Dihydroergotamine	0.5–1 mg SQ/IM	Maximum 2 mg/day and 6 mg/week

9. For how long should prophylactic therapy be continued?

Patients should be maintained on preventive medications for slightly longer than their typical cycles; for example, if the cluster period usually lasts six weeks, we keep patients on their anti-cluster regimen for eight weeks and then gradually taper the preventive medications. Recurrences are treated by adjusting the dosage upward, then re-tapering at a later date.

10. How are acute attacks treated?

The two acute treatment alternatives for cluster are oxygen and sumatriptan. Oxygen is usually administered via face mask or nasal cannula for 10–15 minutes. Subcutaneous sumatriptan 6 mg rapidly aborts attacks of cluster in 5–10 minutes in most patients. Unfortunately, the drug cannot be given more than twice daily, and sufferers may have more than two attacks daily. Dihydroergotamine (DHE) administered IM or SQ is also effective. DHE is not specifically indicated for cluster headache. Sumatriptan has recently received FDA approval for treatment of cluster headaches. For patients with nocturnal attacks, ergot suppositories at bedtime may prevent night-time headaches.

11. If these medications fail to break the attacks, what else can be done?

Medically refractory patients can be treated in a number of ways. Hospitalization and treatment with repetitive dihydroergotamine and metoclopramide every eight hours has been proven to break cluster cycles. Alternatively, ipsilateral occipital nerve blocks may occasionally help. For patients refractory to these treatments, percutaneous glycerol injections into the trigeminal cistern, percutaneous radiofrequency trigeminal rhizotomy, or decompression of the nervus intermedius may be attempted.

BIBLIOGRAPHY

1. Manzoni GC, Terzano TG, Bono G, et al: Cluster headache—Clinical features in 180 patients. Cephalalgia 3:21–30, 1983.
2. Newman LC, Lipton RB, Solomon S: Hemicrania continua: Ten new cases and a review of the literature. Neurology 44:2111–2114, 1994.
3. Solomon S, Lipton RB, Newman LC: Prophylatic therapy of cluster headaches. Clin Neuropharmacol 14:116–130, 1991.
4. Tahu JM, Tew JM: Long-term results of radio frequency rhizotomy in the treatment of cluster headache. Headache 35:193–196, 1995.

11. THE PAROXYSMAL HEMICRANIAS

Lawrence C. Newman, M.D., and Richard B. Lipton, M.D.

1. What are the paroxysmal hemicranias?

The paroxysmal hemicranias are a group of rare, benign headache disorders that resemble cluster headache in most ways but do not respond to anticluster medications. The headaches are characterized by severe, excruciating, throbbing, boring, or pulsatile pain affecting the orbital, supra-orbital, and temporal regions. These pains are associated with at least one of the following signs or symptoms ipsilateral to the painful side:

1. Conjunctival injection
2. Lacrimation
3. Nasal congestion
4. Rhinorrhea
5. Ptosis
6. Eyelid edema

Attacks occur from one to 40 times daily, usually exceeding eight attacks in a 24-hour period. Duration is typically from two to 25 minutes, but, on rare occasions, attacks may last as long as two hours. Headaches may occur any time during the day or night, and there is often a predisposition to nocturnal attacks, in which the patient is awakened from a sound sleep by an incapacitating headache.

2. Are there different clinical variations of the paroxysmal hemicranias?

Sjaastad and colleagues initially described a condition they called chronic paroxysmal hemicrania (CPH). Their patients suffered from recurring episodes of severe hemicranial headaches with autonomic features occurring multiple times a day, every day, without sustained remission. In 1987, Kudrow and associates reported a patient whose headaches were identical to CPH except that the patient had enduring, pain-free remissions lasting weeks or months. The authors termed this condition episodic paroxysmal hemicrania (EPH). Although there has been controversy regarding the nomenclature of the paroxysmal hemicranias, there appear to be three related forms: (1) chronic paroxysmal hemicrania (CPH), in which multiple headaches occur daily for years on end without remission; (2) episodic paroxysmal hemicrania (EPH), in which there are discrete phases characterized by frequent daily attacks separated by long-term, pain-free remissions; (3) pre-CPH, in which an initially episodic form of these headaches ultimately evolves into the chronic unremitting form. Some authors prefer alternative nomenclature. At present, only CPH is recognized in the diagnostic system of the International Headache Society (IHS).

3. What distinguishes EPH from cluster headache?

The major distinguishing features of the paroxysmal hemicranias and cluster headache lie in the frequency of the attack, the duration of the attack, and the response to treatment. In addition, the paroxysmal hemicranias do not show the striking preponderance among males that characterizes cluster headache. In cluster headache, attacks are less frequent and of longer duration (one or two attacks a day with a typical duration of 30 minutes to two hours) than in the paroxysmal hemicranias (more than five attacks a day lasting from two to 25 minutes each).

4. What triggers attacks of paroxysmal hemicranias?

Like cluster headaches, the paroxysmal hemicranias can be triggered by alcohol. Approximately 10 percent of patients with chronic paroxysmal hemicrania report that attacks may be precipitated either by bending or by rotating the head. Headache attacks may also be triggered by exerting external pressure against the transverse process of the C4-C5, the C2 root, or the greater occipital nerve. Headaches may be precipitated within a few seconds of the trigger (range five to 60 seconds), sometimes in rapid succession without any refractory period.

5. Does it matter whether we call these headaches clusters or paroxysmal hemicranias?

The differential diagnosis is exceptionally important, as the paroxysmal hemicranias are often resistant to the medications that typically prevent cluster headaches. The paroxysmal hemicranias are uniquely responsive to treatment with indomethacin. In fact, the International Headache Society has deemed response to indomethacin therapy a sine qua non for establishing the diagnosis. Some headache specialists believe that there are patients with paroxysmal hemicrania refractory to indomethacin.

Differential Diagnosis of the Paroxysmal Hemicranias

	CLUSTER	CHRONIC PAROXYSMAL HEMICRANIA	EPISODIC PAROXYSMAL HEMICRANIA
Age of onset (range)	1–61	6–81	12–51
Gender ratio M:F	6:1	1:2.8	1:1.45
Pain quality	Boring/throbbing	Throbbing	Throbbing/stabbing
Pain severity	Excruciating	Excruciating	Excruciating
Location of maximal pain	Unilateral orbit, temple, jaw	Unilateral temple, orbit, jaw	Unilateral orbit, temple
Autonomic features	Present	Present	Present
Attack frequency (daily)	1–8	1–40	6–30
Attack duration (minutes)	20–120	2–120	1–30
Nocturnal awakenings	Yes	Yes	Yes
Precipitated by alcohol	Yes	Yes	No
Response to indomethacin	Occasionally	Yes	Yes

6. Once the diagnosis of EPH or CPH is established, are any further workups necessary?

Although the paroxysmal hemicranias are benign by definition, there have been patients with organic mimics of the disorder. To date, there have been a number of published cases with CPH-like headaches associated with collagen vascular diseases, malignant brain tumors, arteriovenous malformations, and ischemic stroke. Neuroimaging is therefore recommended in all cases with the presumptive diagnosis of either CPH or EPH to exclude organic causes of these rare headaches. Several of the cases with organic headache also responded to indomethacin.

7. Once the diagnosis is established and neuroimaging is normal, how are these headaches treated?

The paroxysmal hemicranias exhibit unique responsiveness to indomethacin but not to other nonsteroidal anti-inflammatory agents. Initial therapy consists of indomethacin 25 mg/3 times/day. If there is no response or if there is a partial response after one week, the dose should be increased to 50 mg/3 times/day. Complete resolution of the headache is prompt, usually occurring within one to two days of initiating the effective dose. Patients should be advised of the risks of gastritis and ulcer disease as well as the other side effects of indomethacin. In patients with CPH, concurrent treatment with misoprostol or histamine H-2 receptor antagonists should be considered. Rarely, some patients require indomethacin doses as high as 300 mg/day. Recent reports suggest that a need for high indomethacin doses may be an ominous sign pointing to an underlying organic etiology.

Some patients develop breakthrough headaches at the end of dosing intervals. These headaches are usually eliminated by increasing the dose or shortening the dosing interval. For patients with breakthrough headaches in the early morning hours, slow release indomethacin at night may be helpful. Occasionally, suppositories are better tolerated than oral indomethacin.

8. If indomethacin fails to treat the headaches, what then?

Reconsider the diagnosis and make sure there is no underlying cause. If upon further review, the diagnosis of CPH or EPH is still likely, partial response has been demonstrated with verapamil, acetylsalicylic acid, ibuprofen, piroxicam, naproxen, and paracetamol. These agents are not nearly as effective as indomethacin and should not be used as first-line therapy.

BIBLIOGRAPHY

1. Antonaci F, Sjaastad O: Chronic paroxysmal hemicrania (CPH): A review of the clinical manifestations. Headache 29:648–656, 1989.
2. Blau JN, Engel H: Episodic paroxysmal hemicrania: A further case and review of the literature. J Neurol Neurosurg Psychiatry 53:343–344, 1990.
3. Haggag KJ, Russell D: Chronic paroxysmal hemicrania. In Olesen J, Tfelt-Hansen P, Welch KMA (eds): The Headaches. New York, Raven Press, 1993, pp 601–608.
4. Kudrow L, Esperanza P, Vijayan N: Episodic paroxysmal hemicrania? Cephalalgia 7:197–201, 1987.
5. Medina JL: Organic headaches mimicking chronic paroxysmal hemicrania. Headache 32:73–74, 1992.
6. Newman LC, Gordon ML, Lipton RB, et al: Episodic paroxysmal hemicrania: Two new cases and a literature review. Neurology 42:964–966, 1992.
7. Newman LC, Herskovitz S, Lipton RB, et al: Chronic paroxysmal hemicrania: Two cases with cerebrovascular disease. Headache 32:75–76, 1992.
8. Sjaastad O, Dale I: Evidence for a new (?) treatable headache entity. Headache 14:105–108, 1974.
9. Sjaastad O, Stovner LJ, Stolt-Nielson A, et al: CPH and hemicrania continua: Requirements of high indomethacin dosages—An ominous sign? Headache 35:363–367, 1995.

12. SUBARACHNOID HEMORRHAGE

Ronald Kanner, M.D.

1. A 40-year-old woman in the emergency department complains of the worst headache of her life that has its onset during sexual intercourse. On examination, she is slightly sleepy and has a stiff neck but no other signs. What diagnosis should be considered?

This is a classic story for subarachnoid hemorrhage. The sudden onset of "the worst headache of my life" should be the tipoff for subarachnoid hemorrhage. Most commonly, it occurs during the Valsalva maneuver—while straining at stool or during sexual intercourse. Patients commonly demonstrate stiff neck and some alteration of level of consciousness. The absence of localizing signs on neurologic examination does not contradict the diagnosis of subarachnoid hemorrhage. A few specific types of subarachnoid hemorrhage present with localizing signs (see question 3).

2. What are the studies of choice to confirm the diagnosis of subarachnoid hemorrhage?

Computed tomography (CT scan) shows blood in the subarachnoid space in over 95% of patients with subarachnoid hemorrhage. In the remaining 5%, lumbar puncture may be needed to demonstrate blood. Lumbar puncture usually shows an elevated opening pressure and an abundance of red blood cells. If the tap is done early, white blood cells and red blood cells should be in the same proportion as they are in the peripheral blood. Later, irritation of the meninges from the blood may produce a higher proportion of white blood cells. If the CT scan clearly shows a subarachnoid hemorrhage, a lumbar puncture is not necessary.

3. A patient presents to the emergency department with the sudden onset of a severe headache. The patient is awake and alert, but the left eyelid is drooping, the left pupil is dilated, and the left eye is exodeviated. What is the problem?

The patient has a severe headache and a third-nerve palsy. Third-nerve palsy and headache are often thought of as signs of uncal herniation. However, the patient is awake. Furthermore, there is no hemiparesis. An isolated third-nerve paresis with severe headache is a common presentation of a ruptured aneurysm in the posterior communicating artery. The third nerve passes between the posterior communicating artery and the superior cerebellar artery. Rupture of the aneurysm may put pressure on the third nerve, causing ptosis, mydriasis, and exodeviation of the eye.

4. What is a sentinel headache?

Sentinel headaches are brief, severe headaches that may precede a subarachnoid hemorrhage. They are presumed to be due to enlargements of the aneurysm before bleeding. However, there may be tiny hemorrhages that are not seen. If the aneurysm is in the posterior communicating artery, sentinel headaches may be accompanied by a third-nerve paresis, as described in question 3. Sentinel headaches may occur with aneurysms in essentially any cerebral location.

5. A patient presents with a typical history of subarachnoid hemorrhage and the typical severe headache. Lumbar puncture shows blood in the cerebrospinal fluid. However, angiography is negative. What are the possible causes of this syndrome?

Subarachnoid hemorrhage with negative angiography has a number of possible causes. One common cause is that rupture of the aneurysm destroys the aneurysm; therefore, the pouch itself is not seen on angiography. However, there is usually some surrounding vasospasm to point out the area of the original hemorrhage. Another cause is clotting of the aneurysm. An aneurysmal dome filled with clotted blood does not show up on angiography. A much less common cause is a spinal subarachnoid hemorrhage. Finally, severe vasospasm around the aneurysm may cause such low flow that the aneurysm itself is not visualized on angiography.

6. What is the definitive study of choice to establish the cause of a subarachnoid hemorrhage?

At present, selective cerebral angiography is the diagnostic tool of choice. In most cases, it shows whether an aneurysm or an arteriovenous malformation (AVM) is present. As CT angiography and MR angiography become more sophisticated, they may replace this more invasive procedure. At present, however, most surgeons require an angiogram to define clearly the site and cause of the subarachnoid hemorrhage.

7. A patient with a subarachnoid hemorrhage undergoes angiography, which demonstrates multiple aneurysms. What signs are helpful in determining which aneurysm caused the subarachnoid hemorrhage?

In general, larger aneurysms (> 1 cm) are more likely to bleed than smaller aneurysms. If aneurysms are similar in size, a number of signs may point to the offending aneurysm. Small nipples on the aneurysm are a sign that it has ruptured and healed. A smooth-domed aneurysm is less likely to have bled than an aneurysm with small out-pouchings. Arterial spasm is more likely to be present around the site of the ruptured aneurysm. On CT scanning, a clot surrounding an aneurysm is diagnostic of the offending aneurysm. More commonly, however, there is diffuse blood throughout the subarachnoid space.

8. A patient with severe headache from subarachnoid hemorrhage improves over a few days, then experiences another severe headache. What are the possible causes?

The most common cause is rebleeding of the aneurysm, which occurs within the first 2 weeks in up to 30% of patients who have had a subarachnoid hemorrhage. Fifty percent of rehemorrhages are fatal. Less commonly, blood may block either the reabsorptive system or one of the foramina through which cerebrospinal fluid flows. This blockage gives rise to hydrocephalus and headache. Onset is usually much more insidious than onset of headache of repeat subarachnoid hemorrhage.

9. What is the appropriate treatment for the headache of subarachnoid hemorrhage?

The pain of subarachnoid hemorrhage is often severe. As such, it may require potent analgesics. Aspirin and nonsteroidal antiinflammatory drugs are to be avoided because they may increase bleeding and because they are rarely available in a parenteral form. Ketorolac is an exception because it can be administered intramuscularly. In general, however, low doses of opioids administered intravenously usually provide significant headache relief. A balance must be struck among headache relief, obtundation, and respiratory depression. When respiratory depression occurs, it is often accompanied by an increase in cranial pressure. Doses must be titrated carefully. A 2-mg dose of morphine administered intravenously usually provides significant relief.

10. What are the delayed complications of subarachnoid hemorrhage?

Headache is an unusual late complication of subarachnoid hemorrhage. Most commonly, if the arachnoid granulations through which the cerebrospinal fluid is reabsorbed become blocked, a transient period of increased intracranial pressure may lead to mild headaches for weeks to months. As these subside, one theory has it that normal-pressure hydrocephalus may ensue. In such patients, dementia, gait impairment, and urinary incontinence are the classic triad. Patients also may develop seizure disorder, cognitive impairment, and focal deficits.

BIBLIOGRAPHY

1. Biller J, Godersky JC, Adams HP: Management of aneurysmal subarachnoid hemorrhage. Stroke 19:1300–1305, 1988.
2. Brust JCM: Subarachnoid hemorrhage. In Rowland LP (ed): Merritt's Textbook of Neurology, 8th ed. Philadelphia, Lea & Febiger, 1989, pp 235–243.

13. BRAIN TUMOR HEADACHES

Ronald Kanner, M.D.

1. What is the classic brain tumor headache?

Standard texts describe the classic brain tumor headache as a morning headache that may even awaken the patient from sleep in the early hours of the morning. It improves as the day goes on and characteristically responds to aspirin and steroids. At one point, the "steroid test" was used as a diagnostic tool for brain tumor headaches. A dramatic response to steroid administration strengthened the diagnosis, on the theory that peritumor edema was resolving. Over the years, however, it has become increasingly clear that steroids can relieve many types of headaches—not just those due to brain tumors.

2. What was the theoretical basis for the classic brain tumor headache?

It is still believed, to some degree, that the increased intracranial pressure that may occur with sleep and recumbency can increase pain due to brain tumors. Mild CO_2 retention during sleep leads to vasodilatation and increased pressure. Similarly, when the patient is recumbent, venous return from the brain decreases and intracranial pressure increases. As the patient awakens and ambulates, CO_2 drops and venous return increases, thus making the headache improve as the day progresses.

3. How common is the classic brain tumor headache?

The classic syndrome seems to occur in only about 17% of patients with brain tumors and headaches. Most commonly, headaches due to brain tumor are diffuse, nondescript, and "tension-like." They are usually bilateral and commonly affect the vertex.

4. How often are brain tumor headaches unilateral?

In somewhat less than one-half of brain tumor headaches, pain is unilateral. However, when it is unilateral, it is invariably felt on the side of the tumor. A migraine-like presentation is highly unusual.

5. If brain tumor headaches are most commonly tension-like, how can one differentiate between a benign tension-type headache and a brain tumor headache?

There are a number of differentiating factors. The most important is probably the time course. A new-onset headache that progresses over days to weeks is much more suspect of representing a space-occupying lesion than is a chronic headache that has been stable over a long period. Furthermore, abnormalities on the neurologic examination are virtually unheard of in benign headache syndromes (with the exception of Horner's sign in cluster headache) but may occur in more than one-half of patients with brain tumor headaches.

6. How commonly is headache the presenting complaint in patients with metastatic brain tumors?

About 50% of patients with metastatic brain tumor have headache as their presenting complaint. It is the single most common presenting complaint of patients with brain metastases. Of interest, headache without other focal findings is more common in patients with multiple metastases than in those with only a single metastasis.

7. Under what circumstances do brain tumor headaches present with a sudden increase in pain rather than the usual gradual onset?

The two most common causes for a sudden onset of headache in brain tumors are hemorrhage and obstruction of cerebrospinal fluid (CSF) flow. Certain tumors are much more likely than others to hemorrhage. Metastatic melanoma hemorrhages with great frequency. In fact, even in the absence of clinically evident hemorrhage, imaging may show blood density within the tumors. Hypernephroma and choriocarcinoma also hemorrhage with some frequency. The direction of CSF flow is from the lateral ventricles to the third ventricle (through the foramina of Munro) and from the third to the fourth (through the cerebral aqueduct). CSF leaves the fourth ventricle through the foramina of Luschka (laterally) and Magendie (medially) in the cerebellum. Tumors in these areas are particularly prone to causing obstructive hydrocephalus.

8. Why do brain metastases cause headaches?

Brain tissue itself is not pain-sensitive; that is, there are no nociceptors in the gray or white matter of the brain. However, the structures surrounding the brain—i.e., the meninges, tentorium cerebelli, blood vessels, and cranial nerves—are pain-sensitive. As tumors grow, they may invade or put traction on these structures. Inflammation or stretching of nociceptors in these structures causes pain.

9. Which systemic tumors commonly metastasize to the brain?

The most common primary sources are lung, breast, and melanoma. Small cell carcinoma of the lung and adenocarcinoma are particularly likely to metastasize. Breast cancer is a common cause of brain metastases because of its high prevalence in the population. However, given a patient with breast cancer, a patient with lung cancer, and a patient with melanoma, the patient with melanoma is most likely to suffer brain metastasis. Melanoma is also more likely than the other tumors to cause multiple metastases. With other tumors, single metastases occur with the same frequency as multiple metastases.

10. Under what circumstances is a brain tumor likely to produce severe headaches with little or no neurologic focality?

Tumors that involve the frontal lobes may grow to enormous size without producing focal neurologic deficits. Usually, however, there is some change in personality or cognition. Tumors that obstruct CSF flow may cause hydrocephalus and headache without significant neurologic focality. Finally, tumors involving the cerebellum in the midline may cause headaches without much in the way of localizing neurologic signs.

11. Do primary brain tumors cause headaches?

Yes. Gliomas, the most common of the primary cerebral tumors, tend to arise deep in the brain. Initially, they grow in a way that invaginates among brain structures and may cause little in the way of headaches. Eventually, however, they achieve sufficient size to increase intracranial pressure and cause headaches.

12. What is the preferred treatment for brain tumor headaches?

Because most of the headaches are due to increased mass, removal of the tumor usually relieves the headaches. However, with recurrent or growing tumors, ongoing therapy is needed. Steroids reliably relieve brain tumor headaches, but complications generally preclude long-term use. Radiation therapy initially increases the headache because of increased swelling. However, as tumors resolve, the headache tends to resolve pari passu.

13. What is pari passu?

Pari passu is a Latin expression that means walking at the same pace. The headache that results from radiation-induced swelling tends to resolve at the same pace as the swelling resolves.

14. How can a cerebellar metastasis cause retroorbital pain?

The cerebellum lies just under the tentorium cerebelli. Innervation of the tentorium is through the trigeminal nerve. The trigeminal nerve also innervates the orbital structures. Referred pain is fairly common when a given nerve (or nerve roots) innervates two separate structures. As a cerebellar metastasis grows, it can stretch the tentorium cerebelli, stimulating the nociceptors that lie therein. Pain arising there is referred to the eye.

15. What is the Foster-Kennedy syndrome?

Foster-Kennedy syndrome is characterized by optic atrophy in one eye and papilledema in the other eye. It is caused by large tumors of the optic nerve. As the tumor grows, it produces optic atrophy on the affected side. As it grows larger, intracranial pressure increases. Increased intracranial pressure causes papilledema. However, because the ipsilateral optic nerve is compressed, it cannot develop papilledema. Therefore, there is optic atrophy on the affected side and papilledema on the contralateral side.

16. A 60-year-old woman presents with progressive unilateral headache and facial pain. On examination, she shows nystagmus, hearing loss, facial weakness, and ataxia. What is the likely diagnosis?

This constellation of symptoms indicates dysfunction of cranial nerves V, VII, and VIII, along with cerebellar dysfunction, and is typical of a cerebellopontine (CP) angle tumor. Often such tumors are acoustic neuromas or meningiomas. Occasionally, however, a metastasis produces this picture.

17. A patient presents with pain behind one eye and progressive diplopia. The patient initially shows a sixth-nerve palsy but then develops complete external ophthalmoplegia and numbness of the right forehead. What should be considered?

This syndrome involves dysfunction of cranial nerves III, IV, and VI as well as the first division of cranial nerve V. All of these nerves come together in the cavernous sinus, which lies just lateral to the sphenoid sinus. It is a venous sinus through which pass the carotid artery; cranial nerves III, IV, and VI; and the first two divisions of cranial nerve V.

18. A middle-aged man presents with progressive headaches and is found to have a frontal glioma. Headaches become worse, and he develops diplopia that is most pronounced on distant gaze and not present on near gaze. What is a likely explanation?

When diplopia is mainly present on distant gaze, one must consider a sixth-nerve palsy. The sixth nerve abducts the eye. Therefore, for reading or looking at something close, the eyes are converged and do not require sixth-nerve function. At far gaze—for example, watching television—the sixth nerve must keep the eyes focused outward. Therefore, with sixth-nerve dysfunction, diplopia is worse on far gaze. Increased intracranial pressure may lead to mild sixth-nerve dysfunction. The sixth nerve has the longest intracranial course of the cranial nerves. As pressure increases, it may be affected, even without local compression. This phenomenon is called a falsely localizing sixth nerve.

BIBLIOGRAPHY

1. Forsythe PA, Posner JB: Headaches in patients with brain tumors: A study of 111 patients. Neurology 43:1678–1683, 1993.
2. Posner JB: Intracranial metastases. In Posner JB: Neurological Complications of Cancer. Philadelphia, F.A. Davis, 1995, pp 77–110.

14. HEADACHES DUE TO INCREASED OR DECREASED INTRACRANIAL PRESSURE

Ronald Kanner, M.D.

1. What is normal intracranial pressure?

Intracranial pressure is generally measured by lumbar puncture. It is presumed that, because the spinal fluid at the lumbar level is continuous with spinal fluid throughout the brain, pressures are equal. The normal pressure on lumbar puncture is 65–195 mm of cerebrospinal fluid (CSF) or water. This is the equivalent of about 5–15 mmHg.

2. What is the Monro-Kellie doctrine?

The Monro-Kellie doctrine states that an increase in the volume of any component of the calvarium (brain tissue, blood, CSF, or brain fluids) must be accompanied by a decrease in the volume of another component or intracranial pressure will increase markedly because the bony calvarium rigidly fixes the total cranial volume. Under normal circumstances, brief increases in intracranial pressure are associated with the Valsalva maneuver, including coughing, sneezing, or straining at stool. Some of the increased intracranial pressure is mitigated by the fact that the cerebral vessels are somewhat elastic and can be compressed. In patients who already have increased intracranial pressure or irritated meninges, transient rises may produce severe pain.

3. Under what circumstances does the pressure measured by lumbar puncture not reflect true intracranial pressure?

If there is a block in CSF flow at a spinal level above the level of the lumbar puncture but below the foramen magnum, there may be a pressure gradient between the cerebral space and the lumbar space.

4. How is cerebrospinal fluid formed?

CSF fills the four ventricles of the brain, is distributed over the convexity, and also fills the spinal canal. It is secreted by the choroid plexus, a series of capillaries surrounded by epithelial cells. A small amount of CSF is also formed directly by brain capillaries. The direction of flow of CSF is from the lateral ventricles (where the choroid plexuses are located) through the foramina of Monro into the third ventricle. From the third ventricle, CSF flows through the aqueduct of Sylvius to the fourth ventricle. The third and fourth ventricles are single, midline structures, whereas the lateral ventricles are bilateral. From the fourth ventricle, it exits laterally through the foramina of Luschka and medially through the foramen of Magendie. Then it goes down the spinal canal, bathing the spinal cord. The spinal cord itself ends at about the level of the L1 or L2 vertebral body. The dural sac, however, extends to nearly the end of the spinal canal. Thus the space between L2 and the bottom of the canal is filled with some nerve roots and ample CSF. This is the area commonly used for lumbar puncture and measuring CSF pressure.

5. What is benign intracranial hypertension?

The clinical symptoms of benign intracranial hypertension, also known as pseudotumor cerebri, are headache and visual disturbance. No particular clinical characteristic of the headache is pathognomonic. Patients almost invariably demonstrate papilledema. Although it may occur at any age, most cases occur in the third and fourth decades. Women are much more commonly affected than men. Visual acuity is usually normal, but careful examination of the visual fields demonstrates enlarged blind spots. The neurologic examination reveals no other focal abnormalities. If focal abnormalities are present, the diagnosis of pseudotumor should not be entertained. A normal computed tomogram (CT) or magnetic resonance image (MRI) of the brain is mandatory for diagnosis. Pseudotumor cerebri is a diagnosis of exclusion; according to an old axiom, the most common cause of pseudotumor is a real tumor.

6. What studies are important if the diagnosis of pseudotumor is entertained?

First, the patient must meet clinical criteria, including headache and papilledema with no other obvious cause. An imaging procedure must rule out the presence of a structural lesion. Lumbar puncture is then performed to confirm a CSF pressure greater than 200 mm of CSF. In most cases, it is well over 300 mm of CSF. Imaging studies may appear normal; that is, both the ventricles and the sulci appear quite small. An electroencephalogram (EEG) is not necessary. The vast majority of patients have normal EEGs, and even when the EEG is abnormal, it does not help with the diagnosis.

7. What is the pathophysiology of pseudotumor cerebri?

Most cases of pseudotumor are associated with a significant reduction in CSF outflow. The cause of this increased resistance is not clear, but it seems to occur at the level of the arachnoid granulations. There does not seem to be any increase in CSF production, nor is it clear that there is any appreciable cerebral edema. Blood volume appears to be normal, and cerebral blood flow studies have revealed conflicting results. There may be some degree of interstitial edema.

8. What are the most common predisposing factors in benign intracranial hypertension?

The reason is unclear, but most patients with pseudotumor cerebri are obese women. In some cases, oral contraceptives or corticosteroid withdrawal has been implicated. The consumption of tetracyclines and large doses of vitamin A have also been thought to be predisposing factors. Secondary causes of benign intracranial hypertension include venous hypertension, venous sinus thrombosis, and any process that impedes venous drainage from the brain.

9. What are the main complications of untreated pseudotumor cerebri?

Two of the most common complications are visual loss and the empty sella syndrome. Continuous pressure on the optic nerve may lead to optic atrophy. It is unclear whether surgically releasing the optic sheath eliminates this complication.

10. What are the treatments for pseudotumor cerebri?

The first treatment actually occurs at the time of diagnosis. When a lumbar puncture is performed, increased pressure is relieved. Relief is not due only to removal of fluid. Fluid forms so rapidly (0.4 ml/min) that the amount removed is immediately replenished. However, because lumbar puncture causes a rent in the dura, there is some leakage of fluid for a long while after the spinal tap. If a large-bore needle is used, the rent in the dura may be sufficient to serve as a shunt. One of the most accepted medical therapies is acetazolamide, which reduces CSF production. This diuretic, a carbonic anhydrase inhibitor, presumably decreases the mechanism for production of CSF. Other diuretics also may be of value in pseudotumor cerebri. With repeated lumbar punctures, pressure often normalizes over a few weeks. If the pressure does not normalize and cannot be restored to normal with diuretics, a shunting procedure may be necessary. The most common procedure is a lumboperitoneal shunt, which drains CSF into the peritoneal space. Glycerol, a hyperosmolar agent, is sometimes used; however, it is poorly tolerated and may cause further weight gain in already obese patients.

11. Why does increased intracranial pressure cause headaches?

The presumed mechanism is traction on pain-sensitive structures. However, when the pressure is diffuse, this explanation does not necessarily hold. Clearly, with brain tumors or other localized lesions, shifts of intracranial structures cause traction on pain-sensitive structures. With pseudotumor cerebri, however, the increase in intracranial pressure is diffuse, and it is not clear that it is associated with traction on dura or blood vessels. In healthy volunteers, infusions into the CSF, raising pressure up to 600 mm, have not produced significant headaches.

12. What focal neurologic signs can be seen with diffuse increases in intracranial pressure?

A mild palsy of cranial nerve VI may complicate increased intracranial pressure. The sixth cranial nerve (abducens) has a long course in the subarachnoid space, and it may be compromised by diffuse increases in pressure. When compromise occurs, the affected eye is deviated slightly medially. In contrast to tumors that directly compress the sixth nerve, diffusely increased intracranial pressure usually causes mild, rather than complete, compromise. Patients complain of diplopia on far gaze. The diplopia disappears on near gaze because the eyes tend to converge.

13. Other than pseudotumor cerebri, what are the most common intracranial causes of increased intracranial pressure?

In any case of increased intracranial pressure, a space-occupying lesion should be sought. Primary and metastatic brain tumors are among the most common causes.

14. How do brain tumors cause increased intracranial pressure?

1. Growth of the tumor may increase mass so much that intracranial pressure increases. The mass of the tumor is compounded by the surrounding edema.

2. The tumor may obstruct CSF flow. CSF flows from the lateral ventricles into the third ventricle, from the third ventricle to the fourth, and out the fourth ventricle into the subarachnoid space. A tumor obstructing the aqueduct of Sylvius (between the third and fourth ventricles) causes massive dilatation of the third and lateral ventricles, sparing the fourth. This obstructive hydrocephalus presents as rapidly increasing intracranial pressure with headache. Obstruction of CSF outflow at any point may produce hydrocephalus.

15. What are the risks of performing lumbar puncture in patients with increased intracranial pressure?

The greatest fear is that lumbar puncture will produce a pressure gradient between the brain and lumbar subarachnoid space, causing the brain to herniate downward. In diffusely increased intracranial pressure, as seen in pseudotumor cerebri, this risk is minimal or nonexistent. The main concern is with large, laterally placed lesions, which may cause massive shifts in the brain when pressure is relieved from below.

16. What is the uncal herniation syndrome?

Uncal herniation refers to a syndrome in which a large, laterally placed mass pushes the temporal lobe through the incisura. Expansion of the intracerebral mass causes contralateral hemiparesis. As the mass pushes downward, it compresses the third nerve, causing an ipsilateral third-nerve palsy (ptosis, pupillary enlargement, and exodeviation of the eye). The syndrome, therefore, is ipsilateral third nerve palsy and contralateral hemiparesis.

17. What historical data lead to the diagnosis of increased intracranial pressure?

Although no symptom is pathognomonic, headaches due to increased intracranial pressure tend to be worse in the early morning hours and to improve during the day. The supine position leads to more blood pooling in the head. During sleep, mild CO_2 retention may cause vasodilation with increased cerebral blood flow.

18. What are low-pressure headaches?

The CSF serves as a cushion for the brain, buffering its movements within the skull. When CSF pressure is markedly decreased, this cushioning ability is less effective. Patients complain of positional headache. They have severe headaches when sitting or standing, but the headaches are entirely relieved by lying supine.

19. What are the most common causes of low-pressure headache?

CSF leaks are the most common causes. They may occur after lumbar puncture or inadvertent puncture of the dura during an attempted epidural block. Most commonly, they occur after epidural anesthesia for childbirth. The needle used for an epidural block is thicker and blunter than the one used for usual lumbar puncture. Therefore, with an inadvertent dural tear the hole in the dura is larger than the hole caused by lumbar puncture. The results are prolonged CSF leak and postural headache.

20. How can low-pressure headache be diagnosed?

Usually the history is sufficient: lumbar puncture or epidural block, followed by the classic positional headache. To confirm a CSF leak, a radionuclide can be injected into the subarachnoid space, and a scan can be performed to pick up sites of radioactivity outside the column.

21. Other than iatrogenic causes (dural tears), what else may cause decreased intracranial pressure?

Idiopathic causes of decreased intracranial pressure are presumed to be due to insufficient CSF production. Such cases are rare. More commonly, pathologic processes (destructive tumors or infections) invade bone and cause CSF leaks.

22. What is the treatment of choice for low-pressure headaches?

In most cases of low-pressure headache, the causative rent in the dura heals on its own, and normal CSF production raises the pressure to baseline levels. During this process, supportive measures should be used. Patients should be encouraged to increase fluid intake and to use minor analgesics. If this approach fails, intravenous infusion of fluids may be helpful. Intravenous administration of 1 liter of saline with 500 mg of caffeine also has been reported to relieve low-pressure headaches. In particularly refractory cases, blood patches may be used. Autologous blood is injected into the epidural space and patches over the rent in the dura.

BIBLIOGRAPHY

1. Cook NR, Davies MJ, Beavis RE: Bedrest and postlumbar puncture headache— the effectiveness of 24 hours' recumbency in reducing the incidence of postlumbar puncture headache. Anesthesia 44:389–391, 1989.
2. Eggenberger ER, Miller NR, Vitale S: Lumboperitoneal shunt for the treatment of pseudotumor cerebri. Neurology 46:1524–1530, 1996.
3. Kunkle EC, Ray BS, Wolff HG: Experimental studies on headache: Analysis of the headache associated with changes in intracranial pressure. Arch Neurol Psychiatry 49:323–358, 1943.
4. Mann JD, Johnson RN, Butler AB, et al: Impairment of cerebrospinal fluid circulatory dynamics in pseudotumor cerebri and response to steroid treatment. Neurology 29:550, 1979.
5. McCarthy KD, Reed DJ: The effect of acetazolamide and furosemide on CSF production and choroid plexus carbonic anhydrase activity. J Pharmacol Exp Ther 189:194–201, 1974.
6. Poukkula E: The problem of post-spinal headache. Ann Chir Gynaecol 73(3):139–142, 1984.
7. Seeberger MD, Kaufman M, Staender S, et al: Repeated dural punctures increase the incidence of post-dural puncture headache. Anesth Analg 82:302–305, 1996.
8. Disturbances of cerebrospinal fluid circulation. In Adams RD, Victor M (eds): Principles of Neurology. New York, McGraw-Hill, 1989.

15. TEMPORAL ARTERITIS

Robert A. Duarte, M.D.

1. What is giant cell arteritis?

It's a specific form of vasculitis seen primarily in the elderly. It is also known as temporal arteritis, cranial arteritis, and Horton's syndrome. The disease is characterized pathologically by granulomatous inflammation of medium-sized arteries and clinically by headache, malaise, and an elevated erythrocyte sedimentation rate. It should be high on the list of differential diagnosis of any elderly person presenting with new onset headaches.

2. What is the epidemiology of the disease?

Giant cell arteritis is a disease of the elderly. It is very uncommon under the age of 50, and its incidence rises dramatically with increasing age. The mean age at the time of diagnosis is about 70 years. It appears to be more common in northern geographic areas, especially in people of British or Scandinavian heritage. It is rare in Asians and African-Americans.

3. What are the most common symptoms in giant cell arteritis?

Headache is the most common presentation, occurring in about 90% of patients with giant cell arteritis. Patients often complain of head soreness or scalp pain. The skin and hair are sensitive to the touch. Jaw claudication (pain with chewing) is almost pathognomonic. Throat and shoulder pain, as well as generalized malaise, fever, anorexia, and muscle pains, are common concomitants.

4. What are the common physical findings in giant cell arteritis?

Signs in giant cell arteritis depend on the vessels involved and the end organ damage sustained. The term "temporal" arteritis may be a misnomer in that this condition may involve many other arteries. While the temporal artery itself is superficial and may be palpable and hard, the other signs are usually due to infarction or claudication. Carotid bruits are occasionally heard. Papilledema and extraocular muscle paresis are rare.

5. What are the neurologic complications of giant cell arteritis?

The most serious complication is blindness. Amaurosis fugax may precede it, but there are usually no premonitory signs. When blindness occurs, it is the result of the occlusion of the posterior ciliary arteries, with anterior ischemic optic neuropathy. About one-third of patients may develop diplopia or ophthalmoplegia. It is usually said that temporal arteritis does not involve the intracranial arteries. However, cerebral infarctions or transient ischemic attacks have been reported frequently. This may be due to inflammation at the site where the artery pierces the dura. Posterior circulation infarctions are more common than anterior circulation disease.

6. What disease is often associated with giant cell arteritis?

Polymyalgia rheumatica occurs in about 20% of patients with giant cell arteritis. Conversely, about one-half of patients with polymyalgia rheumatica will go on to develop giant cell arteritis. Polymyalgia rheumatica is characterized by morning stiffness and muscle aches. The proximal muscles are most affected, and patients have trouble rising from bed or from a chair. The erythrocyte sedimentation rate is markedly elevated, and there is dramatic relief within four or five days of starting prednisone 10 mg daily. It should be noted, however, that higher doses of prednisone are required for the treatment of temporal arteritis.

7. What laboratory data are helpful in establishing the diagnosis of giant cell arteritis?

Any elderly patient with a new onset headache should be suspected of having giant cell arteritis. The erythrocyte sedimentation rate (ESR) must be done as soon as possible. The ESR is greater than 50 mm/hour in 89% of cases. An elevated C-reactive protein may also be found. Patients may show anemia consistent with chronic disease.

8. What are the problems with biopsy of the temporal artery?

Arterial involvement in giant cell arteritis is not uniform. There are pieces of the artery that are involved and others that are disease free. A given biopsy may miss some of the lesions and give a false-negative diagnosis. A false-positive is unusual.

9. When should treatment be undertaken in suspected giant cell arteritis?

As soon as the diagnosis is suspected, prednisone therapy should be initiated. Therapy should not be withheld pending results of a temporal artery biopsy because these may take days and may be inconclusive. Furthermore, the patient can lose ground very abruptly and irreversibly. Treatment consists of prednisone 80 mg/day, for at least a month or two. After that, gradual tapering of less than 10% of the daily dose per week may be started. Disease activity should be monitored clinically and through the ESR. After a few months, the patient should be kept on the lowest dose of prednisone that does not allow for recurrence of symptoms or elevation of the ESR. On average, patients need to be treated for about one year.

BIBLIOGRAPHY

1. Bengtsson, B-A: Giant cell arteritis. Acta Medica Scand (Suppl. 658):1–102, 1982.
2. Caselli, RJ, et al: Neurological disease in biopsy proven giant cell (temporal) arteritis. Neurology 38: 352–358, 1988.
3. Healy, LA, Wilske K: The Systemic Symptoms of Temporal Arteritis. New York, Grune and Stratton, 1978.
4. Huston, KA, Hunder, GG, Lie, JT et al: Temporal arteritis: A 25-year epidemiologic clinical and pathological study. Ann Intern Med 88:162–167, 1978.
5. Liang, GC, Simkin, PA, Hunder CC, et al: Familiar aggregation of polymyalgia rheumatica and giant cell arteritis. Arthritis Rheum 17:19–24, 1974.
6. Wilkinson, IMS, et al: Arteries of the head and neck in giant cell arteritis: A pathological study to show the pattern of arterial involvement. Arch Neurol 27:378–383, 1972.

16. HEADACHES ASSOCIATED WITH SYSTEMIC DISEASE

Robert A. Duarte, M.D.

1. How often are headaches a manifestation of systemic disease?

While headache is the most common pain complaint for which patients seek medical help, it is rarely of organic origin. The vast majority of headaches seen by practitioners are migraine or tension-type. A smaller number are cluster, and an even smaller number are paroxysmal hemicranias. Fewer than one percent of patients presenting to a clinical practice with a complaint of headache have an underlying systemic disease that caused the headache. Patients with sleep apnea also tend to complain of headaches more commonly than does the general population. These headaches usually are present upon awakening and diminish as the day goes on. They are thought to be due to CO_2 retention during sleep.

2. How do the criteria of the International Headache Society categorize headaches associated with systemic diseases?

These criteria eliminate headaches due to infection of the pericranial structures and divide the headaches into those associated with noncephalic infections and those associated with metabolic disorders.

3. What do patients believe is the most common systemic cause for headaches?

After eliminating local complaints such as "sinuses," patients most often believe that their headaches are due to elevations in blood pressure. This is rarely, if ever, the case. Clearly, in cases of hypertensive encephalopathy, with papilledema and mental status changes, headaches are a common concomitant. However, within the range of autoregulation, headaches due to fluctuation in blood pressure are relatively uncommon and elevations in blood pressure are generally asymptomatic.

4. What is the most common systemic cause of headache?

Febrile illnesses are often associated with headache. Even the common cold is usually associated with a headache. However, when meningitis is superimposed, these headaches become much more severe, may be bursting in character, and rapidly increase over a period of minutes to hours. In severe cases, there is stiff neck, nausea, vomiting, and photophobia. These headaches result from a direct irritation of meningeal nociceptors due to inflammation or infection. With bacterial meningitis, signs are usually fulminant. However, with an aseptic or viral meningitis, signs may be subtle, progressive over hours to days, and the cerebrospinal fluid commonly shows just a few cells (mainly lymphocytes) and increased protein. Pheochromocytoma, malignant hypertension, and systemic lupus erythematosus also have headache as a common symptom.

5. Describe the headache characteristics associated with Lyme disease.

Only rarely is headache the presenting symptom of Lyme disease. When it does occur, the headache tends to resemble migraine or tension-type headaches but is associated with cognitive impairment or focal neurologic dysfunction. These headaches are usually seen as part of a meningitic process or an encephalitic picture, and are accompanied by a CSF pleocytosis. Lyme is an endemic, tick-borne illness with many neurologic manifestations. Patients presenting with new onset headache, focal neurologic deficits, and residence in a Lyme-endemic region should be investigated for CNS Lyme.

6. What percentage of patients with herpes simplex encephalitis present with headache?

The incidence of headache varies with the accompanying presentation. If focal neurologic deficits are present, up to 90% of patients will also have a significant headache. If meningeal signs are present, headache is present in about 60% of cases. When there is only confusion or some obtundation, headache occurs in about 50 or 80% of patients. Overall, headache is a very common presenting symptom in herpes encephalitis but is usually accompanied by focal neurologic deficits, alterations in level of consciousness, and, usually, seizures.

7. What exogenous substances can precipitate a headache?

The most commonly recognized substances are the vasodilators. Amyl nitrite, a substance often used to heighten the sexual experience, is a potent vasodilator and may cause a severe pounding headache, even in patients who do not have a headache diathesis. Similar reactions may occur in patients taking nitrates for cardiac disease. Alcoholic beverages can also cause headaches, both in the acute and the well-known hangover phase. The exact mechanism is unclear. For the acute headache, it appears to be vasodilatation. The hangover may be due to some vasoactive substances that are in the "congeners" in the alcoholic beverage. Caffeine most often causes a headache as a withdrawal symptom. Cocaine, usually a vasorestrictive substance, can also cause headaches. These may be due to transient severe rises in blood pressure or to a cerebral vasculitis. Monosodium glutamate (MSG) is a clear precipitant in patients who are sensitive to the substance. There are a number of other drugs that may exacerbate headache. Nonsteroidal anti-inflammatory drugs, commonly given for pain, may cause headache. Of the hormones, estrogens and oral contraceptives are commonly associated with headaches. Rarely, some antibiotics may cause headaches.

8. What systemic tumors cause headaches without metastases?

Pheochromocytoma is the prototype of this group. These headaches are often paroxysmal, lasting seconds to minutes and occurring in a crescendo pattern. They are usually described as severe, bilateral, throbbing pain, sometimes associated with nausea, truncal sweating, palpitations, and tremor. The headache is usually associated with a sudden rise in blood pressure.

9. In what degenerative diseases of the nervous system is headache a common complaint?

About one-third of patients with Parkinson's disease report headaches. The exact mechanism is unclear, but it appears as a constant, dull pain, usually located over the cervical region. The temptation is to ascribe this to muscular stiffness, but the headaches do not necessarily correlate with the severity of the disease nor do they usually respond to anti-parkinsonian therapy. About ten percent of patients with multiple sclerosis complain of significant headaches. Degenerative disease of the cervical spine can often produce a headache that radiates up from the back of the head to the vertex. This headache is usually more intense in the morning, after the patient has slept on an elevated pillow. Treatment with cervical roll pillow may alleviate some of the pain.

10. What headache patterns are seen in systemic lupus erythematosus?

There are three major types of headache in SLE. They may be vascular, tension-type, or associated with lupus cerebritis. Migraine-type headaches seem most common at the onset of SLE. Later in the disease, tension-type headaches are more likely to develop. The headache of lupus cerebritis is accompanied by a clear-cut picture of cerebritis, with confusion and obtundation.

11. What types of headaches occur in patients with HIV infections or AIDS?

Most patients with HIV infections have an identifiable organic cause for their headaches. Some studies have shown that cryptococcal meningitis is the most common cause. This is a subacute headache, often without fever or significant neurologic findings. CNS toxoplasmosis is also a common cause, usually with multiple toxoplasmosis lesions visible on CT or MRI. These are usually late complications of AIDS. However, at the time of seroconversion, patients may develop an aseptic meningitis with headache.

12. What are three of the more common metabolic disorders associated with headaches?
Remember the 3 H's:

Hypoxia
Hypoglycemia
Hemodialysis

High altitude headaches are the most commonly reported hypoxic headaches. This is the most common clinical manifestation of altitude sickness and becomes more severe with ascents into high altitudes. The headache is most commonly frontal and pounding. They are increased by exertion and improved by intake of cold fluids or carbohydrates. In the most severe cases, cerebral edema may ensue. The theoretical basis for the headache is not entirely understood, but it is believed to be hypoxia leading to markedly increased cerebral blood flow and subsequent excitation of the trigemino-vascular system, similar to migraine. Usually, a partial oxygen pressure of less than 70 mm of mercury is needed to make the diagnosis.

13. Rather than headaches being a manifestation of certain diseases, what diseases are seen more commonly in patients with chronic headache syndromes?
Hypertension, dizziness, gastroesophageal reflux, depression or anxiety, peptic ulcer disease, and irritable bowel syndrome seem to be more common in patients with headache than in patients without headache.

BIBLIOGRAPHY

1. Featherstone HJ: Medical diagnoses and problems in individuals with recurrent idiopathic headaches. Headache 25:136–140, 1985.
2. Solomon GD: Concomitant medical disease and headache. Med Clin North Am 75(3):631–639, 1991.

17. TRIGEMINAL NEURALGIA

Robert A. Duarte, M.D.

1. What are the divisions and functions of the trigeminal nerve?

The three main divisions to the trigeminal nerve are the ophthalmic (V1), maxillary (V2), and mandibular (V3), which supply sensation to the face. The ophthalmic division supplies sensation from the eyebrows to the coronal suture. Note: The sensory distribution does not stop at the hair line, but at the corona, which may help in differentiating anatomic lesions from factitious illness, because patients feigning sensory loss will usually make the divide at the hairline. Innervation of the cornea is divided, being supplied by V1 in its upper half and V2 in its lower half. The cheek bones and the inside of the nares are supplied by V2. The mandibular branch supplies the lower jaw. However, the angle of the jaw is supplied by a cervical root, rather than by the trigeminal nerve. Again, this helps in anatomic differentiation.

The motor functions of the trigeminal nerve include the muscles of mastication. These are the temporalis, masseters, and pterygoids. The first two are involved in vertical closing of the jaw, and the third is involved in lateral motion of the jaw (grinding).

2. Name the exit (or entry) foramina for the branches of the trigeminal nerve.

The ophthalmic branch exits through the superior orbital fissure, along with cranial nerves III, IV, and VI, and the ophthalmic vein. The maxillary branch goes through the foramen rotundum in the base of the skull and the mandibular branch through the foramen ovale.

3. What is the gasserian ganglion, and where does it sit?

The gasserian ganglion is the sensory ganglion for the trigeminal nerve. It sits in Meckel's cave, which is an indentation on the petrous bone. This is an important point to remember because tumors or infections of this bone can cause trigeminal pain (secondary trigeminal neuralgia).

4. What is the classic presentation of trigeminal neuralgia?

Trigeminal neuralgia is characterized by sharp, jabbing sensations, sometimes described as an electrical pain, in the distribution of one or more branches of the trigeminal nerve. The V2–V3 distribution is the most common, followed by V2; the ophthalmic division is involved in only 5% of cases. The attacks are brief, lasting a few seconds, and the patient is pain free in between. By definition, in primary trigeminal neuralgia, there is no persistent sensory loss or motor dysfunction between attacks. Occasionally, the episodes can be so frequent that the pain appears continuous. The pain usually involves only one division of the trigeminal nerve and is almost invariably unilateral.

5. What is the natural history of trigeminal neuralgia?

The peak onset is in middle age. Patients below the age of 30 presenting with true trigeminal neuralgia should be investigated for a demyelinating lesion. Trigeminal neuralgia in the young is often the harbinger of multiple sclerosis. Similarly, if there is bilateral involvement, multiple sclerosis should be suspected.

The disease usually follows an exacerbating but remitting course. There may be months or years when the patient is pain free. Therefore, drug holidays should be attempted to see if the patient is, indeed, responding to the drug or simply having a remission of the disease. In some patients, the attacks become more frequent and may be nearly continuous.

6. What are trigger points?

Trigger points, a characteristic feature of trigeminal neuralgia, are points that, when touched, bring on paroxysms of pain. They are most commonly located around the upper lip or nose. Chewing, brushing teeth, or a breeze can trigger a painful event.

7. What clinical features differentiate an episode of cluster headache from an attack of trigeminal neuralgia?

While both of these pains may exhibit a V2 distribution, cluster pain rarely has the electric-shocklike quality of trigeminal neuralgia. It is a more constant, penetrating pain that lasts for more than 15 minutes. Furthermore, cluster pain is usually accompanied by ptosis, coryza, and lacrimation.

8. What is pre-trigeminal neuralgia?

In unusual cases, the appearance of classic trigeminal neuralgia is preceded, for a number of years, by an aching pain centered on a tooth or the paranasal sinuses. It is triggered by jaw movements or by drinking hot or cold liquids. These patients are sometimes subjected to dental extractions or temporomandibular joint surgery.

9. What is the pathogenesis of trigeminal neuralgia?

Both central and peripheral mechanisms have been invoked to explain the pain of trigeminal neuralgia. The central theory holds that there is a disinhibited pool of neurons in the pons, and spontaneous discharge in these neurons causes pain. The peripheral theory holds that compression of the nerve (primarily by an aberrant blood vessel) sets up an abnormal train of discharges. It is this later theory that has led to treatment of trigeminal neuralgia by surgical decompression of the nerve.

10. What is the difference between primary and secondary trigeminal neuralgia?

Primary trigeminal neuralgia implies no known structural cause for the pain (even though an aberrant vessel may be found in some cases). In secondary trigeminal neuralgia, pain is caused by either compression or demyelination. The clinical pain syndrome is indistinguishable. However, secondary syndromes usually involve dysfunction of the trigeminal nerve between attacks. This may take the form of sensory loss in one of the distributions of the nerve or paresis of one of the muscles of mastication.

11. What is the drug of choice for trigeminal neuralgia?

The primary drug of choice for trigeminal neuralgia is carbamazepine. The usual starting dose is 100 mg twice a day. This can be increased by 100 mg every day or two until the patient is pain free or side effects occur. The usual maintenance dose is between 600 and 1200 mg/day (serum levels of 4 to 10 µg/ml). Carbamazepine is effective in 95% of patients with true trigeminal neuralgia.

12. What are the most common side effects of carbamazepine?

The most feared side effect of carbamazepine is aplastic anemia. However, this is rare. There is usually a mild depression of the white blood cell count, but little else. The most common side effects are the four Ds: drowsiness, dizziness, diplopia, and dyspepsia, which are dose-related.

13. What type of monitoring is necessary for the use of carbamazepine?

A complete blood count and hepatic and renal profiles should be performed before starting treatment with carbamazepine. The blood count should be repeated weekly for the first two months, then every three months. After the first year, blood counts should be performed every six to 12 months. If the white blood cell count drops below 3,000, or if the absolute neutrophil count drops below 1,500, carbamazepine therapy should be discontinued. Aplastic anemia is a very rare complication of carbamazepine therapy, but mild leukopenia and thrombocytopenia occur in about 2% of patients.

14. List the drug interactions of carbamazepine.

Carbamazepine induces microsomal enzymes. Therefore, it increases its own metabolism as well as the metabolism of clonazepam, ethosuximide, oral contraceptives, warfarin, and haloperidol.

This increased metabolism is of particular concern with the oral contraceptives and anticoagulants, since dose adjustments will need to be made to ensure efficacy. Propoxyphene, isoniazid, and erythromycin can inhibit the metabolism of carbamazepine, causing high levels.

15. What are the other pharmacologic alternatives for treating trigeminal neuralgia?

Baclofen (Lioresal), an analog of gamma-aminobutyric acid (GABA) that binds to the GABA-β receptor, should be considered in those patients who do not respond to carbamazepine or who are unable to take carbamazepine. The starting dose is 5 mg/three times/day, with an increase to 5 to 10 mg/day, depending on the patient's response. Maintenance dose is between 50 to 60 mg/day in divided doses, with a recommended maximum of 80 mg/day. Side effects include sedation and nausea. When baclofen and carbamazepine are taken together, side effects are more common.

Phenytoin (Dilantin), like carbamazepine, depresses the response of spinal trigeminal neurons to maxillary nerve stimulation in laboratory animals. Phenytoin has been shown to be effective in up to 60% of patients with trigeminal neuralgia. However, it should be considered in patients who did not respond to baclofen or carbamazepine. The initial starting dose is 300 to 500 mg/day. Dose-dependent side effects include nystagmus, ataxia, and dysarthria. Higher levels may produce ophthalmoplegia and cognitive impairment. The advantage of phenytoin is that it can be given intravenously if a patient presents with severe, intractable trigeminal neuralgia, whereas baclofen and carbamazepine cannot.

16. Which surgical procedures have been used successfully for trigeminal neuralgia?

Surgical procedures for trigeminal neuralgia are divided into two groups: decompressive and destructive. The most commonly employed decompressive lesion is based on the theory that an aberrant vessel (often one of the cerebellar arteries or veins) compresses the nerve near its entry zone. Through a small posterior fossa craniotomy, the vessel is lifted and a cushion is placed between the nerve and the vessel. While success rates of over 90% have been reported, there have been no double-blind studies (for obvious reasons), and pain may recur, possibly from slippage of the sponge.

The offending branches of the nerve may be lesioned percutaneously, either with radiofrequency devices or alcohol injection. The procedures involve inserting a needle through the skin, into the foramen of the nerve where it exits the skull. Anesthesia dolorosa (pain in the numb area previously supplied by the nerve) is a bothersome complication.

Percutaneous injection of glycerol around the gasserian ganglion is also effective. While these destructive lesions are less invasive than a craniectomy for decompression, they have a higher incidence of side effects and failures.

17. What is Raeder's syndrome?

This syndrome is characterized by paroxysmal pain in the first division of the trigeminal nerve and is often accompanied by ptosis and miosis. It seems to be a crossover syndrome between true trigeminal neuralgia and cluster headache. The mechanism is unknown, but some cases may be due to local inflammation around the eye or the carotid artery.

BIBLIOGRAPHY

1. Brisman R: Bilateral trigeminal neuralgia. J Neurosurg 67:44–48, 1987.
2. Dalessio DJ: Diagnosis and treatment of cranial neuralgias. Med Clin North Am 75:605–615, 1991.
3. Fromm GH: Trigeminal neuralgia and related disorders. Neurol Clin 7:305–319, 1989.

18. GLOSSOPHARYNGEAL AND OTHER NEURALGIAS

Robert A. Duarte, M.D.

1. What are the classic features of glossopharyngeal neuralgia?

Glossopharyngeal neuralgia is similar in many ways to trigeminal neuralgia. It presents with paroxysms of lancinating pain that involve the glossopharyngeal and vagus nerves. Therefore, pain is felt around the jaw, throat, ears, larynx, or base of the tongue. The pain is usually unilateral and lasts for about one minute. Multiple attacks can occur throughout a day and may even awaken the patient out of a sound sleep. The usual triggers are talking and chewing. Pain on swallowing (odynophagia) is a specific trigger in glossopharyngeal neuralgia that is rarely, if ever, seen in trigeminal neuralgia. When glossopharyngeal neuralgia is not caused by an underlying tumor, spontaneous remissions often occur.

2. Is glossopharyngeal neuralgia a common disorder?

The incidence of glossopharyngeal neuralgia is about 1/100 that of trigeminal neuralgia, making it a relatively rare disorder. The average age of onset is about 50.

3. A patient presents with odynophagia and sudden loss of consciousness. What is a likely explanation?

Swallow syncope is an odd syndrome of unclear mechanism that occurs in patients with glossopharyngeal neuralgia. It is thought that a barrage of impulses from the glossopharyngeal nerve, through the tractus solitarius, to the dorsal motor nucleus of the vagus nerve produces bradycardia or brief asystole. This is most commonly seen in patients with tumors of the neck and, in previously operated patients, usually represents tumor recurrence.

4. What is the difference between idiopathic glossopharyngeal neuralgia and secondary glossopharyngeal neuralgia?

The difference is a clearly identified underlying cause. Clinically, idiopathic glossopharyngeal neuralgia rarely, if ever, shows objective sensory impairment on physical examination. However, if the pain syndrome is caused by tumor involvement, secondary glossopharyngeal neuralgia (sensory loss on the soft palate) is much more common. In fact, if sensory loss is found, an imaging procedure of the neck is imperative. Even in patients without an obvious sensory loss, it is probably wise to perform an MRI of the head and neck with gadolinium to exclude a structural cause for the pain.

5. A patient presents with severe pain in the ear, followed by ipsilateral facial weakness. What extremely important physical sign should be sought?

In any case of facial palsy, the search for a causative lesion is imperative. When there is severe ear and face pain, the lesion to be sought is a herpetic eruption. This may involve the ear, palate, or pharynx. The syndrome of facial nerve palsy with a herpetic eruption is called Ramsay Hunt syndrome, a particularly painful neuralgia.

6. What is the most common presentation of herpes zoster in the face?

Ophthalmic zoster (a V1 distribution) is the most common and most troublesome. The forehead and upper lid are involved with a vesicular eruption. Pain may precede the eruption for as much as three or four days. Viral vesicles may involve the eye itself. Aside from the general symptomatic treatment for zoster, the eye must be protected from secondary infection. The complication of postherpetic neuralgia is far more common in the elderly than in the young and seems to be more common when the zoster rash affects the V1 distribution. A further description of postherpetic neuralgia and its treatment is given in Chapter 27.

7. Describe the clinical features of occipital neuralgia.

In this syndrome, a sharp pain originates at the base of the skull and shoots up the back of the head. It may go as far forward as the coronal suture. It is generally unilateral and stabbing in nature. In idiopathic cases, there is no sensory loss, and some of the triggering mechanisms may be the same as those in other cranial neuralgias. However, occipital neuralgia may be a harbinger of more serious disease. Metastases to the occipital condyle can reproduce this syndrome, as can lesions at the C2–3 level of the spine. In these cases, local pressure will reproduce the pain, and there may be some accompanying sensory loss. Computerized tomography with overlapping cuts and bone windows can usually demonstrate the lesion. Occasionally, lesions around the foramen magnum can also produce this type of syndrome. Trauma is also a common cause; infection and chronic compression are less frequent causes.

8. How is occipital neuralgia treated?

In general, idiopathic cases respond to carbamazepine. In refractory cases, occipital nerve blocks may be curative. However, occipital nerve blocks may also relieve pain in migraine and other types of atypical facial pain. Therefore, it should not be used as a diagnostic tool. In particularly severe or refractory cases, neurectomy may be needed.

9. What is superior laryngeal neuralgia?

The superior laryngeal nerve, a branch of the vagus nerve, innervates the cricothyroid muscle of the larynx. This muscle stretches, tenses, and adducts the vocal cord. Superior laryngeal neuralgia usually appears as a postsurgical complication. There are paroxysms of unilateral submandibular pain, sometimes radiating to the eye, ear, or shoulder. This pain may be indistinguishable from glossopharyngeal neuralgia. It lasts from seconds to minutes and is usually provoked by swallowing, straining the voice, turning the head, coughing, sneezing, yawning, or blowing the nose.

10. What is sphenopalatine neuralgia?

This syndrome has been given a number of names, including lower half headache, greater superficial neuralgia, Sluder's neuralgia, and atypical facial pain. It is an uncommon form of facial neuralgia. The key clinical features include unilateral pain in the face (usually around the nasal region) lasting for days and associated with nasal congestion, otalgia, and tinnitus. By contrast to trigeminal and glossopharyngeal neuralgia, sphenopalatine neuralgia is usually not associated with a trigger zone. Some authors believe that this is not a separate syndrome and may simply be a variation of cluster headache. Sphenopalatine ganglion blocks have been advocated, but this treatment remains controversial.

11. What is Charlin's syndrome?

This is the clinical syndrome of "ciliary neuralgia." It is characterized by unilateral paroxysms of pain in the eye, profuse watery rhinorrhea, keratitis, iritis, and congestion of the nasal mucosa. The keratitis and pain disappear immediately after instillation of cocaine into the anterior half of the lateral wall of the affected nostril.

BIBLIOGRAPHY

1. Bogduk N: Greater occipital neuralgia. In Long DM: Current Therapy in Neurological Surgery. St. Louis, CV Mosby, 1985, pp 175–180.
2. Chalmers AC, Olson JL: Glossopharyngeal neuralgia with syncope and cervical mass. Otolaryngol Head Neck Surg 100:252–255, 1989.
3. Ferrannini G: Charlin's syndrome. Ann Ophthalmol 95:807–811, 1969.
4. Peet J: Glossopharyngeal neuralgia. Ann Surg 101:120–122, 1975.

19. LOW BACK PAIN

Ronald Kanner, M.D.

1. What are the most common causes of acute back pain?

In most cases of acute back pain, no clear pathophysiologic mechanism is defined, and patients are diagnosed as having "back strain." Episodes are usually preceded by minor trauma, heavy lifting, or a "near fall." Direct trauma is rarely a cause. A small minority of patients have acute medical illnesses that cause back pain. The first urgent crossroad in the diagnosis of low back pain is to decide whether the patient has a medically emergent condition (tumor, infection, or trauma) or a benign back pain. The signs and symptoms that should alert the clinician to impending disaster are focal spine tenderness, fever, weight loss, or bowel or bladder dysfunction.

2. Why does the back hurt?

Erect posture forces the spine into a position in which it is constantly exposed to minor trauma and to stress on pain-sensitive structures. These pain-sensitive structures are the supporting bones, articulations, meninges, nerves, muscles, and aponeuroses. The vertebral body, despite being short, is actually a long bone with endplates of hard bone and a center of cancellous bone. It is innervated by the dorsal roots. The periosteum is markedly pain-sensitive. (This is why banging the shin is so painful: the periosteum is unprotected). The articulations (facet joints) are true diarthrodial joints and have a capsule and meniscus. The capsule and bones are richly innervated with nociceptors and are subjected to stress every time the spine turns or bends.

3. What are the characteristics of pain arising from the back?

The type of pain suffered varies with the structure involved. Pain originating in a vertebral body (from osteoporosis, tumor, or infection) tends to be local and aching. It is somatic, nociceptive pain, made worse by standing or sitting and relieved by lying supine. Even though it is usually local, it may refer to other sites. Characteristically, the L1 vertebral body refers pain to the iliac crests and hips. When facet joints are involved, pain is most pronounced when the back is extended. Limitation of active range of motion is a hallmark of facet pain.

4. How do the intervertebral discs ("slipped discs") contribute to back pain?

The intervertebral disc is composed of a firm anulus fibrosus, with a more spongy nucleus pulposus inside. The fibrous ring is innervated by nociceptors, but the nucleus pulposus is not. When strong vertical stress is applied to the spine, the nucleus pulposus bulges outward through the anulus fibrosus. Stretching of the fibrous ring is painful; in general, it produces localized low back pain. Once the anulus breaks, disc material may extrude and press against a nerve. Pressure on the nerve root is felt as radicular pain ("sciatica"). Of interest, as the anulus bursts, the intense low back pain tends to subside and is replaced by radicular pain. A bulging disc in itself is usually not painful. Anything that increases pressure on the spine increases pain from a disc. Thus, pain is exacerbated by standing, sitting, and the Valsalva maneuver.

5. What is the usual outcome of a patient with acute low back pain?

The vast majority of the general population will have acute back pain at some point in their lives. Over 90% of cases resolve, without specific therapy, in less than 2 weeks. As mentioned earlier, in most cases no specific diagnosis is made.

6. How helpful are radiographs in determining the etiology of acute low back pain?

Most patients with acute low back pain require no imaging procedures. It may not be easy to convince a patient who is writhing in pain that no radiographs are needed. However, plain radiographic findings of degenerative disease are as common in asymptomatic patients as in patients with acute back pain. Furthermore, magnetic resonance imaging (MRI) is far too sensitive and nonspecific to be used as a screening procedure. More than one-half of adults with no history of back pain may show asymptomatic bulging of discs at one or more lumbar levels, and fully one-fourth show disc protrusion. Imaging procedures should be reserved for patients in whom the diagnosis is in question. Specifically, if fever or point tenderness on the spine raises the suspicion of infection or tumor, an imaging procedure is imperative.

7. A patient complaining of left lower back pain stands with his buttocks protruding and with his shoulders tilted to the left. What does this stance indicate?

The spine has a number of normal curvatures. With the patient standing erect, the normal position of the spine shows cervical lordosis, thoracic kyphosis, and lumbar lordosis. In low back pain with muscle spasm, the lumbar lordosis may be lost or hyperaccentuated. If the patient tilts toward one side, there may be muscle spasm or foraminal encroachment. With lateral tilt, the ipsilateral intervertebral foramen narrows. Therefore, if there is nerve root compression in the foramen, pain increases. Conversely, when the patient tilts away from an affected side, the foramen on that side opens, lessening neural pain but possibly accentuating pain from muscle spasm. In lateral disc herniations, patients tend to lean away from the side of the herniation.

8. What is the normal range of motion of the spine?

The lumbar spine should be able to flex forward between 40° and 60° from the vertical. As the patient extends backward, range is somewhat smaller (about 20–35°). Severe pain on extension of the spine may indicate pathology in the articular facets.

9. What is the significance of the straight leg-raising maneuver?

Straight leg-raising is used to diagnose nerve root compression from disc disease. It is most commonly used to look for lower lumbar root pathology. The patient lies supine, and the leg is elevated from the ankle, with the knee remaining straight. Normally, patients can elevate the leg 60–90° without pain. In disc herniations, elevations of 30–40° produce pain. Ipsilateral straight leg-raising is more sensitive but less specific than contralateral straight leg-raising. That is, nearly all patients with herniated discs have pain on straight leg-raising on the affected side. However, straight leg-raising elicits pain in many other conditions—for example, severe hip arthritis. However, contralateral straight leg-raising does not produce pain on the affected side if the pain is not due to root disease. To differentiate between hip and lumbar root pathology, Patrick's maneuver can be used. The thigh is flexed on the abdomen and the knee is externally rotated, putting stress on the hip joint but not on the nerve root. Therefore, the patient with hip pathology experiences pain, but the patient with root pathology does not.

10. What is the significance of pain on percussion of the spine?

Benign disease (disc protrusion and muscle spasm) rarely, if ever, produces pain on percussion of the spine. This sign usually indicates bone disease, most often metastases or infection; it requires immediate investigation with imaging procedures.

11. What historical data should raise suspicion of infection or tumor rather than benign disease?

Most patients with herniated discs or other benign mechanical causes of back pain state that the pain improves with bed rest. When they are no longer weight-bearing, pain is relieved. Patients with tumor or infection often say that their worst pain is at night when they are in bed. Nocturnal exacerbation is a clear danger signal.

12. What is the most common presentation for a herniated intervertebral disc?

Patients report severe back pain after lifting something heavy, and a few days later pain radiates down the leg. This sequence of events is due to the pathologic process underlying a herniated disc. With the initial exertion, the nucleus pulposus pushes against the anulus fibrosus, causing it to distend. This distention causes local back pain. As the anulus ruptures, the back pain is relieved, but the nucleus then presses against a nerve root, causing radiated pain down the leg.

13. What is the most common presentation for vertebral metastases?

Vertebral metastases almost invariably present as localized back pain. More than 95% of patients with malignant epidural spinal cord compression have pain as their first complaint. Pain is usually described as deep, localized, and aching. As neural structures become involved, the pain radiates in the distribution of the affected nerves. Because the thoracic spine is the site most commonly affected, pain radiates in a band around the chest. As time progresses, further neurologic problems ensue. If epidural spinal cord compression progresses, patients present with paraparesis, sensory loss, and bowel and bladder involvement. Epidural spinal cord compression from tumor is a medical emergency. With the administration of high doses of dexamethasone, pain usually resolves fairly quickly. Definitive treatment with radiation therapy or surgery is then undertaken.

14. What is the radiographic appearance of spinal metastases?

On plain films one of the earliest signs of spinal metastasis is erosion of a pedicle. As time progresses, the vertebral body begins to lose height. MRI reveals a change in signal intensity in the vertebral body. As tumor progresses, it may be seen invading the epidural space and compressing the spinal cord.

15. Both vertebral metastases and vertebral osteomyelitis can cause destruction of vertebral bodies and changes on MRI signal. How can they be differentiated?

When tumors affect the vertebral bodies, they tend to spare the disc spaces. Even though two or three adjacent vertebral bodies may be destroyed by tumor, the disc spaces between them tend to be preserved. In the case of vertebral osteomyelitis, the disc space is generally destroyed by the infection and the adjacent vertebral bodies appear to form a block of infection.

16. What is the difference between an osteoporotic vertebral collapse and vertebral collapse due to tumor involvement?

Clinically, the pain from an osteoporotic collapse is almost invariably relieved by a brief period of bed rest. Tumor, on the other hand, is often unrelieved by bed rest. Pathologically, an osteoporotic collapse is essentially an accordion of the vertebral body. A hollow body collapses on itself. With tumor involvement, collapse of the vertebral body causes extrusion of tumor material, which may then compress the spinal cord. Spinal cord compression from osteoporosis, on the other hand, is exceedingly rare.

17. What treatment should be used for the pain from metastatic destruction of a vertebral body?

Pain from vertebral metastases is due to destruction of bone trabeculae, expansion of the periosteum, and stretching of the dura. This is a classical somatic nociceptive pain syndrome. As such, it is well treated by a combination of either nonsteroidal antiinflammatory drugs (NSAIDs) or steroids and an opioid. As bone metastases grow, they elaborate prostaglandin E_2, which continues destruction of bone trabeculae. The administration of an NSAID or steroids decreases production of prostaglandin E_2 and slows destruction.

18. Why is osteoporosis painful?

In general, osteoporosis is not painful in the absence of fractures. In weight-bearing bones, microfractures may occur with minor trauma. Unfortunately, this type of pain generally makes a patient take to bed. The absence of weight-bearing leads to further demineralization of the bone and further fractures with weight-bearing. In such patients, progressive exercise is of paramount importance. Weight-bearing leads to greater bone density and fewer fractures. Of interest, when a vertebral body collapses completely, it is painful at first, but the pain subsides once the fracture is complete.

19. How should pain from an osteoporotic vertebral collapse be treated?

The first issue is to be sure that the pain is due to benign osteoporotic collapse. Although postmenopausal women and patients treated with corticosteroids are at high risk, it should not necessarily be assumed that the osteoporosis is idiopathic. Serum protein electrophoresis, sedimentation rate, alkaline phosphatase, phosphorus, serum calcium, and plain films should be evaluated to rule out a secondary cause for the osteoporosis. Once a secondary cause has been ruled out, the patient should be treated with therapy directed at reversing the osteoporosis and with analgesics and exercise.

20. What is the most common presentation of vertebral osteomyelitis?

Vertebral osteomyelitis usually presents as subacute back pain that increases over days to weeks. Progressive pain is felt in the low back and, if untreated, focal weakness and bowel and bladder problems ensue. Focal tenderness is present, and usually another source of infection is found. Although previously the most common presentation was in the lumbar spine and in men over 50, the AIDS epidemic has changed the epidemiology somewhat. Younger men are affected, and the cervical spine is becoming a more common site of vertebral osteomyelitis.

21. What is the most common cause of vertebral osteomyelitis?

In immunocompetent hosts, *Staphylococcus aureus* infection is the most common causative agent. Infection involves the vertebral bodies, endplates, and disc spaces but generally spares the posterior elements. In the rare cases of actinomycosis or coccidioidomycosis, the posterior elements may be involved, and the spine becomes unstable.

22. What is sciatica?

The term *sciatica* has come into rather broad usage and usually refers to any sharp pain that radiates down the posterior aspect of the leg. Its initial formulation was for pain in a sciatic nerve distribution. However, it is used to describe pain of L5 root compromise, S1 root compromise, and true sciatic neuropathy.

23. What is piriformis syndrome?

The sciatic nerve passes through the piriformis muscle as it exits the pelvis. Occasionally, the muscle has a fibrous band or area of contraction. Pain is felt in the distribution of the sciatic nerve, but there is no back pain. Pain radiates from the buttocks down the posterior aspect of the thigh. Deep palpation of the piriformis muscle, either through the buttocks or through a rectal examination, exacerbates the pain and reproduces the patient's clinical syndrome. Therapy involves repeated stretching of the piriformis muscle or, in extreme cases, injection of lidocaine and steroids into the piriformis.

24. What are the common areas of radiation of pain with lumbar and sacral radiculopathies?

L1 pain radiates into the iliac crest and inguinal canal. L2 goes to the inguinal canal. L3 radiates to the anterior thigh. L4 radiates to the anterior thigh and medial calf. L5 radiates to the buttocks and the lateral aspect of the shin. S1 radiates down the buttocks to the posterior thigh.

25. If a patient presents with severe back pain radiating into the anterior thigh, accompanied by weakness of the leg, how can one differentiate between an L4 radiculopathy and a femoral nerve lesion?

The L2, L3, and L4 roots split into anterior and posterior divisions. The anterior divisions come together to form the obturator nerve, and the posterior divisions come together to form the femoral nerve. The quadriceps muscle is innervated by the femoral nerve, and the adductors of the thigh are innervated by the obturator nerve. In an L4 radiculopathy, both the quadriceps and the adductors are affected. In a femoral nerve lesion, the quadriceps are affected, but the adductors are spared.

26. Which nerve roots subserve the knee jerk reflex?

The L2–L3 and L4 roots, through the femoral nerve, form the afferent and efferent arc of the knee jerk. When the patellar tendon is tapped, the quadriceps contract.

27. Which nerve root subserves the Achilles reflex?

The Achilles reflex is mediated through the S1 nerve root. Tapping of the Achilles tendon produces contraction of the gastrocnemius muscle.

28. What is the role of MRI in the diagnosis of herniated discs?

The MRI scan is highly sensitive for disc pathology. Even slight bulges in the disc can be picked up with an appropriate MRI; however, it may be overly sensitive. The fact that a disc is seen to be bulging or herniated on MRI does not mean that it causes the pain syndrome. Nearly one-half of a sample of asymptomatic patients were shown to have disc bulges on MRI. The advantage of MRI over CT scan is that the nerve root can be seen.

29. In a patient with low back pain and a previously operated herniated disc, how can one differentiate between a new disc herniation and scar tissue?

This distinction can be a particularly vexing clinical problem. On MRI scan, discs do not enhance with gadolinium, but inflammatory tissue may.

30. If a patient presents with acute low back pain and no findings on clinical examination, how much bed rest is required?

No evidence indicates that bed rest influences the ultimate outcome of low back pain. In general, patients with acute pain feel more comfortable with a day or two in bed. However, more prolonged bed rest leads to deconditioning and may prolong recovery time.

31. What weight of traction should be used for low back pain?

The theoretical benefit of traction is to lower intradiscal pressure. Simply lying supine reduces pressure, and no evidence indicates that traction significantly alters the outcome of low back pain. Traction from five pounds to total body inversion has been used without clear demonstration of lowering pressure beyond the levels achieved by recumbency.

32. What is the role of myelography in low back pain?

Myelography has been almost completely supplanted by MRI scanning in low back pain. However, in cases in which the exact location or morphology of a disc herniation is in doubt, myelography can be combined with CT scanning to provide exquisite anatomic images.

33. What is meant by a facet syndrome?

The articular facets are the means by which the vertebral bodies articulate with each other. When these joints become inflamed or arthritic, range of motion is diminished. Maximal stress is put on these joints when the spine is hyperextended. Thus, when the patient reports no pain on anterior flexion but severe pain on extension, a facet syndrome is believed to be present. The diagnosis is confirmed by CT scanning of the affected area with demonstration of marked arthritic changes of the specific facet. In some cases, direct instillation of a steroid solution and lidocaine into the affected facet produces dramatic relief.

34. What is meant by degenerative disease of the spine?

The term *degenerative joint disease* (DJD) is probably overused. Most joints, after age 40, show osteophytes or other signs of deterioration. In the spine, these signs are particularly common and may not correlate with pain states.

35. What is spondylolisthesis?

Spondylolisthesis refers to slippage of one vertebral body on the adjacent one. It is fairly common in the elderly (10–15% of even asymptomatic patients over the age of 70). Most cases are caused by lysis of the posterior elements, which may be due to advanced age or trauma. When pain is markedly exacerbated by movement, imaging should be performed with flexion and extension views, which show whether there is any increase in movement at the abnormal joint.

36. What is meant by a lateral recess syndrome?

The lumbar spine contains a triangular space bordered by the pedicle, vertebral body, and superior articular facet. Facet hypertrophy or a disc fragment may encroach upon this triangular space (the lateral recess) and compress a nerve root on its way to exit at the next lower level. Pain is often neuropathic and is characterized by lancinating jabs or by a burning, dysesthetic pain in the distribution of the affected nerve root.

37. What is lumbar arachnoiditis?

Lumbar arachnoiditis refers to thickening of the arachnoid lining around the nerve roots. It is most commonly iatrogenic, produced by repeated myelography or by surgery. Nerve roots may become matted in an inflamed arachnoid or by scar tissue. On MRI, the nerve roots appear matted together. They may form a clump in the center of the canal or be matted to the sides of the canal.

38. What is spinal stenosis?

Spinal stenosis is a narrowing of the spinal canal. Facet hyerptrophy, ligamentous hardening, and spondylolisthesis can narrow the diameter of the lumbar canal as a result of normal aging. In some cases, this may lead to a syndrome called neurogenic claudication, in which patients are pain-free at rest but develop pain upon walking. The pain is felt as an ache in both legs. Patients characteristically say that they get relief after stopping for a few minutes and leaning forward at the waist. According to one theory, compromise of the radicular arteries gives rise to the claudication.

39. What is the role of epidural steroid injections in low back pain?

There are not enough well-controlled clinical trials in select patient populations to define accurately the indications for epidural steroid injection. However, clinical experience shows that many patients may have dramatic responses. A small amount of a corticosteroid is mixed with a small amount of lidocaine, and the mixture is instilled into the epidural space. In good responses, patients report early pain relief from the lidocaine, exacerbation of pain in the evening, and then gradual diminution of pain as the steroids take effect. In good hands, epidural steroid injections are a relatively low-risk procedure. In any case, no more than three injections should be performed in any 6-month period, because epidural steroid injections may lead to ligamentous laxity.

40. What are the indications for laminectomy and discectomy?

The indications are open to great dispute. Some surgeons believe that the only cure for lumbar radiculopathy is surgical removal of the causative disc. However, in many cases of low back pain, the herniated disc may not be the causative factor. A conservative approach dictates that progressive pain with neurologic impairment is an indication for surgical intervention.

41. What is meant by failed low back syndrome?

Patients who undergo one or more operative procedures for low back pain without resolution of pain are often said to have failed low back syndrome. There are a number of causes. The single most important factor is probably poor patient selection for the initial operative procedure. The problem may be as simple as inattention to psychological factors that complicate pain. Overinterpretation of radiologic procedures may lead to surgery in a patient in whom a herniated disc is not the cause of the pain syndrome. Incorrect surgery is possible a less common cause. When pain persists from the time of surgery, efforts should be made to uncover persistent pathology or to determine whether the indication for surgery was incorrect. If a patient has initial relief from surgery and then recurrence of pain, a structural cause should be sought. However, postoperative imaging is complicated because new lesions may look much the same as the old lesions. Rarely, a complication of surgery may cause failed low back syndrome. Arachnoiditis, resulting in chronic neuropathic pain, is one such cause. Occasionally, removal of the posterior element leads to spinal instability, which gives rise to mechanical, nociceptive pain.

42. What is the paintbrush sign?

In patients with large herniated lumbar discs, the disc may flatten the cauda equina. On myelography, the multiple roots of the cauda equina are seen to be flattened and parallel, giving the appearance of large bristles on a paintbrush.

43. Which tumors commonly metastasize to the vertebral bodies?

Lung, breast, and prostate tumors are three of the most common causes of vertebral metastases. They generally produce osteolytic lesions and local pain. If the tumors progress, they may cause epidural spinal cord compression with paraparesis, sensory level compromise, and bowel and bladder dysfunction. Occasionally, tumors that grow paraspinally (lymphoma and lung tumors) may invade the epidural space through the intervertebral foramen without affecting the bone. In such cases, epidural spinal compression may occur in the presence of normal bone radiographs.

44. What is the usual radiographic appearance of bone metastases in the vertebral bodies?

As noted earlier, washout of a pedicle is a common early sign. Most vertebral metastases have a lytic appearance, with a punched-out appearance on plain films. In rare cases, lesions may be blastic and appear hyperdense; this variation characteristically occurs in myeloma and in some breast and prostate tumors.

45. What are the most common levels at which herniated discs occur?

The L4–L5 and L5–S1 interspaces are the most common sites. They produce, respectively, L5 and S1 radiculopathies.

46. With an L5 radiculopathy, what is the most common pattern of weakness?

The muscles most commonly affected by an L5 lesion are the extensor hallucis longus (the extensor of the great toe) and the dorsiflexors of the foot. Invertors of the foot also may be affected, but both invertors and evertors have a combination of L5 and S1 innervation. In severe cases, the dorsiflexors may be affected so much that the foot cannot be elevated (foot drop).

47. Why may it be difficult to assess weakness in an S1 radiculopathy?

Among the main muscles innervated by S1 are the plantarflexors, which are normally extraordinarily strong, capable of exerting many hundreds of pounds of pressure. If they are tested manually, they can lose 20–30% of their strength without showing weakness. To assess these muscles properly, testing must be done in a functional manner; that is, the patient should be asked to stand on tip-toes.

48. What is the best treatment for back pain?

Back pain is a multifactorial disease. It may be something as straightforward as an arthritic joint or as complex as multiple nerve lesions in a patient with significant psychopathology. No single treatment modality is best for all cases. Careful patient selection and follow-up may lead to more accurate definition of treatment modalities in the future. Outcome assessment has been a major problem; currently under way is a study by the Back Pain Outcome Assessment Team (BOAT).

BIBLIOGRAPHY

1. Boden SD, David DO, Dina MD: Abnormal magnetic-resonance scans of the lumbar spine in asymptomatic subjects. J Bone Joint Surg 72A:403–406, 1990.
2. Cole AJ, Herring SA: The Low Back Pain Handbook. Philadelphia, Hanley & Belfus, 1997.
3. Deyo RA: Conservative therapy for low back pain: Distinguishing useful from useless therapy. JAMA 250:1057–1063, 1983.
4. Kanner RM: Low back pain. In Portenoy RK, Kanner RM (eds): Pain Management: Theory and Practice. Philadelphia, F.A. Davis, 1996, pp 126–144.
5. Loeser JD, Volinn E: Epidemiology of low back pain. Neurosurg Clin North Am 2:713–718, 1991.
6. Long DM: Failed blow back syndrome. Neurosurg Clin North Am 2:899–912, 1991.
7. Portenoy R, Lipton R, Foley K: Back pain in the cancer patient: An algorithm for evaluation and management. Neurology 37:134–138, 1987.

20. NECK AND ARM PAIN

Ronald Kanner, M.D.

1. Who had the first case of neck pain?

In his book on neck and arm pain, Dr. Rene Cailliet cites writings in the Papyrus, over 4,600 years ago, describing cervical vertebral dislocation and sprains. He goes on to say that Tutankhamen described what may have been the first cervical laminectomy. At any rate, it appears that cervical pain has been present since man walked erect.

2. Why does the neck hurt?

As in the lumbar spine, there are a number of pain-sensitive structures in the cervical spine. These include the vertebral bodies, laminae, dura, and surrounding muscles. Inflammation or destruction of any one of these structures produces pain.

3. What is the normal configuration of the cervical spine?

In the pain-free, normal cervical spine, there is a gentle lordosis from C1 to T1. As the head flexes forward, this lordosis normally disappears. Anterior flexion should be pain-free, even with the chin touching the chest. On lateral flexion, the ears should come within a few centimeters of the shoulder. Flexion and extension have a combined excursion of about 70 degrees. Rotations about the vertical axis (left and right) are approximately 90 degrees in each direction. Lateral flexion should be about 45 degrees in each direction. When testing range of motion of the cervical spine, always have the patient try active range of motion before passive range of motion is attempted. If there are structural abnormalities, the patient will guard the area.

4. What is the prevalence of neck pain?

Neck pain appears to be less common than low back pain in the general population. There are very few demographic studies of neck pain in the literature. The vast majority of pain prevalence studies have been done on low back pain. Acute attacks of stiff neck appear to be relatively common, occurring in anywhere from 25 to 50% of workers. Chronic neck pain, however, is less prevalent.

5. How many cervical vertebrae and roots are there?

There are seven cervical vertebrae and eight cervical spinal nerves. C1, however, has no sensory root and innervates the muscles that support the head.

6. What is the difference in the exiting characteristics of the nerves in the cervical spine from those in the rest of the spine?

In the thoracic and lumbar spines, the spinal nerves exit through the intervertebral foramen subjacent to the vertebral body numbered for that root. Therefore, the L1 root exits between the L1 and L2 vertebral bodies, L2 between L2 and L3, and so on. The root is numbered for the body under which it exits. In the cervical spine, however, the numbering is somewhat different. The C8 root exits between the 7th cervical and the first thoracic vertebrae. C7 exits between C6 and C7, and so on in a cephalad direction.

7. On which articulations in the neck do most of the anterior and posterior flexions depend?

Fifty percent of the AP flexion of the neck is centered on the atlanto-occipital joint. The other fifty percent is divided relatively evenly among the other cervical vertebral articulations. Therefore, even with relatively severe cervical spondylosis, some degree of nodding ability is maintained.

8. How does movement of the head affect the intervertebral foramina through which cervical roots exit?

Anterior flexion of the head opens the neuroforamina. As the head turns from side to side or tilts from side to side, the ipsilateral intervertebral foramen closes. If there is nerve root compromise, tilting or turning the head toward that side increases radicular pain.

9. What is the most benign cause of cervical pain?

Stress, with accompanying muscle tension, can produce neck pain and tenderness. With tension and anxiety, the shoulders are held shrugged and muscle pain ensues. The ideal treatment for this would be removal of the stress, though this is rarely possible. More practically, local applications of heat or cold or relaxation techniques may be useful.

10. What is meant by spondylosis?

Spondylosis refers to pathologic changes in the spinal column. It is also called degenerative disc disease and osteoarthritis of the spine. Radiographically, there is hypertrophy of the facet joints, narrowing of disc spaces, and osteophyte formation. All of these changes narrow the spinal canal and compromise nerve roots as they exit through the intervertebral foramina. Neurologic compromise may be at the root or cord level.

11. What is whiplash injury?

This term refers to acceleration/deceleration of the head, whipping the neck. It most commonly occurs in motor vehicle accidents, usually when a car is struck from behind. Patients complain of soreness and tenderness in the neck, usually occurring a day or two after the initial injury. In most cases, pain resolves spontaneously. In some, it can go on for many months or years. Some of these patients are suspected of having "litigation neurosis," but there is little evidence to support this contention, despite the fact that it is almost invariably the car struck, rather than the car striking, in which injuries occur. On examination, there is tenderness of the neck muscles and limitation of range of motion. Focal neurologic dysfunction is uncommon.

12. What is a central cord injury?

In severe trauma to the neck there may be hemorrhage into the central canal of the spinal cord. With time, this may progress to form a true syrinx. Patients initially complain of burning in the hands. With time, they may develop atrophy of the hand muscles and a "suspended sensory loss." This suspended sensory loss or cape distribution of loss of pinprick and temperature sense is due to the anatomy of the crossing, second order, nociceptive fibers. As noted in the chapter on neuroanatomy, the second order neurons that are going to form the lateral spinothalamic tracts cross anterior to the central canal in the spinal cord. An injury at that level will produce suspended sensory loss, without sensory loss below or above the point of injury.

13. What are the signs and symptoms of cervical epidural spinal cord compression?

The first symptom is almost invariably pain. It is usually local pain with some radicular radiation. The particular radiation depends upon the level at which the compression occurs. With compression of the spinal cord, myelopathy ensues. Myelopathic changes are characterized by sensory loss below the level of compression and paraparesis. There is hyperreflexia, along with Babinski signs. With cervical cord compression, bowel and bladder involvement are common.

14. What are the common causes of cervical cord compression?

The most common causes are trauma, infection, and tumor. Cervical spondylosis can produce spinal cord compression, but it is usually insidious and progresses over many years. Prognosis in spondylitic cord compression is poorest in the elderly and in patients with sphincter disturbances.

15. What roots form the brachial plexus?

Cervical roots 4, 5, and 6 form the upper trunk of the brachial plexus, C7 forms the middle trunk, and C8 and T1 form the lower trunk.

16. What is the sensory distribution of the cervical nerve roots?

C1 has no sensory representation.

C2 covers the occiput.

C3 and 4 cover part of the neck and trapezius.

C5 goes over the cap of the shoulder and part of the lateral arm.

C6 produces sensory symptoms over the lateral forearm, lateral hand and the first and second digits.

C7 mainly affects the 3rd and 4th digits.

C8 covers the medial part of the forearm and the 5th finger.

17. What reflex changes are commonly seen with cervical nerve root compression?

C5 lesions commonly lead to diminished biceps and brachioradialis reflexes, while C7 affects the triceps. There is some C6 contribution to the biceps and brachioradialis, but isolated C6 lesions are unusual and they tend not to affect the reflexes, because C5 is the main innervation.

18. What muscles are innervated by the C5 root?

The main muscles are supraspinatus, infraspinatus, deltoid, biceps, and brachioradialis.

19. What is the thoracic outlet syndrome?

This refers to compression of the neurovascular bundle as it crosses the first rib and enters the arm. It may be compressed by a cervical rib, by the scalenus muscle, or by fibrous bands. Pain is usually felt in the forearm and is exacerbated by movement and by elevation and abduction of the arm.

20. What is Adson's sign?

This is disappearance of the radial pulse when the arm is abducted and the head is turned contralaterally. It is thought to be a sign of vascular compression at the thoracic outlet.

21. A 19-year-old man presents with severe pain in the shoulder and upper arm. Pain resolves over a few days but is replaced by weakness in the deltoids, biceps, brachioradialis, and triceps. What is the most likely diagnosis?

Brachial plexitis is a relatively common syndrome in young men. Inflammation of the brachial plexus produces severe pain that gradually subsides and is replaced by weakness that depends upon the distribution of the inflammation of the plexus. Commonly, it is just the upper plexus, affecting the deltoids, biceps, and brachioradialis. Occasionally, it can be more widespread.

22. What is Pancoast syndrome?

Tumors affecting the superior pulmonary sulcus can grow upward into the brachial plexus. This causes severe pain in the arm, with weakness of the muscles subserved by the lower trunk of the brachial plexus. These are primarily the intrinsic muscles of the hand. Early in the disease, pain may be the only symptom. As the disease progresses, the full syndrome is characterized by an ipsilateral Horner's syndrome (ptosis, myosis, and anhydrosis), atrophy of the muscles of the hand, decreased reflexes, and sensory loss in a C8–T1 distribution. If the tumor progresses further, it can involve the entire brachial plexus and spread medially to invade the epidural space. In very advanced cases, epidural spinal cord compression occurs. On the average, pain is present for 7–12 months before an accurate diagnosis is made.

23. What is tennis elbow?

Lateral epicondylitis is a very common clinical condition that produces pain on the extensor surface of the lateral forearm. It is referred to as tennis elbow. It is usually thought to be an inflammatory lesion at the insertion of the extensor tendons, mainly of the extensor carpi radialis brevis.

24. What is carpal tunnel syndrome?

Carpal tunnel syndrome is characterized by numbness and tingling over the thumb, index, and middle fingers. It is most pronounced upon awakening. Patients state that they have to "shake the hand to wake it up." Sensory loss maps out to the distribution of the median nerve. It affects the thumb, index finger, and radial side of the ring finger. It is due to entrapment of the median nerve as it passes under the ligamentous canal in the wrist (see figure). Weakness, when it occurs, is in the muscles innervated by the median nerve. These are the opponens and the abductor pollicis brevis (APB). Initial treatment is with nighttime splints. If treatment fails and weakness progresses, surgical decompression of the nerve at the wrist may be necessary.

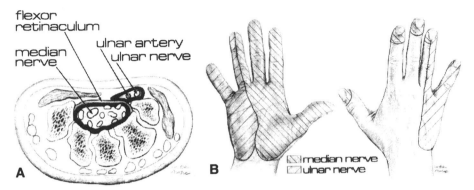

A, Wrist anatomy showing the median nerve through the carpal tunnel in close proximity to Guyon's canal, where the ulnar nerve passes. *B,* Median and ulnar nerve sensory distributions. (From West SG (ed): Rheumatology Secrets. Philadelphia, Hanley & Belfus, 1997.)

25. What is the value of electrodiagnostic studies in the evaluation of radicular pain in the neck and arm?

Electromyography (EMGs) and nerve conduction velocities (NCVs) help in localizing lesions and quantifying their severity. They can be used to determine which level is involved and at what point that nerve or root is injured. In lesions proximal to the dorsal root ganglion, sensory nerve action potentials (SNAPs) are preserved. Signs of denervation in a group of muscles innervated by a single root and their absence in other muscles are indicative of compression of that root. However, it takes up to three weeks after nerve injury for those signs to appear.

26. What are some of the EMG signs of denervation?

Normal muscles show electrical silence at rest. After denervation, there is increased insertional activity (spontaneous electrical discharges after an EMG needle is inserted into the muscle). Fibrillations and sharp waves may also be seen.

27. Clinically, how can a root lesion be differentiated from injury to a peripheral nerve?

A number of muscles may be innervated by the same root, but through different nerves. For example, the biceps, brachioradialis, and deltoids are all innervated by the C5 nerve root, but also by the musculocutaneous, radial, and axillary nerves, respectively. A root injury at the C5 level produces changes in all three muscles, while injury to one of the peripheral nerves produces weakness only in the muscle supplied by that nerve.

28. What is the value of NCVs in carpal tunnel syndrome?

With median nerve compression at the wrist (as in carpal tunnel syndrome), nerve conduction is locally slowed.

BIBLIOGRAPHY

1. Bovim G, Schrader H, Sand T: Neck pain in the general population. Spine 19(12):1307–1309, 1994.
2. Brazis PW: The localization of spinal and nerve root lesions. In Brazis PW, Masdeu JC, Biller J (eds): Localization in Clinical Neurology. Boston, Little, Brown, 1990.
3. Cailliet R: Neck and Arm Pain. Philadelphia, F.A. Davis Company, 1991.
4. DiPalma JR, DiGregorio GJ: Management of low back and neck pain by analgesics and adjuvant drugs: An update. Mt Sinai J Med 61(3):193–196, 1994.
5. Matthews JA: Neck pain. In Klippel JH, Dieppe PA (eds): Rheumatology. St. Louis, Mosby, 1994.
6. Strausbaugh LJ: Vertebral osteomyelitis. How to differentiate it from other causes of back and neck pain. Postgrad Med 97(6):147–154, 1995.

21. ABDOMINAL PAIN

Ronald E. Greenberg, M.D.

1. Which three afferent relays mediate appreciation of abdominal pain?
1. Visceral or splanchnic pathway
2. The somatic or parietal pathway
3. The referral pathway

Visceral abdominal pain is produced by activation of nociceptors located in the walls of the abdominal viscera. Somatic abdominal pain is produced by activation of nociceptors located in the parietal peritoneum and intra-abdominal supporting structures. Referral pain occurs when strong visceral impulses enter the spinal cord at the same level as afferents from other areas; this is mistakenly "read" as pain arising from the second area (e.g., shoulder pain is gallbladder disease).

2. How can visceral, somatic, and referred abdominal pain be clinically distinguished?
Visceral pain tends to be poorly localized, felt in the midline, and is often felt as a dull soreness that fluctuates in severity. Visceral pain may be very difficult for patients to describe and may be referred to as an aching, gnawing, burning, or cramping discomfort or as pain commonly attended by restlessness and associated symptoms of autonomic disturbance (i.e., nausea, vomiting, diaphoresis, and pallor). In contrast, somatic pain is typically more acute, intense, sharp, localized, and aggravated by movement. Referred pain combines features of both visceral and somatic pain and is well localized in areas distant from the precipitating stimulus. Referred pain is commonly associated with cutaneous hyperesthesia, and the skin may be the dominant location where pain is perceived.

3. Can the location of abdominal pain be useful in determining the origin of the problem?
The location, depth, and radiation of pain can provide both helpful and, at times, misleading clues. Pain mediated along visceral afferent pathways tends to be poorly localized and referred to the midline, regardless of the lateral location of the pathologic process. However, the level of midline pain can provide helpful clues. Pain from gastroduodenal and hepatobiliary structures is usually perceived in the epigastrium; pain from the small bowel is usually periumbilical; and pain from the colon tends to be perceived in the lower abdomen.

4. What four classes of stimuli generate abdominal pain?
The abdominal visceral organs are insensitive to many stimuli that would ordinarily provoke cutaneous pain such as burning, pinching, stabbing, and cutting. The abdominal visceral organs will generate pain in response to four general classes of stimuli:
1. Distention and contraction
2. Traction
3. Compression and torsion
4. Stretch

5. Abdominal pain is poorly localized and usually midline because of the paucity of visceral afferent nerves and the bilateral symmetric innervations of most abdominal organs. What is the significance of abdominal pain that is clearly lateralized?
Clearly lateralized abdominal pain may arise either from one of the few intra-abdominal organs with predominant one-sided innervation (e.g., kidney, ovary, ureter) or from structures with somatic rather than visceral innervation.

6. What determines where in the abdomen pain is experienced?
Afferent nerves from the abdominal viscera enter the spinal cord at different levels, and the level of entry governs where within the abdomen pain is experienced. Foregut structures, including

the distal esophagus, stomach, duodenum, pancreas, liver, and biliary tree, are innervated by spinal segments T5–T6 to T8–T9 and manifest pain between the xyphoid process and umbilicus. Midgut structures, including the small bowel, appendix, and colon up to the distal transverse part, are innervated by spinal segments T8–T11 and L1 and manifest pain in the periumbilical region. Hindgut structures, including the distal colon and rectum, are innervated by spinal segments T11–L1 and result in pain between the umbilicus and pubic symphysis.

7. What historical attributes must always be assumed when obtaining the history from a patient with abdominal pain?

The mnemonic **PQRST** provides a framework that ensures a full exploration of a given patient's abdominal pain.

P   P refers to factors that either palliate or provoke abdominal pain. For example, pain relieved by defecation suggests a colonic origin.

Q   Q refers to the qualities of the pain (i.e., burning, sharp, crampy).

R   R refers to radiation of pain. For example, biliary tract pain radiates to the right periscapular region; pancreatic pain radiates to the back; and subdiaphragmatic pain may be referred to the shoulder tips.

S   S refers to the severity of the pain.

T   T refers to temporal events associated with the pain (i.e., duration of pain, constant or intermittent, association with eating or defecation).

In addition, any relationship to other associated gastrointestinal symptoms (e.g., vomiting, diarrhea) or dysfunction of other contiguous organ systems (e.g., genitourinary or thoracic) must be sought.

8. What historical symptoms suggest the presence of an uncomplicated peptic ulcer?

Peptic ulcer pain is commonly described as a burning or gnawing pain in the midepigastric or subxyphoid region. Occasionally patients with peptic ulcer deny any pain and complain of discomfort and distress with a "hunger" or "empty stomach feeling" in the epigastrium. Peptic ulcer pain may vary from patient to patient but is commonly classic for a given patient and occurs in an episodic and rhythmic fashion. The episodic pattern refers to the way in which ulcer pain recurs over a long period of weeks, months, and years. Rhythm refers to the pattern in which pain recurs during a 24-hour period, typically adhering to the sequence of pain-food-relief. Ulcer pain typically occurs when the stomach is empty and is relieved by eating or drinking, especially for ulcers located at or near the pyloroduodenal junction. Pain from more proximal ulcers may be exacerbated by eating.

9. A 39-year-old man with a history of duodenal ulcer experiences sudden severe pain throughout the abdomen. What may have happened?

Any alteration in the previous pattern of pain in a patient with a peptic ulcer should raise the suspicion of perforation. Acute free perforation occurs suddenly and with almost immediate peak intensity. Severe pain may be felt throughout the abdomen and may be referred to the shoulders or flanks and lower abdomen. Physical examination demonstrates abdominal wall rigidity and involuntary guarding due to peritoneal irritation. In extreme cases of peritonitis, a boardlike rigid abdomen is detected. Palpation for muscular rigidity and guarding must be gentle. The practice of eliciting "rebound tenderness" should not be attempted as it can be misleading, may cause the patient significant discomfort, and provide no more information than can be obtained using gentle palpation for underlying muscular rigidity.

10. What clinical features suggest the complication of ulcer penetration?

Ulcer penetration connotes the presence of a confined perforation where the ulcer crater has extended beyond the stomach or duodenum but is walled off by an adjacent structure (as opposed to acute free perforation). For example, a posterior wall bulbar duodenal ulcer may penetrate into the head of the pancreas. The complication of ulcer penetration must be considered when a patient's previous typical pattern of pain-food-relief is disrupted, giving way to more constant and unrelenting pain. In addition, pain that is not relieved by previously effective measures (e.g., antacids), pain that radiates to the upper lumbar back, occurrence of night pain, and change in the location, radiation, and intensity of anterior epigastric discomfort should also raise the suspicion of ulcer penetration.

11. A 68-year-old woman with a long history of duodenal ulcer has recently been experiencing her typical intermittent discomfort of epigastric burning and gnawing relieved by food but recurring two hours later. However, for the last week she notes an upper abdominal cramping spasm, early satiety, and postprandial vomiting. What complication of ulcer disease may have ensued?

Peptic ulcer disease, especially at or near the pyloroduodenal junction, may be complicated by gastric outlet obstruction. Symptoms of gastric stasis include upper abdominal distention, crampy spasm, early satiety, loss of the usual rhythm of ulcer pain, and postprandial vomiting.

12. What are some of the characteristics of small bowel pain?

Pathologic processes of the small bowel typically give rise to pain felt in the periumbilical and midabdominal regions. The pain is poorly localized and varies in quality depending on the underlying pathologic process. Small bowel obstruction resulting in spasm of small intestinal smooth muscle provokes cramping pain. Mucosal inflammatory or ulcerative processes result in a vague soreness and ache. An inflammatory or neoplastic process that extends through to the serosa and adjacent parietal peritoneum will stimulate somatic pain pathways and become manifest as more sharply localized pain at the site of the lesion (i.e., characteristic parietal pain). Small bowel pain, as opposed to peptic ulcer pain, is typically precipitated by eating and palliated by fasting. Progressive vomiting and obstipation occur with small bowel obstruction. In severe cases, vomitus may be feculent. The most common causes of small bowel obstruction are adhesions, external hernias, internal hernias, Crohn's disease, and primary or metastatic carcinoma.

13. You are called to examine an 88-year-old woman with a history of atrial fibrillation, peripheral vascular disease, and diabetes who now complains of severe, diffuse, constant abdominal pain. She is quite distressed. Examination reveals the abdomen to be soft and nontender without guarding or peritoneal signs. What is the likely diagnosis?

The diagnosis is acute mesenteric ischemia secondary to an embolism to the superior mesenteric artery. Acute mesenteric ischemia typically manifests as severe, acute abdominal pain out of proportion to physical findings. The absence of peritoneal signs must not deter this diagnosis from being considered because potentially reversible vasospasm precedes bowel infarction and necrosis. Acute mesenteric ischemia may result from embolization, thrombosis, or a low flow to the superior mesenteric artery. Thrombosis of the superior mesenteric vein produces a similar syndrome. Colonic ischemia due to atherosclerotic disease of the inferior mesenteric artery results in crampy lower abdominal pain and bloody diarrhea. The syndrome of chronic, postprandial, periumbilical crampy pain and weight loss due to anorexia and aversion to eating is sometimes referred to as abdominal angina.

14. What is the pelvic floor tension syndrome?

A syndrome of chronic pelvic pain that occurs predominantly in women. It presents as chronic, unremitting lower abdominal pain aggravated by standing or walking. It is commonly associated with dysmenorrhea, dyspareunia, and depression.

15. A 72-year-old man with severe tricuspid valve regurgitation complains of a chronic right upper quadrant pain felt as a constant, nonradiating dull ache. Physical examination reveals tender hepatomegaly with a soft, blunted, pulsatile liver edge. What is the likely diagnosis?

This case typifies the type of pain that originates from the liver. The hepatic parenchyma is insensitive to pain. However, Glisson's capsule (around the liver) is rich in nociceptors and readily gives rise to pain in response to penetration, stretching, or distention. The pain is felt in the subcostal area but especially in the right hypochondrium because of the larger size of the right hepatic lobe. The severity and intensity of hepatic pain depends on the rapidity with which the liver capsule is stretched. Abrupt distention can cause sudden, sharp pain that may mimic gallstone disease whereas more gradual distention typically causes a dull ache.

16. Why is the commonly used term biliary colic a misnomer?

Biliary tract pain is not colicky but is typically a sustained pain that steadily rises to a peak that may be sustained for several hours and then subsides (crescendo/decrescendo). Although biliary tract pain may fluctuate in intensity and severity, it does not remit and recur as would the colic of small bowel obstruction.

17. A 42-year-old woman with abdominal pain reports a history of chronic, intermittent, recurrent attacks of severe dull epigastric pain that typically occurs during the night, radiates to the right periscapular region, and lasts four to six hours. She has had approximately four such episodes several months apart with intervening periods during which she was asymptomatic. She now complains of severe right upper quadrant pain, nausea, and nonbloody emesis, and she is noted to have right upper quadrant abdominal tenderness that is accentuated on inspiration. What is the likely diagnosis?

This patient is suffering from symptomatic gallstones. Her previous episodes typify biliary colic where a gallstone is transiently impacted in the cystic duct or bile duct, stimulating nociceptors served by visceral afferent pathways. As is typical of visceral pain, this is poorly localized to the epigastrium. Her current episode is notable for more localized right upper quadrant pain with marked tenderness and a positive Murphy's sign compatible with a diagnosis of acute cholecystitis. Continued obstruction of the cystic duct provokes an inflammatory process in the gallbladder wall, which may progress to involve the serosal surface of the gallbladder and parietal peritoneum, resulting in a more intense, localized somatic type of pain.

18. How might a patient with chronic pancreatic disease describe his or her pain?

Chronic pancreatic pain results from stimulation of visceral afferent pathways and is a midline, midepigastric deep, dull ache, which may spread to the right or left hypochondrium. It characteristically penetrates to the back. Patients with chronic pancreatic pain report that lying in the fetal position or sitting up and leaning forward decreases the severity of the pain and hyperextension of the back typically exacerbates it. Chronic pancreatic pain from either carcinoma or chronic pancreatitis is provoked by eating and is often associated with significant weight loss, diarrhea, steatorrhea, and diabetes.

19. Which diagnostic technique can help distinguish chronic abdominal pain due to disease of the abdominal wall from that of intra-abdominal origin?

Carnett's test can help make this distinction. The site of maximum tenderness is identified, and the patient is asked to assume a partial sitting position with arms crossed, which causes the abdominal wall muscles to generate increased tension. Carnett's test is positive if increased tenderness on repeat palpation is noted. The differential diagnosis of chronic abdominal wall pain includes rectus sheath hematoma, rib tip syndrome, abdominal wall hernia, myofascial pain syndrome, and cutaneous nerve entrapment syndromes.

20. What is the significance of differing pain patterns in patients with chronic abdominal pain?

Two general distinct patterns should be recognized because these patterns have implications with regard to the differential diagnosis and response to therapy. Abdominal pain that occurs in intermittent discrete attacks with intervening asymptomatic periods can usually be explained by specific pathophysiologic disorders (e.g., symptomatic cholelithiasis). In contrast, chronic abdominal pain lasting days to weeks may have no clear pathophysiologic explanation and may be deemed functional in origin. Examples include nonulcer dyspepsia, which presents with chronic epigastric ulcerlike pain but without any ulcer; and irritable bowel syndrome, which presents with lower abdominal cramping pain, bloating, and disordered bowel function (most notably alternating diarrhea and constipation). Chronic abdominal pain that lasts longer than six months, remains undiagnosed, and lacks features of nonulcer dyspepsia and irritable bowel syndrome is termed chronic intractable abdominal pain. In all of these patients a detailed psychosocial history is crucial. Recognition of depression or anxiety may be key.

21. Patients with chronic abdominal pain commonly exhibit many of the same psychologic responses that other chronic pain patients exhibit. What are they?

Many patients with chronic abdominal pain will also suffer from depression, insomnia, loss of libido, fatigue, withdrawal, and anxiety. The predisposition to these responses is in part mediated by social and family circumstances, culture, and the patient's psychologic state. Many patients with chronic intractable abdominal pain, the majority of whom are women, report a history of childhood physical or sexual abuse.

22. What clinical features suggest the presence of chronic idiopathic abdominal pain?

Patients with chronic idiopathic abdominal pain commonly have nearly constant discomfort and pain that is relatively unchanging in location, character, and intensity. The pain follows no consistent pattern and cannot be explained by known pathophysiologic mechanisms. Patients rarely show weight loss or fever, commonly have a history of other chronic pain, and may show associated psychopathology.

23. What are some of the well-recognized disorders of organs in the thorax that can present as abdominal pain?

Abdominal pain can occur in patients with disorders at extra-abdominal sites. Thoracic pathologic processes that can cause abdominal pain include pneumonia, myocardial infarction, pulmonary embolism, pneumothorax, esophagitis, emphysema, and myocarditis.

24. What are some of the caveats about atypical presentations of abdominal pain?

In certain circumstances, such as in elderly or immunosuppressed patients or in those receiving corticosteroids, common abdominal disorders may present in an atypical fashion. Fever may be absent or low grade, signs of peritoneal irritation may be blunted, and an altered mental status (e.g., dementia) may modify the history and physical examination.

25. Not all abdominal pain is caused by gastrointestinal pathologic processes. In particular, especially in women, disorders of the pelvic organs must always be considered in the differential diagnosis of either chronic or acute lower abdominal pain. What are some diagnostic considerations?

A full history and physical is required of all women with lower abdominal pain, including a detailed sexual and menstrual history, pelvic examination, and pregnancy test (for women of child-bearing age). Pelvic disease causes lower abdominal pain. Diagnostic considerations include pelvic inflammatory disease, endometriosis, ectopic pregnancy, uterine obstruction, ovarian cyst torsion, ovulatory pain (mittelschmerz), ruptured ovarian cyst, and dysfunction of pelvic floor muscles. Pain occurring at monthly intervals suggests endometriosis or ovulatory pain.

BIBLIOGRAPHY

1. Beard RW, Reginald PW, Wadsworth J: Clinical features of women with chronic lower abdominal pain and pelvic congestion. Br J Obstet Gynaecol 95:153–161, 1988.
2. Gallegos NC, Hobsley M: Abdominal wall pain: An alternative diagnosis. Br J Surg 77:1167, 1990.
3. Haubrich WS: Abdominal pain. In Berk JE, Haubrich WS, (eds): Gastrointestinal Symptoms: Clinical Interpretation. Philadelphia, BC Decker Inc., 1991, pp 23–58.
4. Klein KB: Approach to the patient with abdominal pain. In Yamada T, (ed): Textbook of Gastroenterology, 2nd ed. Philadelphia, JB Lippincott Co., 1995, pp 750–771.
5. Thompson WG, Creed F, Drossman DA, et al: Functional bowel disease and functional abdominal pain. Gastroenterol Int 5:75, 1992.

22. CHRONIC PELVIC PAIN

Helen Greco, M.D.

1. What is chronic pelvic pain?

Pain that is recurrent or persistent for six months or longer. There may or may not be an identifiable causative lesion.

2. What are some other hallmarks of chronic pelvic pain?

Pain and disability appear out of proportion to physical abnormalities. There may be signs of depression, such as loss of appetite, weight change, and sleep disturbance. Pain interferes with daily lifestyle, causing inability to perform normal household or job-related tasks, exercise, or sexual intercourse. A history of physical or sexual abuse may be elicited.

3. What impact does chronic pelvic pain have on family interaction?

Pain may become an "interpersonal device" through which family members communicate. Caregivers may infantalize the patient, and, in turn, the patient may use the pain to manipulate the family.

4. Identify important information that can be obtained from the history.

1. What may aggravate or alleviate the pain. Whether it is related to the menstrual cycle or stress. Continuous or intermittent. Characteristics such as quality, severity, and region, as well as radiation of the pain are all important factors to elicit.

2. Age, parity, and use of contraception are important in respect to the ovulatory cycle as well as the possibility of prolapse of the uterus.

3. Menstrual history may give insight as to duration of discomfort and at which point of the menstrual cycle it occurs.

4. A history of endometriosis may be significant, since this may cause scarring and adhesions that give rise to pain.

5. Sexual history may reveal introital pain, dyspareunia, or sexual abuse. Vaginal spasm may be due to an inflammatory reaction or scarring or may have a psychologic origin. A history of sexually transmitted infection or pelvic inflammatory disease is relevant because these may lead to adhesions.

6. Is there associated pain in other areas of the body, including the lower back, gastrointestinal tract, and the urinary tract? Radiation of pain may be important in ruling out other etiologies of pain, including a neuropathy or radiculopathy.

7. Previous operative procedures or abdominal or pelvic infections may be significant for adhesions and scarring in the area.

5. How can the physical examination contribute to the diagnosis?

A vaginal, rectal, and rectovaginal examination should be performed in an attempt to reproduce the pain. A Pap smear and cervical cultures for *Chlamydia trachomatis* and *Neisseria gonorrhoeae* are done as well as a pregnancy test, if warranted. During bimanual and rectovaginal examination, areas of tenderness should be evaluated by assessing the thickness of the uterosacral ligaments, which are commonly thick and tender in endometriosis. Adnexal or uterine tenderness, as well as mobility, should also be assessed. Infection and scarring from endometriosis can affect normal mobility, as well as thicken and damage tissue.

6. Is a retroflexed uterus a cause for pain?

Approximately 20% of normal women have a uterus in the retroflexed position. A retroflexed uterus may be due to adhesions from postoperative or postinflammatory process or endometriotic lesions. Pain in these cases is not due to the position of the uterus, but rather the primary disease. On occasion, anterior displacement of the uterus may alleviate the pain. In this case, a pessary or uterine suspension may be considered.

7. What are the common signs and symptoms of endometriosis?

Pain tends to follow the menstrual cycle. Pain on defecation as well as intercourse may occur because the disease affects the cul-de-sac and/or uterosacral ligament. In severe cases, the bowel wall may be involved, causing cramping or even obstruction.

8. What is the pelvic congestion syndrome?

This syndrome is due to pelvic vascular engorgement that presents as a heaviness and pain and that starts after arising in the morning and worsens as the day continues. This diagnosis is made by laparoscopy. The uterus looks dusky with a mottled appearance. The broad ligament veins demonstrate varicosities.

9. What is the relationship among bowel habits, menstrual cycle, and lower abdominal pain?

Lower abdominal cramping pain that is intermittent in nature may be due to constipation or irritable bowel syndrome (IBS). IBS is characterized by bouts of abdominal cramping and frequent bowel movements. Pain due to IBS may be aggravated in the luteal phase of the menstrual cycle. Progesterone has a slowing effect on visceral contractions and may relieve IBS but exacerbate constipation.

10. What medications may contribute to lower abdominal pain?

Anticholinergic drugs, opioids, antipsychotic agents, antihypertensives, cold relief preparations, and over-the-counter diuretics.

11. When is a urinary tract evaluation necessary?

Urinary tract evaluation is necessary when symptoms such as urgency, discomfort in the suprapubic area, colicky flank pain, or hematuria are present.

12. What are the various gynecologic causes of chronic pelvic pain?

1. Mittleschmerz describes mid-cycle pain due to peritoneal irritation from follicular fluid or blood that has been released from the ovary at the time of ovulation.

2. Any inflammatory process that can irritate the peritoneal lining, such as endometriosis or acute chronic salpingitis.

3. Adenomyosis can create cramping with a mildly boggy, enlarged, tender uterus, especially during menses.

4. Myomata can create pressure as well as degeneration, thereby causing inflammation.

5. Uterine anomalies as well as cervical stenosis can create an obstruction of menstrual outflow.

6. Prolapse of reproductive organs can cause significant lower abdominal pressure.

7. Primary dysmenorrhea may have no organic pathology. It is usually due to prostaglandin-induced uterine contractions with ischemia. Secondary dysmenorrhea is due to an organic pathology.

8. A fallopian tube prolapsed through the vaginal cuff after a hysterectomy, residual ovarian syndrome with one or both ovaries adherent to the vaginal apex, or a chronically infected vaginal cuff with granulation tissue can cause deep dyspareunia.

9. Pelvic malignancy may compress or invade various organs as well as cause severe adhesions.

13. What are the common extragenital causes of chronic pelvic pain?

Gastrointestinal causes include colitis, diverticulitis, appendicitis, pancreatitis, perihepatitis, obstruction, and irritable bowel syndrome. Urinary tract dysfunction, such as an infectious process, obstruction, calculus, tumor, or adhesions, may be a cause. Orthopedic conditions, such as arthritis or disk lesions, may also be a cause.

14. What associated symptoms may suggest a gynecologic etiology of pain?

Dyspareunia, menorrhagia, amenorrhea, any other type of menstrual disturbance, as well as vaginal/cervical discharge or pain related to ovulation suggest a gynecologic etiology. If pain occurs when changing from a combination oral contraceptive to one that does not suppress ovulation, the pain is likely to be of gynecologic origin.

15. What are the most common causes of pelvic pain in a woman who is of postreproductive age?

Gastrointestinal problems can create lower abdominal pain. Bladder dysfunction, pelvic relaxation, and genital atrophy can be other etiologies. Muscular spasm, pressure pain, and easily inflamed tissue further complicate the problem.

16. How does knowledge of a woman's parity contribute to the assessment of pelvic pain?

Patients who are parous are more likely to have pelvic relaxation with symptomatic cystocele, rectocele, or enterocele than are nulliparous women.

17. Why would a patient who is anovulatory or oligo-ovulatory experience pelvic pain?

Patients with this condition may develop enlarged ovaries from multiple cysts. There may be chronic pain due to enlargement or adhesions or acute pain due to rupture.

18. What laboratory tests may aid in making a diagnosis?

An elevated white blood count and erythrocyte sedimentation rate may reveal an inflammatory process. An abnormal urinalysis or positive urine culture may point to a kidney stone, urinary tract infection, or other urologic etiology. Stool positive for blood may reveal an inflammatory or infectious process of the bowel. An elevated serum amylase may indicate pancreatitis.

19. What special diagnostic procedures, where appropriate, can help in diagnosing the etiology of pain?

Lidocaine infiltration in areas of pain may be not only diagnostic but therapeutic as well. Pain from wound neuromas, vestibulitis, and the uterosacral ligament may be relieved. Laparoscopy can give the definitive diagnosis for chronic pelvic pain after noninvasive evaluation has been exhausted. Social and psychologic evaluation may add further insight to the patient's complaints.

20. If no apparent organic cause can be demonstrated, what other possibility could there be for chronic pelvic pain?

Levator ani muscle spasm or spasm of other local pelvic muscle groups may occur. Digital palpation must reproduce the pain and local anesthetics may relieve it before the diagnosis can be made with assurance. Interstitial cystitis is another possibility.

21. How do you approach the patient with chronic idiopathic pelvic pain?

Psychologic and pharmacologic approaches can be used. There should be careful questioning to identify underlying depression, anxiety, or somatoform disorder (see Chapter 7). Cognitive/behavioral techniques may be helpful. In addition, antidepressant medications may be used but in lower doses than used for chronic depression. The long-term use of narcotics is not effective nor appropriate for this condition.

22. Does a response to nonsteroidal anti-inflammatory drugs (NSAIDs) mean there is no structural cause for dysmenorrhea?

No. Endometriosis may respond to NSAIDs because the dysmenorrhea experienced with endometriosis is in part due to prostaglandin release by the ectopic endometrium and the intrauterine endometrium. Therefore, it should not be immediately assumed that endometriosis is not present just because there is a response to NSAIDs.

23. How do fibroids cause chronic pelvic pain?

In general, they do not. However, when they are large, they may create pressure on other organs or tissues or outgrow their blood supply and degenerate. If they compress the anterior vaginal mucosa, they may cause dyspareunia. Partial bladder obstruction may cause incomplete emptying of the bladder, leading to recurrent urinary tract infections. Direct bladder pressure may cause urgency.

24. How can the diagnosis of adenomyosis be made?

Patients with adenomyosis usually develop dysmenorrhea in their thirties, and it tends to be unresponsive to NSAIDs or ovulation-suppression agents. Sonography can demonstrate a globular, boggy type of uterus, which may also be felt on pelvic examination. Definitive diagnosis can only be made histologically.

25. If no organic condition has been found through extensive evaluation, can a hysterectomy help?

The patient often insists on having a hysterectomy out of desperation to feel better. However, the physician must keep in mind that hysterectomy often does not relieve the pain and may aggravate it because of the formation of new scar tissue from a laparotomy. Chronic pain of unknown etiology should rarely, if ever, be addressed surgically.

26. What other medical approach can be used for adenomyosis?

Combination estrogen-progestin oral contraceptives may be effective in suppressing ovulation as well as in decreasing the amount of menstrual blood flow, thereby decreasing the amount of prostaglandins released. Sometimes the use of continuous oral contraceptives without withdrawal bleeding may alleviate the pain. NSAIDs are usually ineffective.

27. What is the next step when medical management of chronic pelvic pain has failed?

A laparoscopic evaluation is in order. Direct visualization of not only the pelvic organs but also the abdominal cavity may provide a diagnosis. Endometriosis can be identified this way, as can adhesions.

28. Is a laparoscopy only a diagnostic tool?

No. It may be used as a therapeutic measure whereby adhesions may be lysed, endometriosis ablated with laser or electrocautery, and other pathology handled in an appropriate manner.

29. If chronic pelvic pain due to endometriosis that has been treated with both medical and conservative surgical intervention continues, what is the next step?

A hysterectomy with removal of both fallopian tubes and ovaries is usually the next step. However, there is no guarantee of improvement of pain, since adhesions may contribute to this disease process. Furthermore, extragenital deposits of endometriosis (on the bowel or peritoneum) can be an ongoing source of pain.

BIBLIOGRAPHY

1. The American College of Obstetricians and Gynecologists: Precis V: An update in obstetrics and gynecology, 68–71, 1994.
2. ACOG Technical Bulletin. Chronic Pelvic Pain, No. 129. June 1989.
3. Andrews MC: Pelvic pain. In Rosenwaks Z et al (eds): Gynecology Principles and Practices. New York, Macmillan Publishing Company, 1987, pp 587–595.
4. Herbst AL et al: Comprehensive Gynecology, 2nd ed. St. Louis, Mosby, 1991, pp 169–172.
5. Julian TM: Chronic pelvic pain part 1: Workup and diagnosis. Female Patient 14:19–31, February, 1989.

23. FIBROMYALGIA AND MYOFASCIAL PAIN

Mark Thomas, M.D., and Ronald Kanner, M.D.

1. What is the myofascial pain syndrome?

Myofascial pain is a regional pain syndrome characterized by trigger points and taut bands. It was described by Travell and later elaborated on by Travell and Simons. It can occur at most points on the body, but is most common in the cervical and lumbar regions. Trigger points are defined as tender points which, when palpated, produce pain at a distant site. The syndrome is often caused by minor trauma, "near falls," or degenerative osteoarthritis.

2. What are "taut bands"?

In patients with myofascial pain, deep palpation of muscles may reveal an area that feels tight. Stretching this band of muscle produces pain. Those areas are called taut bands. Trigger points are characteristically found within taut bands of muscle. The exact etiology and pathogenesis are unclear. They do not seem to be due to muscle spasm in the usual sense of the word, because the EMG findings are not universally abnormal. Rolling the taut band under the fingertip at the trigger point (snapping palpation), may produce a local "twitch" response. This is shortening of the band of muscle and was held to be one of the cardinal signs of fibromyalgia.

3. What is fibromyalgia?

Fibromyalgia is a clinical syndrome characterized by chronic, diffuse pain and multiple tender points. Characteristic features also include fatigue, sleep disturbance, stiffness, paresthesias, headaches, irritable bowel syndrome, Raynaud's-like symptoms, depression, and anxiety. Widespread pain must be above and below the waist, bilateral, and affect at least 11 of the 18 designated tender points.

4. What are some of the most common sites of tender points in fibromyalgia?

These include the upper border of the mid-trapezius, the lower part of the sternocleidomastoid muscle, the lateral part of the pectoralis major muscle, the mid-supraspinatus muscle, the upper outer quadrant of the gluteal region, the trochanteric region and the medial fat pad of the knee.

5. What syndromes are commonly associated with fibromyalgia?

Depression, anxiety, insomnia, and the chronic fatigue syndrome are common concomitants. Some authors believe that these may simply represent different points on the same spectrum of disease and that fibromyalgia is a psychosomatic disorder.

6. Is there gender difference in fibromyalgia?

In most reported series, 80–90% of patients with fibromyalgia were female.

7. What laboratory investigations are useful in fibromyalgia?

All laboratory values in this syndrome are used for exclusionary purposes. There are no characteristic laboratory abnormalities, neither chemical, electrical, nor radiographic. Sleep studies are often abnormal, but the abnormalities are seen in other painful conditions as well.

8. What treatments are commonly used for fibromyalgia and for myofascial pain?

A combination of physical, anesthesiologic, and pharmacologic techniques are commonly used. Some of the earliest techniques involved injection or dry-needling of trigger points. This was based on a concept that these trigger points represented areas of local muscle spasm. The efficacy of trigger point injections has never been fully substantiated, although transient relief may be obtained in some patients. Physical techniques, such as stretching, spray and stretch, massage, heat, and cold have all been advocated, but none fully documented in well-controlled studies. Tricyclic antidepressants are the most widely used drugs for this syndrome. It is not clear whether they are affecting a chronic pain syndrome, a clear underlying pathophysiology, or depression. Nonsteroidal anti-inflammatory drugs are also used, but again their role is unclear.

9. Are the diagnoses of fibromyalgia syndrome and myofascial pain syndrome universally accepted?

No. Two interesting statements are quoted by Dr. Bohr in a *Neurologic Clinics* dedicated to malingering and conversion reactions. He quotes Drs. Wolfe and Moldofsky as making the following two statements, respectively:

"Fibromyalgia may or may not be a useful concept, and objective vs. subjective data may or may not be better."

"With fibromyalgia, the entity became defined, criteria were established, and now it is legitimate! Whether it is truly legitimate or not is another question."

10. What are the American College of Rheumatology 1990 criteria for the classification of fibromyalgia?
  1. History of widespread pain.
  Definition: Pain is considered widespread when all the following are present—pain in the left side of the body, pain in the right side of the body, pain above the waist, and pain below the waist. In addition, axial skeletal pain (cervical spine, anterior chest, thoracic spine, or low back) must be present. In this definition, shoulder and buttock pain is considered as pain for each involved side. "Low back pain" is considered lower segment pain.
  2. Pain in 11 of 18 trigger point sites on digital palpation.
  Definition: On digital palpation, pain must be present in at least 11 of the following 18 (9 pairs) tender point sites:
  Occiput—Bilateral, at the suboccipital muscle insertions
  Low cervical—Bilateral, at the anterior aspects of the intertransverse spaces at C5 to C7
  Trapezius—Bilateral, at the midpoint of the upper border
  Supraspinatus—Bilateral, at origins, above the scapular spine near the medial border
  Second rib—Bilateral, at the second osteochondral junctions just lateral to the junctions on upper surfaces
  Lateral epicondyle—Bilateral , 2 cm distal to the epicondyles
  Gluteal—Bilateral, in upper outer quadrants of buttocks in anterior fold of muscle
  Greater trochanter—Bilateral, posterior to the trochanteric prominence
  Knee—Bilateral, at the medial fat pad proximal to the joint line
  Digital palpation should be performed with an approximate force of 4 kg.
  For a tender point to be considered "positive," the subject must state that the palpation was painful. "Tender" is not to be considered "painful."

11. What are the proposed pathophysiologic mechanisms for fibromyalgia?
  As in many other syndromes of somewhat nebulous origin, pathophysiologic explanations have ranged from primarily central, to a combination of central and peripheral, to primarily peripheral. It has been thought to be a variation of an affective disorder, primarily based on its common association with depression, irritable bowel syndrome and chronic fatigue syndrome. Another central theory holds that the sleep abnormality is the main disturbance, later altering pain perception. Peripheral factors, such as musculoskeletal derangements, have been thought to be most important, with all of the emotional factors coming as a result of the chronic pain. Travell and Simons believed that the muscle problem was primary, rejected any psychosomatic definitions, and dubbed this a "somato-psychotic illness."

12. How is sleep disturbance related to fibromyalgia?

This is one of the most common complaints and, indeed, was one of the criteria for diagnosis. It was initially described as "nonrestorative sleep." Some of the patients studied were shown to have an intrusion of alpha rhythms into their stage IV sleep. However, the same electroencephalographic pattern is often seen in other chronically painful conditions. The incidence of sleep disturbance seems more related to the duration of pain than to a specific diagnosis.

13. What is a "spray and stretch" technique?

This technique is based on the theory that trigger points for taut bands are the principle cause of pain in fibromyalgia or myofascial pain syndromes. A taut band in the muscle is identified and then a vapo-coolant spray (ethylchloride or fluoromethane) is applied directly to the tender point. Once the point is cooled, the appropriate muscle is stretched from both ends.

14. What controlled studies are available to determine the efficacy of the various treatments used for fibromyalgia?

There is a paucity of controlled studies with adequate outcome measures. Studies have been performed using tricyclic antidepressants, EMG biofeedback, education, and physical training, hypnotherapy, and a variety of drug combinations. In 145 reports of outcome measures, only 55 were able to differentiate the active treatment from placebo. Even in trials of amitriptyline, no clinical outcome has been shown to be consistent.

BIBLIOGRAPHY

1. Bohr WT: Fibromyalgia syndrome and myofascial pain syndrome. Do they exist? Neurol Clin 13(2):365–384, 1995.
2. Braddom RL: Physical Medicine and Rehabilitation. Philadelphia, W.B. Saunders, 1996.
3. Klippel JH, Dieppe PA: Rheumatology. St. Louis, Mosby-Year Book, 1994.
4. Moldofsky H: Fibromyalgia, sleep disorder and chronic fatigue syndrome. In Bock C, Whelan J (eds): Chronic Fatigue Syndrome. CIBA Foundation Symposium 173. Chichester, Wiley, 1993.
5. West SG: Rheumatology Secrets. Philadelphia, Hanley & Belfus, 1997.
6. White KP, Harth M: An analytical review of 24 controlled clinical trials for fibromyalgia syndrome (FMS). Pain 64:211–219, 1996.
7. Wolfe F: Litigation–chronic pain syndrome. Am J Pain Management 3:53, 1993.

IV. Syndromes in Which Pain Is a Significant Component

24. POSTOPERATIVE PAIN MANAGEMENT

Michael Hanania, M.D.

1. What is the pathophysiology of acute postoperative pain?

Postoperative pain is mainly nociceptive (see chapter 2). There is also central sensitization. At the periphery, inflammatory mediators (prostaglandins, histamine, serotonin, and bradykinin) increase the sensitivity of nociceptors. Central sensitization is a result of functional reorganization in the dorsal horn of the spinal cord. Both of these processes result in an exaggerated response to noxious stimuli, spread of hyperresponsiveness to noninjured tissue, and a reduced threshold for producing pain.

2. What are the deleterious physiologic effects of postoperative pain?

Muscle splinting secondary to pain in the abdomen or chest results in a decreased vital capacity and ultimately decreased alveolar ventilation. Atelectasis is therefore a common postoperative complication. If coughing is very painful and performed with minimal effort or infrequently, retention of secretions and subsequent pneumonia may result. Release of stress hormones and catecholamines secondary to pain may cause persistent tachycardia and hypertension, resulting in increased cardiac work and myocardial oxygen consumption. Increased sympathetic activity decreases intestinal motility and prolongs recovery.

3. What is pre-emptive analgesia?

Pre-emptive analgesia provides pain relief prior to surgery and throughout the perioperative period. Acute postoperative pain is associated with alterations in synaptic function and nociceptive processing within the spinal cord dorsal horn, neuroendocrine responses, and sympathoadrenal activation. Theoretically, pre-emptive analgesia would minimize these responses and prevent the spinal cord "wind-up phenomenon" (central sensitization), which is more resistant to treatment and is associated with chronic pain conditions. Clinically, pre-emptive analgesia results in reduced opioid requirement and improved pain scores, but whether it also decreases morbidity has not yet been determined.

4. What is intravenous PCA?

Intravenous patient-controlled analgesia (PCA) is a system of opioid delivery that consists of an infusion pump interfaced with a timing device. The PCA device allows the patient to titrate the analgesic dose required for optimal control of pain. The patient presses a button, and a preset dose of analgesic is delivered. A programmed "lock-out" period (usually 6 to 15 minutes) prevents inadvertent overdoses and excessive sedation. This system may be used on top of a baseline continuous infusion.

5. What are the advantages of a PCA system over nurse-administered intramuscular opioids?

There are three main problems with the traditional nurse-administered intramuscular opioids given on a PRN basis.

1. Lack of knowledge regarding analgesic pharmacodynamics and overconcern about respiratory depression and addiction liability.

2. A long lag period between the onset of pain and the administration of opioid, because of the process involved in calling for a nurse, obtaining and recording narcotics, and administration of the drug. This lag period is extended by the time required for absorption of an intramuscular dose and further complicated by the pain of IM administration. Intravenous PCA eliminates these factors.

3. Patients and staff often think it's better to wait and tolerate pain as much as possible before taking pain killers.

6. Is a background continuous infusion necessary with intravenous PCA?

A continuous background infusion does not improve pain scores and is even associated with more side effects, such as sedation and respiratory depression, when used after less painful abdominal surgeries such as cesarean section. It's usually not necessary with other abdominal procedures but probably serves a useful role in extensive abdominal and thoracic operations, although definitive data are not available. Certainly, if a patient has been taking opioids preoperatively, the daily equivalent dose in the opioid being used should be administered as a continuous infusion in addition to the PCA bolus.

7. What opioids and doses are commonly used for intravenous PCA?

Morphine is most commonly used because it is relatively inexpensive and has an intermediate duration of action. The typical adult bolus dose is 1 mg with a 6- to 10-minute lockout. Other opioids used include meperidine (10 mg bolus dose), hydromorphone, and fentanyl. Ultralong-acting opioids, such as methadone, would require very long lockout intervals; ultrashort-acting opioids, such as alfentanil, would require a very short lockout with a basal infusion, making them suboptimal choices for PCA. An agonist-antagonist such as butorphanol may be used when pain is not severe, since a ceiling effect for analgesia is characteristic of this drug. However, mixed agonist-antagonists cannot be used with pure agonists.

8. What is the youngest age for which PCA is appropriate?

Patients over the age of 7 do very well with PCA and those age 5–6 have variable success. Patients ages 4 and under did not use PCA successfully. Preoperatively, each patient has to be evaluated individually, but it would seem that PCA is inappropriate for those under 5 years of age.

9. What is spinal or neuraxial opioid analgesia?

This is a technique of managing postoperative pain by epidural or intrathecal delivery of opioids. Epidural opioids can be delivered through an indwelling epidural catheter by intermittent injections or continuous infusion or both (i.e., epidural PCA). Intrathecal or subarachnoid opioid delivery is usually a single bolus injection via a spinal needle, but it can be given through a catheter placed in the subarachnoid space. These techniques have become widely accepted for the management of moderate to severe postoperative pain, because of their ability to provide prolonged and profound analgesia.

10. What is the mechanism of action of spinal opioids?

Epidural or intrathecal administration of opioids provides analgesia at least in part through opioid receptor binding in the dorsal horn of the spinal cord. Binding to opioid receptors occurs in Rexed's laminae I and II (substantia gelatinosa). Some analgesia is a result of systemic absorption and rostral flow of drug acting at the level of the brain.

11. How does opioid lipophilicity play a role in spinal analgesia and systemic side effects?

Lipophilicity determines how much drug will cross the dura or stay within the cerebrospinal fluid (CSF). Therefore, the spinal action of lipophilic opioids is local and brief, but they may cause side effects as a result of their systemic absorption. Lipophilic opioids such as fentanyl and sufentanil cross the dura rapidly and are also systemically absorbed to a significant degree via the epidural vasculature. Morphine, on the other hand, is hydrophilic and crosses the dura poorly and slowly. It stays in the CSF for a long time. Therefore, small doses of intrathecal morphine will result in prolonged analgesia. However, there is a higher risk of delayed respiratory depression because of the eventual spread cephalad in CSF.

12. List some of the commonly used epidural opioids in order of most hydrophilic to most lipophilic.

Drug	Lipid Solubility*
Morphine	1
Hydromorphone	6
Meperidine	30
Methadone	100
Fentanyl	800
Sufentanil	1500

* Partition coefficient relative to morphine.

13. How do side effects differ between spinal and systemic opioid administration?

Nausea, pruritus, and urinary retention occur slightly more frequently with spinal opioids. Respiratory depression may occur slightly more frequently with spinal administration of morphine. Delayed gastric emptying was shown to be greater when systemic opioids were used after abdominal surgery.

14. What are the advantages of delivering opioids using a thoracic vs. lumbar epidural catheter?

When lipophilic opioids are used for pain in the abdominal area, it is advantageous to place the catheter at the level of the nerve roots involved in the afferent transmission of pain. For example, a thoracic epidural catheter for fentanyl infusion would provide excellent analgesia for abdominal surgical pain. Adding a dilute concentration of local anesthetic may reduce opioid requirement and improve analgesia. If a hydrophilic opioid such as morphine is used, it is less important where the catheter is located because the drug will spread. Good analgesia will be obtained with a lumbar catheter for abdominal pain. Hydrophilic opioids such as morphine and hydromorphone must be used cautiously at the thoracic level, since respiratory depression as a result of cephalad spread is a possibility.

15. What are the advantages of combining regional anesthetic techniques with postoperative spinal analgesia for lower extremity orthopedic and vascular surgery?

There is a decreased incidence of thromboembolic events after lower extremity orthopedic surgery and a decreased incidence of graft thrombosis after vascular procedures when regional anesthesia is used. Postoperative pain management is then usually provided by epidural opioid and local anesthetic. In the case of amputations, phantom limb pain is less likely to develop if pre-emptive spinal analgesia is provided and a regional technique is used for the procedure.

16. What are the side effects of spinal opioids?

The most common are urinary retention, pruritus, nausea and vomiting. Less frequent side effects are hypotension, oversedation, and respiratory depression. Ready et al. found an incidence of 0.2% for respiratory depression in over 1100 patients in a postoperative study of epidural morphine. A recent Swedish study by Rawal documented an incidence of 0.09% following epidural morphine and 0.36% following intrathecal morphine.

17. How should respiratory depression be monitored on a surgical ward?

Hourly respiratory rate checks are ordered for the first 24 hours after a bolus of epidural of intrathecal morphine. The level of sedation should also be assessed, although less frequently. In severely sick and debilitated patients or those who had extensive surgery of the upper abdomen or thorax, monitoring is usually done in the intensive care unit with pulse oximetry and respiratory rate monitors.

18. Explain the early and late respiratory depression associated with spinal opioids.

The early respiratory depression is a reflection of vascular absorption and is typically seen one to two hours after injection of morphine. The late respiratory depression is thought to be due to rostral migration of drug in the CSF affecting the respiratory centers in the brain. These phenomena are more common with large doses of opioid, advanced age, and the Trendelenburg position.

19. What is the most sensitive marker of respiratory depression?

Pulse oximetry is most sensitive. Changes in respiratory rate and level of alertness may lag behind.

20. How does analgesia differ between epidural and intrathecal opioid administration?

Intrathecal opioid administration results in much higher CSF concentrations of opioid and potent analgesia so that a reduced dose is required ($\frac{1}{10}$ the dose of epidural morphine). Onset of analgesia is also faster with intrathecal administration.

21. What are contraindications to epidural or intrathecal injection?

Absolute contraindications include significant coagulopathy, septicemia, local skin infection at the insertion site, and the patient's refusal to have the procedure. Relative contraindications include presence of dural puncture (because of the risk of inadvertent spread to CSF after epidural injection), central sleep apnea (because of increased risk of respiratory depression), and history of latent herpes simplex labialis (reactivation in obstetric population).

22. How is the side effect of pruritus treated?

The typical axial pruritus seen with spinal opioids involves mainly the face and torso. An antihistamine such as diphenhydramine should be tried first, and in extreme cases, a low-dose intravenous infusion of naloxone may be started (1 to 3 µg/kg/hr). The analgesia of spinal opioids (especially morphine) is usually not lost with such a low-dose infusion of naloxone. Propofol has also been reported to relieve pruritus, but repeated dosing may be necessary.

23. How is the side effect of nausea and vomiting treated?

Metoclopramide, droperidol, prochlorperazine, and ondansetron are commonly used to treat nausea and vomiting associated with opioids. Transdermal scopolamine has also been shown to be effective after epidural morphine. Nausea is also somewhat related to position, so telling the patient to remain still reduces nausea.

24. How is the side effect of respiratory depression treated?

Naloxone should be kept at the bedside and may be administered intravenously as 0.4 mg bolus for severe respiratory depression and in increments of 0.04 mg for mild to moderate depression. An infusion of naloxone may be required with long-acting opioids, since naloxone has a relatively short half-life. If the patient has had significant exposure to opioids, naloxone may precipitate withdrawal. Some other form of analgesia will be needed because naloxone reverses the opioids.

25. Why are local anesthetics used in spinal analgesia?

Bupivacaine is a long-acting local anesthetic that provides greater sensory than motor blockade and is often used in conjunction with an opioid in epidural analgesia. When infused with an opioid at the level of the nerve roots involved in pain transmission, a synergism is observed resulting in improved pain relief associated with decreased opioid requirement and sometimes decreased side effects. The stress response associated with postoperative pain is better blunted when a local anesthetic is added. Bowel motility may also return earlier when local anesthetic is used. However, the disadvantage of potential motor and sympathetic blockade must be realized, and restrictions on ambulation and precautions against hypotension must be implemented.

26. How are epidural opioids cleared from the CSF?

Opioid that has gained access to CSF may remain there or bind to opioid receptors in the substantia gelatinosa. Removal of opioid from the dorsal horn primarily occurs through local spinal cord blood flow, including uptake into epidural veins in close proximity to the arachnoid granulations. Highly lipid-soluble agents are rapidly absorbed into blood vessels, and epidural fat from receptor sites, and analgesic duration is short. Hydrophilic opioids preferentially remain in CSF and diffuse more slowly into blood vessels, and thus, analgesia is prolonged.

27. Where is the site of action for local anesthetics when used epidurally for management of postoperative pain?

Local anesthetics, when injected epidurally, pass through arachnoid granulations of the dural cuff region to enter the CSF and nerve roots. Local anesthetics block the sodium channels of nerve axons and therefore block nerve conduction. Small-diameter nerve fibers are more susceptible than larger ones. Therefore, sympathetic blockade occurs at low concentrations followed by sensory and eventually motor blockade.

28. What are other modalities of postoperative pain management?

Regional nerve blocks such as intercostal nerve blocks may be used for one-sided abdominal or thoracic postoperative pain. Upper or lower extremity regional nerve blockade may be performed as a one-time injection or intermittent blockade via a catheter (i.e., continuous axillary catheter). An interpleural catheter may be used for prolonged intercostal nerve blockade.

29. Name some adjuvant drugs (nonopioids) and techniques that may be used in conjunction with opioids for postoperative analgesia.

Nonsteroidal antiinflammatory drugs (NSAIDs) are often used and can act to reduce opioid requirement and improve pain relief. Ketorolac is an example of a popular NSAID that may be administered intravenously. Acetaminophen acts synergistically with opioids through a peripheral mechanism to improve analgesia. Antiemetics such as hydroxyzine and droperidol have been shown to reduce opioid requirement, possibly as a result of their sedative effect. Transcutaneous nerve stimulation (TENS) has been shown to be effective to some degree after less painful operations.

BIBLIOGRAPHY

1. Bailey PL, Rondeau S, Schafer PG, et al: Dose response pharmacology of intrathecal morphine in human volunteers. Anesthesiology 79:49–59, 1993.
2. Bennet RL, Batenhorst RL, Bivins BA, et al: Patient controlled analgesia. Ann Surg 195:700–704, 1987.
3. Bennet RL, Baterhorst RL, Foster TS, et al: Postoperative pulmonary function with patient controlled anesthesia. Anesth Analg 96:171, 1982.
4. Bonica JJ: Management of Pain, 2nd ed. Philadelphia, Lea & Febiger, 1990, pp 461–480.
5. Christopherson R, Beattie C, Frank SM, et al: Perioperative morbidity in patients randomized to epidural or general anesthesia for lower extremity vascular surgery. The perioperative ischemia randomized anesthesia trial study group. Anesthesiology 79:422–434, 1993.
6. Cuschieri RJ, Morran CG, Howie JC, McArdle CS: Postoperative pain and pulmonary complications: Comparison of three analgesic regimens. Br J Surg 72:495–498, 1985.
7. deLeon-Casasola OA, Parker BM, Lema MJ, et al: Epidural analgesia versus intravenous patient controlled analgesia. Reg Anesth 19:307–315, 1994.
8. Frank ED, McKay W, Rocco A, Gallo JP: Intrapleural bupivacaine for postoperative analgesia following cholecystectomy: A randomized prospective study. Reg Anesth 15:26–30, 1990.
9. George KA, Chisakuta Am, Gamble JA, Browne GA: Thoracic epidural infusion for postoperative pain relief following abdominal aortic surgery: Bupivacaine, fentanyl, or a mixture of both? Anaesthesia 47:388–394, 1992.

10. Gourlay GK, Murphy TM, Plummer JL, et al: Pharmacokinetics of fentanyl in lumbar and cervical CSF following lumbar epidural and intravenous administration. Pain 38:253–259, 1989.

11. Kambam JR, Hammon J, Parris WC, Lupinetti FM: Intrapleural analgesia for post-thoracotomy pain and blood levels of bupivacaine following intrapleural injection. Can J Anaesth 36:106–109, 1989.

12. Katz J, Kavanagh BP, Sandler A, et al: Preemptive analgesia. Clinical evidence of neuroplasticity contributing to postoperative pain. Anesthesiology 77:439–446, 1992.

13. Loper KA, Ready LB, Downey M, et al: Epidural and intravenous fentanyl are clinically equivalent after knee surgery. Anesth Analg 70:72–75, 1990.

14. Marks RM, Sachar EJ: Undertreatment of medical inpatients with narcotic analgesics. Ann Intern Med 78:173–181, 1973.

15. Marlowe S, Engstrom R, White P: Epidural patient-controlled analgesia (PCA): An alternative to continuous epidural infusions. Pain, 37:97–101, 1989.

16. Parker RK, Holtmann B, White PF: Effects of nighttime opioid infusion with PCA therapy on patient comfort and analgesic requirements after abdominal hysterectomy. Anesthesiology 76:362–367, 1992.

17. Parker R, Holtzmann B, White P: Patient-controlled analgesia. Does a concurrent opioid infusion improve pain management after surgery? JAMA 266(14):1947–1952, 1991.

18. Parker RK, Holtzmann B, White PF: Effects of a nighttime opioid infusion with PCA therapy on patient comfort and analgesic requirements after abdominal hysterectomy. Anesthesiology 76 (3):362–367, March 1992.

19. Rawal N, Arner S, Gustafsson LL, Allvin R: Present state of extradural and intrathecal opioid analgesia in Sweden. A nationwide follow-up survey. Br J Anaesth 59:791–799, 1987.

20. Rawal N, Arner S, Gustafsson LL, Allvin R: Present state of extradural and intrathecal opioid analgesia in Sweden. A nationwide follow-up survey. Br J Anesth 59:791–799, 1987.

21. Rawal N, Wattwill M: Respiratory depression following epidural morphine. An experimental and clinical study. Anesth Analg 63:8-24, 1984.

22. Ready LB, Loper KA, Nessly M, Wild L: Postoperative epidural morphine is safe on surgical wards. Anesthesiology 75:452–456, 1991.

23. Rosenfeld BA, Faraday N, Campbell D, et al: Hemostatic effects of stress hormone infusion. Anesthesiology 81:1116–1126, 1994.

24. Sinatra R, Chung KS, Silverman DG, et al: An evaluation of morphine and oxymorphone administered via PCA or PCA plus basal infusion in post cesarean-delivery patients. Anesthesiology 71:502–507, 1989.

25. Stevens RA, Petty RH, Hill HF, et al: Redistribution of sufentanil to cerebrospinal fluid and systemic circulation after epidural administration in dogs. Anesth Analg 76:323–327, 1993.

26. Tuman KJ, McCarthy RJ, March RJ, et al: Effect of epidural anesthesia and analgesia on coagulation and outcome after major vascular surgery. Anesth Analg 73:696–704, 1991.

27. Yeager MP, Glass DD, Neff RK, Brinck-Johnson T: Epidural anesthesia and analgesia in high-risk surgical patients. Anesthesiology 66:729–736, 1987.

25. CANCER PAIN SYNDROMES

Gilbert R. Gonzales, M.D.

1. What are the most common causes of pain in patients with cancer?

Pain may be due to tumor involvement of pain-sensitive structures, to complications of therapy, or to processes not directly related to the cancer. The most common cause of pain in cancer is bone metastases. This is a nociceptive pain syndrome.

2. Name some neuropathic pain syndromes commonly seen in patients with cancer.

Tumor invasion of the brachial or lumbosacral plexus is the most common. Postherpetic neuralgia (PHN), phantom limb pain, and peripheral neuropathy also occur frequently.

3. Which factors predispose a patient to develop postherpetic neuralgia (PHN)?

Advancing age is the most important factor. The incidence of PHN rises exponentially after age 70. It is also more common in cancer and immunosuppressed patients than it is in the normal population. It commonly occurs in irradiated parts of the body.

4. Are opioids known to increase the risk of acute herpes zoster eruptions? Are opioids known to increase the subsequent development of postherpetic neuralgia in patients who get acute zoster eruptions?

Opioids are not known to either increase the risk of acute zoster eruptions or increase the risk of postherpetic neuralgia.

5. Describe the pain syndrome associated with metastases to the clivus.

Pain is characterized by a vertex headache and exacerbated by neck flexion. There may be associated abnormalities of the lower cranial nerves, most commonly dysphagia from involvement of the glossopharyngeal nerve (IX). Occasionally, there is weakness of the trapezius from involvement of the spinal accessory nerve (XI).

6. Which types of malignancies are *least* likely to be painful?

Leukemias. In general, solid tumors of viscera and metastatic, invasive, destructive, and nerve-compressing cancers are more painful than leukemias. Bone metastases are the most common cause of pain in patients with cancer.

7. Is phantom-limb sensation common after amputation?

All amputees, including those with cancer-related amputations of limbs and some other parts (i.e., breast, penis, anus, nose, ears) almost invariably experience phantom sensations the day after surgery. These sensations are not always painful and may not be reported spontaneously. A small proportion of these patients go on to experience phantom-limb pain. The rest have sensations that subside.

8. What is meant by incident pain?

When a mass, metastatic lesion, or pathologic fracture results in pain when there is movement such as repositioning, deep breathing, or ambulation, this is known as incident pain. This may be a very difficult pain to control, and it may be necessary to immobilize the injured structure. Anesthesiologic or ablative procedures may be required if analgesics are not helpful.

9. What is the postthoracotomy pain syndrome?

There are two types of postthoracotomy pain: (1) immediate postoperative pain, which clears in three months and is associated with sensory loss in the area of scar, and (2) postoperative pain that lasts longer than three months *or* the recurrence of pain in the surgical area following resolution of the initial postoperative pain. When pain recurs after a pain-free interval, tumor recurrence or infection should be suspected. When these are not found, the pain is most likely neuropathic.

10. Cancer patients with new onset of progressive headaches should undergo imaging studies, even if there are no objective findings on exam. True or false?

True. Headache is the most common presenting symptom in patients with brain metastasis, and it is the most common neurologic complication or symptom of systemic cancer and carcinomatous meningitis. Headaches may appear to be of the tension type, but tend to progress in duration and severity. (See Chapter 13.) Eventually, focal neurologic deficits develop in most patients.

11. What are the clinical differences between radiation injury to the brachial plexus and tumor involvement of the plexus?

A woman with breast cancer treated with mastectomy and radiation of the brachial plexus region may develop ipsilateral pain with arm and hand weakness (a brachial plexopathy) after her treatments. If the symptoms are referable to the lower brachial plexus (i.e., lower trunk), it is most likely due to tumor recurrence. Radiation is more likely to cause a panplexopathy (i.e., involvement of all three trunks of the brachial plexus). Horner's syndrome is more common in tumor involvement.

12. Why do women treated with radical mastectomy have a numb area just distal to the axilla on the inner upper part of the arm?

Injury to the intercostobrachial nerve is common in mastectomy patients and results in numbness in the area shown in the illustration. In some patients, neuropathic pain develops in the same area.

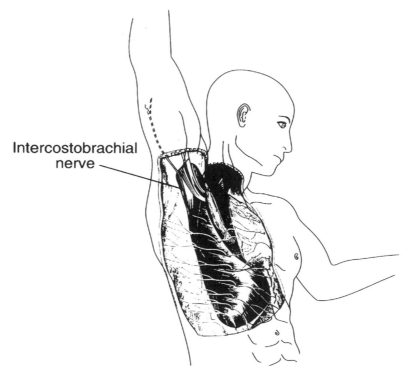

Intercostobrachial nerve

13. Painful peripheral neuropathies can be seen with which of these agents: cisplatin, vinca alkaloids, procarbazine?

All of the listed agents and several others can produce a painful peripheral neuropathy. Less often, motor and autonomic dysfunction can also occur. With cisplatin and the vinca alkaloids, neuropathy seems to be dose-related. Only about 10 to 20% of patients treated with procarbazine (an MAO inhibitor) develop neuropathy.

14. What is steroid pseudorheumatism?

A syndrome that may occur after either slow or rapid withdrawal of steroid medication in patients taking these medications for any length of time. It is characterized by arthralgias, diffuse myalgias, muscle and joint tenderness on palpation, and diffuse malaise without objective inflammatory signs on examination. These symptoms revert with reinitiation of the steroid medication.

15. What is the most common cause of lumbosacral plexopathy?

Direct tumor extension into the plexus (by lymphoma or colon carcinoma) is more common than metastatic involvement or radiation injury. Pain radiates down the leg in a radicular distribution.

16. Mucositis pain from chemotherapy or radiation therapy may be exacerbated by which of the following: secondary fungal infections, secondary viral infections, lack of saliva secretion, secondary bacterial infections, nonopioid analgesics?

All of the above may exacerbate mucositis-induced pain except the nonopioid analgesics. Nonopioid analgesics, such as acetaminophen and the topical anesthetics, are used to treat mucositis pain along with opioid analgesics. Infections and dry mucous membranes may exacerbate the mucositis and the pain.

17. In what percentage of patients with cancer is the pain unrelated to cancer or its treatment?

Ten percent of patients with cancer pain have a pre-existing, painful condition such as degenerative arthritis, diabetic peripheral neuropathy, migraines, or other nonmalignant pain conditions.

18. What are the pain-sensitive structures in bones and joints?

The periosteum and all the components of joints, except cartilage, are pain-sensitive. Articular cartilage is not a pain-sensitive structure. In the intervertebral discs, the annulus fibrosus has nociceptors, but the nucleus pulposus does not. (See Chapter 3.)

19. Do nonsteroidal anti-inflammatory drugs (NSAIDs) have direct tumor effects?

Yes. The NSAIDs are useful for tumor-induced pain partially because of their effects on the margins of the tumor and the inflammation that can exist there. Furthermore, bone metastases require prostaglandin E_2 for growth, and the NSAIDs inhibit prostaglandin synthesis.

20. What is the most common site for tumor infiltration of the brachial plexus?

The site may vary somewhat by tumor type, but the lower plexus is most commonly involved. This leads to hand weakness and pain in a C7–T1 distribution. The classic example is Pancoast tumor.

21. What is the first sign of metastases to the base of the skull?

Pain is the first symptom. Cranial nerve dysfunction occurs later and depends upon which part of the base is involved.

22. What symptoms and signs characterize parasellar metastases?

Most often, patients show unilateral, supraorbital, or frontal headache and ocular paresis without proptosis. The facial nerve is not affected by a parasellar metastasis, as it is not anatomically located in or near the parasellar region (it leaves the cranium by way of the internal acoustic meatus).

Cranial nerves III, IV, V, and VI (oculomotor, trochlear, trigeminal, and abductus) pass through the cavernous sinus, adjacent to the sella. The mandibular division of V exits before the sinus.

23. What signs or symptoms characterize the jugular foramen syndrome?

Hoarseness, dysphagia, glossopharyngeal neuralgia, syncope, and multiple lower cranial nerve abnormalities are the most common abnormalities. Cranial nerves IX, X, and XI (glossopharyngeal, vagus, and accessory spiral) pass through the jugular foramen.

24. What are the five cancer pain groups?

The usefulness of grouping cancer patients into these five groups is to help health care workers to manage the multidimensional issues that can occur in these patients.

Group I: Patients with acute cancer-related pain
               Associated with the diagnosis of cancer
               Associated with cancer therapy (surgery, chemotherapy, radiotherapy)
Group II: Patients with chronic cancer-related pain
               Associated with cancer progression
               Associated with cancer therapy (surgery, chemotherapy, radiotherapy)
Group III: Patients with preexisting chronic pain and cancer-related pain
Group IV: Patients with history of drug addiction and cancer-related pain, including patients:
               Actively involved in illicit drug use
               In a methadone maintenance program
               With a past history of drug abuse
Group V: Dying patients with cancer-related pain.

25. What characterizes the sphenoid sinus syndrome?

Severe bifrontal headache, nasal stuffiness, diplopia, and intermittent retro-orbital pain.

26. What is the most dangerous complication of tumor invasion of the brachial plexus?

Tumor of the brachial plexus commonly spreads along the nerve root into the epidural space. As it does so, pain worsens, and epidural spinal-cord compression can produce paraparesis and bowel and bladder dysfunction.

27. How does epidural spinal-cord compression present?

Epidural tumor from infiltration of bone causing spinal cord compression causes pain in the vast majority of patients (95% have pain as the initial symptom). There is local back pain with tenderness to percussion (most commonly in the thoracic region), and there may be radicular radiation of pain.

28. What are the characteristics of lumbar vertebral metastasis?

Dull, aching mid-back pain exacerbated by lying or sitting and relieved by standing is the usual complaint. Benign pain is usually relieved by recumbency.

29. What is the usual clinical presentation for tumor infiltration of a peripheral nerve?

There may be constant burning pain, hypesthesia, dysesthesia, or sensory loss. There may also be motor dysfunction. Lancinating pains are more common with nerve root involvement.

30. The World Health Organization has developed the Cancer Pain Relief Program and has advocated the three-step approach to the pharmacologic treatment of cancer pain. What are these three steps?

Step 1: Nonopioids with or without adjuvant medications
Step 2: Weak opioids with or without nonopioids and adjuvant medications
Step 3: Strong opioids with or without nonopioids and adjuvant medications

The first step is indicated for mild pain, the second for moderate, and the third for severe. Therapy may be initiated at any step, depending on the severity of the pain.

31. In the terminally ill patient with a malignancy considered nonresponsive to radiation, may radiation still be used in some cases to reduce pain caused by the malignancy?

Yes. A tumor that is not radiosensitive may still be radioresponsive if the response sought is pain reduction. Size reduction is not always necessary to provide analgesia.

32. Hypophysectomy has been used in the terminally ill patient for pain control in which types of cancers?

Metastatic bone pain caused by estrogen-positive breast cancer and prostate cancer have been treated with hypophysectomy, although this procedure is rarely used today in the United States. Other types of cancer pain may respond to this dramatic therapeutic modality as well.

33. What are the most common primary tumors that cause painful vertebral metastases?

Lung, breast, and prostate are the most common. Colon and lymphoma are also seen frequently.

34. What is the first step in assessing pain?

Believe the cancer patient's complaints of pain. Although social and cultural factors and psychologic influences can impact on pain experiences, the complaint of pain in the cancer pain patient can rarely, *if ever*, be assigned to psychologic influences alone. The physician and nurse caring for the patient must start with a belief in the patient's complaint of pain.

35. What is an opiate, and what is an opioid?

1. Opiate—a product such as morphine and codeine specifically derived from the juice of *Papaver somniferum*, the opium poppy.

2. Opioid—a compound that possesses morphine-like activity but that may not necessarily be derived from the juice of *Papaver somniferum*. Opioids are antagonized by naloxone. An example is meperidine, which is a synthetic morphine-like analgesic. Morphine is, by definition, an opioid and an opiate. (See Chapter 32.)

36. There are three primary groups of opioids (Offermeier's classification); what are they and which are used in cancer pain patients?

1. Opioid agonists—the mainstay for the treatment of cancer pain. Morphine is the prototypical agonist and is the preferred drug for severe cancer pain.

2. Opioid agonist-antagonists—used for patients with cancer pain in some parts of the world where pure agonists are not available because of governmental restrictions. They are rarely, if ever, used for chronic cancer pain.

3. Opioid antagonists—Narcan (naloxone) is not used for management of cancer pain except to reverse an opioid agonist intoxication, i.e., it reverses respiratory depression, sedation, *and* analgesia.

37. Are nonopioid analgesics useful for patients with mild cancer pain? Are they useful for moderate and/or severe cancer pain?

The nonopioid analgesics are used in cancer patients whose pain is mild or moderate but they can also be used as an adjunct to a strong opioid to enhance the opioid's effects. Tolerance and physical dependence do not occur with the nonopioid analgesics, but ceiling effects do.

BIBLIOGRAPHY

1. Bach S, Noreng MF, Tjellden NV: Phantom limb pain in amputees during the first 12 months following limb amputation, after preoperative lumbar epidural blockade. Pain 33:297–301, 1988.
2. Cavaletti G, Bogliun, Morzorati L, et al: Peripheral neurotoxicity of taxol in patients previously treated with cisplatin. Cancer 75:1141–1150, 1995.
3. Elliot K, Foley KM: Neurologic pain syndromes in patients with cancer. Neurol Clinics 7:333–360, 1989.

4. Foley KM: Pain syndromes in patients with cancer. In Bonica JJ, Ventafridda V (eds): Advances in Pain Research and Therapy, Vol 2. New York, Raven Press, 1979, pp 59–75.

5. Glass JP, Pettigrew LC, Maor M, et al: Plexopathy induced by radiation therapy. Neurology 35:1261, 1985.

6. Granek I, Ashikari R, Foley KM: Postmastectomy pain syndrome: Clinical and anatomic correlates. Proc Am Soc Clin Oncol (abstract). 3:122, 1983.

7. Greenberg JS, Deck MDF, Vikram B, et al: Metastasis to the base of the skull: Clinical findings in 43 patients. Neurology 31:530–537, 1981.

8. Kori SL, Foley KM, Posner JB: Brachial plexus lesions in patients with cancer: Clinical findings in 100 cases. Neurology 31:45–50, 1981.

9. Portenoy RK, Duma C, Foley KM: Acute herpetic and postherpetic neuralgia: Clinical review and current management. Ann Neurol 20:651–664, 1986.

10. Rotstein J, Good RA: Steroid pseudorheumatism. Arch Intern Med 99:545–555, 1957.

11. Thyagarajan D, Cascino T, Harms G: Magnetic resonance imaging in brachial plexopathy of cancer. Neurology 45:421–427, 1995.

12. Weiss HD, Walker MD, Wiernik PH, et al: Neurotoxicity of commonly used antineoplastic agents. N Engl J Med 291:75–81, 1974.

13. Wood KM: Intercostobrachial nerve entrapment syndrome. South Med J 76:662–663, 1978.

26. PAIN IN RHEUMATOID ARTHRITIS AND OSTEOARTHRITIS

David S. Pisetsky, M.D., Ph.D.

1. What are the causes of pain in rheumatoid arthritis?

Pain in rheumatoid arthritis (RA) is multifactorial and varies in origin with duration and severity of disease. In the initial phases of RA, pain results from inflammation as evidenced by tenderness and swelling of the joint as well as laboratory findings (e.g., increased sedimentation rate, anemia, thrombocytosis). The presence of a rheumatoid factor is also consistent with inflammation. As RA progresses, pain may result not only from inflammation but the damaging effects of erosion of cartilage and bone. Patients with this disease may also develop pain from fibromyalgia and complications such as osteoporosis, with fracture of vertebral bodies leading to acute symptoms. All of these pain syndromes are classified as somatic nociceptive.

When pain in RA occurs disproportionately in a single joint, it is important to exclude septic arthritis, since pre-existing arthritis predisposes to joint-space infection.

2. What is the significance of synovitis?

Synovitis is inflammation of the synovium, which is the lining tissue of the joint. It is the clinical hallmark of RA and produces pain, swelling, and tenderness of the joint. The synovium is richly innervated with nociceptors, which are sensitized by inflammation. In RA, dramatic proliferation accompanies inflammation, and the synovium can become visible and easily palpable. The synovial lining is filled with a dense infiltrate of inflammatory cells and increases to many times its normal size, producing a structure called pannus. The inflammatory cells within the pannus release toxic products such as proteases, which erode cartilage and bone and lead to deformity and pain. While the synovium in RA is filled with lymphocytes, joint space effusions have a predominance of neutrophils and are turbid and almost purulent in appearance.

3. Is joint enlargement always painful?

Synovial inflammation and proliferation can occur discordantly in RA. Thus, some patients have exquisitely painful joints without palpable synovium while others show marked tissue proliferation in the absence of tenderness and pain. In patients with long-standing disease that has "burnt out," synovial masses may be only minimally tender.

4. What joints are commonly affected in rheumatoid arthritis?

The disease is usually insidious in onset and affects both large and small joints in a symmetric pattern. The small joints of the hands and feet, as well as the wrists, elbows, shoulders, knees, and ankles are characteristic sites of inflammation.

5. Is spinal pain common in rheumatoid arthritis?

The cervical spine is commonly affected in RA. Pain may radiate to both arms. It is often complicated by a C1–C2 subluxation. The thoracic and lumbar spines are generally spared.

6. How is the diagnosis of rheumatoid arthritis made?

RA is diagnosed on the basis of history and physical findings. The joint pattern has already been described. The diagnosis of RA is supported by the presence of a rheumatoid factor, which is an IgM anti-IgG antibody. It is important to note, however, that only about 80% of patients with RA display a rheumatoid factor, which can also occur in other clinical settings. The presence of nodules and characteristic deformities (e.g., ulnar deviation, swan neck, and boutonnière deformities of the hands and fingers) substantiate the diagnosis, although these findings indicate more advanced disease and are not invariable.

7. What are the x-ray findings in rheumatoid arthritis?

The usual radiographic findings of RA are soft-tissue swelling, juxta-articular osteopenia, symmetric narrowing of the joint spaces, and bony erosion. X-rays are performed to substantiate the diagnosis of RA, evaluate sources of pain, and stage disease. Bony erosions are indicative of tissue destruction and signify serious prognosis.

8. What painful secondary syndromes occur in patients treated for rheumatoid arthritis?

X-rays of joints in RA may also show evidence of osteoarthritis, which can occur secondary to joint destruction. With sustained disease activity, impaired mobility, and corticosteroid therapy, osteoporosis also occurs and can be demonstrated by x-ray as well as by bone densitometry.

9. What is a flare?

A flare is a painful exacerbation of RA. RA, like other rheumatic diseases, varies in intensity over time and shows periods ("flares") in which signs of inflammation increase dramatically. These flares, which can occur without cause or which may follow infection and other stresses, are associated with increased joint pain and swelling; symptoms such as prolonged morning stiffness, weakness, malaise, and weight loss; and laboratory findings of inflammation. Since RA is a systemic disease, flares are usually polyarticular. The sudden onset of severe pain and swelling in a single joint, however, should raise the suspicion of infection.

10. What is morning stiffness?

Morning stiffness is a very common complaint of patients with RA and is experienced as soreness upon awakening associated with restricted movement. This feeling is generalized in distribution and does not simply affect the joints. While a form of pain, patients may not describe it as such. The duration of morning stiffness is a good indicator of disease activity, and physicians should record this value as part of the clinical assessment. Many patients take a hot shower to relieve the sensation. The "gel phenomenon" is a related symptom and is associated with stiffness and soreness that develops after a period of immobility, for example, sitting in a chair.

11. What are the major differences between rheumatoid arthritis and osteoarthritis?

RA and osteoarthritis (OA) are the two most common forms of arthritis and, because of their predilection for similar joints, can sometimes be confused. The underlying pathophysiology of these diseases is quite distinct, however. RA is inflammatory and initially involves the synovium whereas OA is noninflammatory and results from degeneration of articular cartilage. Furthermore, although OA can be polyarticular in nature, many patients have involvement of only single joints such as the knee or hip. The usual course of RA is symmetric involvement of multiple joints.

In RA, joint fluid is inflammatory and contains neutrophils in abundance (up to 50,000/mm^3) while in OA joint fluid shows few cells (less than 1,000). Another difference between these two diseases concerns the impact on bone. In OA, the hypertrophic changes cause bony enlargement, spurs, or osteophytes, whereas inflammation in RA lacks a bony reaction. In the hands, these bone enlargements are called Heberden's and Bouchard's nodes. Because of the pattern of cartilage and bone involvement, OA is also denoted as degenerative joint disease (DJD) or hypertrophic arthritis.

12. What is inflammatory osteoarthritis?

Some patients with OA show evidence of more prominent inflammation with joint pain, tenderness, and redness. These patients are considered to have inflammatory or erosive osteoarthritis. This condition can be distinguished from RA on the basis of joint distribution, radiographs, and laboratory signs of inflammation.

13. What are the radiographic findings of osteoarthritis?

Typical radiographic findings are asymmetric joint space narrowing, subchondral sclerosis, cysts, and spur formation. Spurs or osteophytes represent bony outgrowths around the joint. OA and RA can be distinguished radiographically, since RA causes symmetric narrowing of the joint space and lacks hypertrophic changes.

14. Is the degree of joint involvement always correlated with the intensity of pain?

No. A painful joint may show only limited change. Furthermore, pain may be referred, necessitating radiographic study of a nearby joint to establish cause. Knee pain, for example, may be referred from the hip.

15. What are the differences in the joint distribution of OA and RA?

These diseases affect many joints in common (e.g., proximal interphalangeal [PIP] joints of the hands, hips, knees, and cervical spine), but there are important differences that have diagnostic significance. In the hands, OA, but not RA, affects the distal interphalangeal (DIP) joints, whereas RA, but not OA, affects the metacarpophalangeal (MCP) joints. Other sites routinely affected by RA, but not OA, include the wrists, elbows, shoulder, ankles, and small joints of the feet. In contrast, OA, but not RA, involves the lumbar spine. The distribution of joints in OA suggests that this disease is not simply the result of joint use or weight bearing but may rather reflect particular mechanical properties of joints.

16. What are the classes of drugs used to treat rheumatoid arthritis?

Therapy can be conveniently divided into four main categories based on steps in the pathophysiologic process that are modified: nonsteroidal anti-inflammatory drugs (NSAIDs); corticosteroids, which are anti-inflammatory and immunosuppressive; analgesics; and remittive agents. Remittive agents are also termed disease modifying antirheumatic drugs (DMARDs) or slow-acting antirheumatic drugs (SAARDs). Therapy in RA frequently involves the simultaneous administration of drugs from more than one category, and there is considerable discussion concerning the timing and duration of therapy as well as relative toxicity and efficacy of different agents.

17. What is a remittive agent?

A drug that reduces the signs and symptoms of rheumatoid arthritis in the absence of conventional analgesic or anti-inflammatory action of an NSAID or corticosteroid. The most commonly used remittive agents are methotrexate, gold salts, penicillamine, hydrochloroquine, and azathioprine.

18. What is the mode of action of NSAIDs?

NSAIDs inhibit the enzyme cyclo-oxygenase and thus block the generation of prostaglandins from arachidonic acid. Because of the physiologic actions of prostaglandins, NSAIDs are anti-inflammatory, analgesic, and antipyretic. These activities make the NSAIDs among the most commonly used drugs in all of medicine, whether by prescription or over-the-counter. Currently available NSAIDs differ in chemical structure as well as half-life, although in general they have similar potency. (See Chapter 31.) Examples include aspirin, ibuprofen, indomethacin, piroxicam, sodium naproxen, and diclofenac. Individuals may differ in their response to different NSAIDs, and it's useful to try more than one before considering this mode of therapy successful. Since NSAIDs are analgesic as well as anti-inflammatory, they are used in both OA and RA.

19. What are the side effects of NSAIDs?

NSAIDs block prostaglandin production and have predictable side effects on the basis of this action. These side effects include bleeding, especially gastrointestinal; gastric irritation and ulceration; fluid retention, edema; and renal insufficiency.

20. Which patients are at greatest risk for renal side effects of NSAIDs?

The elderly and other patients with reduced renal blood flow are at greatest risk. They produce prostaglandins as a compensation for decreased renal blood flow. With prostaglandin production blocked by NSAIDs, these patients can suffer from deterioration in renal function. The common conditions associated with this complication include chronic renal insufficiency, congestive heart failure, use of diuretics, and cirrhosis of the liver.

21. What is the therapeutic dose of aspirin?

The pharmacologic actions of aspirin vary with dose. Low doses (e.g., a single 325-mg tablet or even a baby aspirin [68 mg]) can produce antiplatelet effects. In contrast, analgesic effects are usually achieved with two 325-mg tablets four times/day. Anti-inflammatory effects occur at a blood level of 20 to 25 mg/dl, which requires titration for each patient and verification by determination of a serum salicylate level. For most adults, at least 12 325-mg aspirin tablets are required for a stable therapeutic level, although sometimes more than 20 tablets are needed. Since the metabolism of aspirin involves a pathway that becomes saturated, small increases in aspirin dose can be reflected in large changes in salicylate levels and the occurrence of side effects.

22. What is salicylism?

Aspirin (acetylsalicylic acid) is an NSAID with characteristic side effects called salicylism. These side effects are manifest initially by tinnitus (ringing and roaring in the ears) at blood levels that overlap the therapeutic levels. As blood levels increase further, metabolic acidosis, respiratory alkalosis, disturbances in consciousness, and coma and death may ensue. Aspirin remains a leading cause of drug-related death because of both intentional ingestion for suicide and inadvertent overdosing from simultaneous use of more than one aspirin-containing product. There are hundreds of over-the-counter preparations with aspirin as an ingredient. In a patient on a full salicylate program, additional ingestion of aspirin can lead to toxic levels.

In older patients, aspirin can cause reversible deafness and should be avoided in those with hearing impairment.

23. What is Samter's syndrome?

This condition is marked clinically by asthma, nasal polyps, and sensitivity to salicylates. A proposed mechanism is the shunting of arachidonate metabolites through the lipoxygenase pathway when the cyclo-oxygenase pathway is inhibited by aspirin.

24. What is NSAID gastropathy?

Prostaglandins promote the integrity of the gastric lining, and when their production is inhibited by NSAIDs, bleeding, superficial irritation, and erosion ensue. These lesions are frequently transient, small, and asymptomatic, with endoscopy required for their detection. This condition should be distinguished from peptic ulcer disease, which can also occur in patients on NSAIDs. Many patients on NSAIDs also experience simple dyspepsia, in the absence of signs of erosion.

25. How is NSAID gastropathy prevented?

The frequency of this complication appears to differ among available NSAIDs, although it occurs with all. To reduce their gastric complications, NSAIDs should be taken with food or antacids. If aspirin is used, a buffered or enteric coated preparation may be less toxic for the GI tract. Other preventive measures include the use of H-2 blockers such as cimetidine or ranitidine. Misoprostol is a synthetic prostaglandin approved for use in patients who have had documented GI complications of NSAIDs.

26. What are the differences between acetaminophen and NSAIDs?

Acetaminophen is an analgesic without anti-inflammatory effects. Since it does not inhibit cyclo-oxygenase, acetaminophen lacks some of the complications of NSAIDs. Acetaminophen is commonly used in the treatment of OA, where an anti-inflammatory effect is not essential. In RA, acetaminophen is prescribed as an adjunct to other measures to reduce pain.

27. What are the complications of therapy with remittive drugs?

Each of the remittive agents is associated with significant toxicity that necessitates surveillance for safety. The agents and their common side effects are methotrexate (mucositis, hepatic toxicity); hydroxychloroquine (retinal toxicity); injectable gold salts (rash, cytopenias, proteinuria); oral gold (diarrhea, cytopenias, proteinuria); penicillamine (cytopenias, proteinuria, and autoimmune syndromes); and azathioprine (immunosuppression). Myochrysine (gold thiomalate) can also provoke hypotension in susceptible individuals, causing a nitritoid reaction. Although this reaction is rare, some physicians who use injectable gold prefer to use Solganal (aurothioglucose) in older individuals as well as patients with cardiovascular disease.

28. Why are corticosteroids administered in rheumatoid arthritis?

Because of their potent anti-inflammatory and immunosuppressive actions, corticosteroids effectively reduce joint pain and swelling in RA. These drugs interfere with the inflammatory process at various steps. An important action appears to be blockade of the release of arachidonic acid from the cell membrane, limiting substrate for both the lipoxygenase and cyclo-oxygenase pathways and reducing leukotrienes as well as prostaglandins. Modulation of leukocyte function, including inhibition of cytokine production, contributes to the therapeutic effect.

29. How are corticosteroids used in rheumatoid arthritis pain?

By three routes: (1) Administration of high doses with rapid tapers to treat flares and reduce inflammation as a "bridge" therapy while remittive therapy is instituted. (2) Chronic low-dose administration for treatment of active synovitis that does not respond adequately to NSAIDs or remittive agents. (3) Intra-articular administration to reduce persistent synovitis in single joints. High-dose steroids refers to doses of prednisone, the most commonly prescribed corticosteroid, of 0.5–1.0 mg/kg daily while low dose denotes doses in the range of 5 to 7.5 mg daily. Such intra articular treatment can produce a "chemical synovectomy" and lead to prolonged reduction in pain.

30. What are side effects of corticosteroids?

Therapy with corticosteroids is complicated by hypertension, glucose intolerance, cushingoid features, adrenal suppression, osteoporosis, weight gain, infection, cataracts, and central nervous system changes such as depression and psychosis. Intra-articular steroids can lead to infection and cartilage damage.

31. What is the role of opioid (narcotic) analgesics in the therapy of rheumatoid arthritis?

The goals of therapy in RA are to decrease inflammation, reduce pain, prevent deformity, promote general health, and increase the quality of life. When pain persists despite conventional therapy and detracts from the quality of life, opioid pain relievers may be prescribed. (See Chapter 34.) Opioids are frequently used in patients awaiting joint replacement or in patients for whom joint replacements are indicated but cannot be performed because of co-morbid conditions.

32. How can assistive devices reduce pain in arthritis?

Assistive devices are valuable adjuncts in the care of patients with all forms of arthritis and can decrease pain and facilitate activities of daily living. These devices include splints, canes, and walkers, as well as a diversity of implements to perform activities ranging from buttoning a shirt, to opening a jar, to reaching items in a cupboard, to eating. Canes, used in the hand opposite the affected joint, can decrease pain on ambulation and forestall the need for surgery. Consultation with a physical or occupational therapist is an essential component in the total management of a patient with advanced arthritis.

33. What are the surgical procedures to reduce pain in arthritis?

Although total joint replacement is performed frequently for both RA and OA, it is actually only one of the several procedures available in the treatment of these diseases. In RA, synovectomy can reduce pain and delay total joint replacement. This procedure involves removal of proliferated synovium; arthroscopy is increasingly used for this purpose to avoid the greater trauma of arthrotomy. A useful procedure in osteoarthritis is an osteotomy, in which a wedge of bone is removed to correct joint alignment and improve biomechanics. Joint fusions are performed for both OA and RA; this procedure reduces pain but sacrifices motion.

Pain is the major consideration for replacement of large joints such as the hip or knee. Pain that lasts all day, pain that awakens the patient from sleep, or pain that requires frequent or continuous opioid analgesics usually indicates a need for surgery. Neither radiographic evidence of joint destruction nor functional impairment alone is sufficient.

34. How does the surgical approach to rheumatoid arthritis of the hands differ from that for the large joints?

In contrast to total joint replacement of the knees or hips, surgery of the hands in RA is undertaken to prevent or correct deformity and improve function. Pain is less often the primary indication for hand surgery, which entails synovectomy and rerouting of tendons in addition to joint replacement.

35. What are the complications of total joint replacement?

The major complications of joint replacement are infection, dislocation, fracture, and loosening. Infections of prosthetic joints differ from ordinary joint-space infections in their more indolent course and less dramatic signs of inflammation. Loosening causes pain and can be diagnosed by radiographs.

36. What is the approach to the treatment of foot pain in rheumatoid arthritis?

RA commonly affects the small joints of the feet, causing erosive synovitis and deformity similar to the involvement of the small joints of the hand. The metatarsophalangeal (MTP) heads become subluxed, leading to exquisite pain on walking, callus formation, and ulceration on the soles of the feet. This condition can be treated by use of metatarsal bars on the bottom of shoes to reduce the impact of walking on the MTPs; extra-depth, extra-width shoes and molded shoes to accommodate the deformities and reduce the likelihood of ulceration; and surgery.

37. What is the surgical approach to rheumatoid arthritis of the feet?

The most commonly used procedure is the resection of the metatarsal heads, which removes the painful joints and foreshortens the foot. Frequently, corrective surgery of the feet is the initial procedure performed for a patient with RA with serious involvement of lower extremity joints.

38. What is the treatment of painful ankle in rheumatoid arthritis?

The ankle is commonly involved in RA, with both tibial-talar and subtalar joints subject to erosive damage. Rather than the use of a prosthesis, ankle disease is usually treated with fusion, which can be accomplished by either prolonged immobilization or surgery. A triple arthrodesis can eliminate motion of the ankle and thereby reduce the pain on walking.

39. What is the difference in outcome of total joint replacement in osteoarthritis and rheumatoid arthritis?

Patients with OA, although they may be older and have co-morbid conditions, are not systemically ill with their arthritis and need replacement of isolated joints. The bone stock of patients with OA is frequently good. Because of these favorable factors, results of surgery are excellent. In contrast, patients with RA have polyarticular involvement, are systemically ill, and frequently have low bone reserve because of their disease, immobility, and the use of medications such as corticosteroids. Surgery can eliminate pain and increase mobility in the replaced joint, but patients nevertheless still experience the consequences of disease in their other joints. Not surprisingly, patients with RA, while benefiting greatly from surgery, do not show comparable restoration of function.

40. What is the pseudothrombophlebitis syndrome?

Acute pain and swelling in the calf can result from rupture or dissection of a Baker's cyst and mimic thrombophlebitis. A Baker's cyst is an expansion of the synovial space posterior to the knee joint and can be detected by palpation when the patient is standing. The usual cause is RA, although effusions in OA can produce the same lesion. Diagnostic evaluation includes studies (e.g., venogram or Doppler flow) to exclude deep vein thrombosis as well as ultrasound or arthrogram to demonstrate the cyst. The usual treatment is injection of intra-articular steroids into the knee joint.

41. What are the causes of head pain in rheumatoid arthritis?

Headache is common in patients with RA and usually results from arthritis of the cervical spine, which is the only region of the axial skeleton involved in this disease. Patients with RA can also have pain originating in the temporomandibular joints, which are diarthrodial joints subject to erosive synovitis. Inflammatory disease of the eyes can cause ocular pain, while arthritis of the cricoarytenoid joint is associated with sore throat and hoarseness. Any elderly patient with a systemic "rheumatoid" illness and headache should be investigated for temporal arteritis. (See Chapter 15.)

42. What is C1–C2 subluxation?

The joints of the cervical spine, like other synovial joints, can undergo erosive damage and instability, especially as ligaments are destroyed. Subluxation of the C1–C2 joint (atlantoaxial subluxation) occurs commonly in patients with erosive disease (RA) and can be demonstrated by flexion-extension x-rays of the spine; a separation greater than 2.5 to 3 mm is considered significant. This condition is associated with neck pain, headache, shooting pains in the arms and legs and, when advanced, myelopathy with long tract signs. In the presence of progressive lower extremity weakness and disturbances of bowel and bladder function, fusion of the spine is performed emergently to stabilize the spine and prevent cord damage. In the vast majority of cases, however, treatment is symptomatic, including collars for immobilization.

43. What is spinal stenosis?

Spinal stenosis refers to narrowing of the spinal canal, usually a consequence of degenerative disease. This condition can produce lower extremity pain, which is termed neurogenic claudication. Pain from spinal stenosis is worsened by walking and relieved by bending forward, causing a characteristic posture of these patients.

44. What is DISH?

DISH, or disseminated idiopathic skeletal hyperostosis, is an exaggerated form of osteoarthritis characterized by prominent spine involvement in association with exuberant spur formation. The spine shows calcification of the anterior spinal longitudinal ligament that appears to flow from one vertebra to another in a pattern termed "toothpaste" calcification. In this condition, the disk spaces are preserved. While DISH is commonly associated with back pain, it can also be an incidental finding on chest x-ray.

45. Which conditions are associated with atypical degenerative osteoarthritis?

OA uncommonly involves joints such as the metacarpophalangeal (MCP) joints, wrists, elbows, or ankles. In the absence of a history of trauma or excessive joint usage, OA of these joints suggests the presence of calcium pyrophosphate dihydrate deposition, or CPPD, disease.

This condition can be demonstrated by radiographic findings of chondrocalcinosis or calcification within the articular cartilage. The presence of CPPD suggests an underlying metabolic problem such as hemochromatosis, hyperparathyroidism, or acromegaly. Indeed, degenerative disease of the MCP joints is a classic presentation of hemochromatosis.

46. What are the findings in pseudogout, and how is this condition treated?

Pseudogout is one of the presentations of CPPD and causes acute monarticular arthritis, which, like gout, is extremely painful. Pseudogout is diagnosed by the presence of inflammatory joint fluid containing crystals that are rhomboidal in shape and positively birefringent by polarizing microscopy; in contrast, monosodium urate crystals in gout are needle-shaped and negatively birefringent. This condition can be treated by joint aspiration, NSAIDs, and, sometimes, intraarticular steroids. Attacks of pseudogout can be provoked by metabolic changes and occur commonly after stressful events such as surgery.

47. What is PMR?

PMR, or polymyalgia rheumatica, is a painful condition that is frequently acute in onset and causes pain in the shoulder and limb girdles in the absence of other signs of arthritis. It occurs in older individuals (greater than 50 years of age), shows signs of inflammation with an elevated sedimentation rate (greater than 50 mm/hr), and responds dramatically to low-dose corticosteroids. Since rheumatoid arthritis and systemic lupus erythematosus can present with a similar pattern, these conditions must be excluded by appropriate serologic tests (rheumatoid factor and antinulcear antibody) before the diagnosis of PMR is made. Many patients with PMR have an underlying temporal (giant cell) arteritis. (See Chapter 15).

48. What is fibromyalgia?

Fibromyalgia is characterized by diffuse myalgic pain in the absence of synovitis and other signs of inflammation. Tender points are the cardinal feature of this disease, and pressure on these areas elicits pain. Patients, usually women, with fibromyalgia, frequently report other symptoms such as fatigue, poor exercise tolerance, headache, irritable bowel, and jumpy legs. Sleep disturbance is common among patients with fibromyalgia and may provoke a neuropsychologic disturbance.

Fibromyalgia may occur alone or may be secondary to another condition, such as RA, OA, or SLE. The diagnosis of fibromyalgia in the setting of another musculoskeletal disease is based primarily on the presence of tender points. Therapy for fibromyalgia involves NSAIDs, tricyclic antidepressants to promote sleep, and exercise programs.

49. Which conditions cause a painful shoulder?

In addition to inflammatory diseases such as RA, SLE, and PMR, pain in the shoulder can result from degenerative disease, tendinitis, bursitis, adhesive capsulitis, and impingement syndromes. Nerve root entrapment from cervical spine arthritis can also cause pain. Since pain in the shoulder can also be referred from intrathoracic lesions, evaluation of this condition may necessitate a chest x-ray.

50. What is avascular necrosis?

Avascular necrosis (AVN) or ischemic necrosis of the bone results from vascular insufficiency to bone and causes painful infarction. AVN can occur in the setting of other forms of arthritis (e.g., SLE or RA), although more commonly it results from the effects of corticosteroids, which may increase marrow fat and impede blood flow. The femoral head is the usual site of involvement, although other bones can be affected. Alcohol can produce a similar condition, sometimes called alcoholic osteonecrosis.

X-rays in AVN demonstrate collapse, fracture, and bone irregularity, although early diagnosis of this condition requires magnetic resonance imaging. Treatment involves surgery with total joint replacement in more advanced disease.

BIBLIOGRAPHY

1. Abramson SB, Weissman G: The mechanisms of action of nonsteroidal anti-inflammatory drugs. Arthritis Rheum 32:1, 1989.
2. Bradley JD, Brandt KD, Katz BP, et al: Comparison of an anti-inflammatory dose of ibuprofen, an analgesic dose of ibuprofen, and acetaminophen in the treatment of patients with osteoarthritis of the knee. N Engl J Med 325:87, 1991.
3. Brandt KD: Should osteoarthritis be treated with nonsteroidal anti-inflammatory drugs? Rheum Dis Clin North Am 19:697, 1993.
4. Buckelew SP, Parker JC: Coping with arthritis pain. A review of the literature. Arthritis Care Res 2:136, 1989.
5. Felson DT, Anderson JJ, Meenan RF: The comparative efficacy and toxicity of second-line drugs in rheumatoid arthritis. Results of two metaanalyses. Arthritis Rheum 33:1449, 1990.
6. Fries JF, Williams CA, Ramey DR, et al: The relative toxicity of alternative therapies for rheumatoid arthritis: Implications for the therapeutic progression. Semin Arthritis Rheum 23:68, 1993.
7. Gerber LH, Hicks JE: Surgical and rehabilitation options in the treatment of rheumatoid arthritis resistant to pharmacological agents. Rheum Dis Clin North Am 21:19, 1995.
8. Harris WH, Sledge CB: Total hip and knee replacement. N Engl J Med 323:801, 1990.
9. Lichtenstein DR, Syngal S, Wolfe MM: Nonsteroidal anti-inflammatory drugs and the gastrointestinal tract: The double edge sword. Arthritis Rheum 38:5, 1995.
10. Schumacher HR Jr, Klippel JH, Koopman WJ: Primer on the Rheumatic Diseases, 10th ed. Atlanta, Arthritis Foundation, 1993.
11. Weinblatt ME, Weissman BN, Holdsworth DE, et al: Long-term prospective study of methotrexate in the treatment of rheumatoid arthritis 84-month update. Arthritis Rheum 35:129, 1992.
12. Weiss MM: Corticosteroids in rheumatoid arthritis. Semin Arthritis Rheum 19:9, 1989.
13. Wiske KR, Healy LA: Remodeling the pyramid—A concept whose time has come. J Rheumatol 16:565, 1989.
14. Wolfe F: When to diagnose fibromyalgia. Rheum Dis Clin North Am 20:485, 1994.

27. NEUROPATHIC PAIN

Russell K. Portenoy, M.D.

1. What is neuropathic pain?

The term neuropathic pain is applied to any acute or chronic pain syndrome in which the mechanism that sustains the pain is inferred to involve aberrant somatosensory processing in the peripheral or central nervous system (CNS). Neuropathic pain is commonly distinguished from two other inferred pathophysiologies, which are commonly labeled nociceptive pain and psychogenic pain. The sustaining mechanisms of nociceptive pain are inferred to involve ongoing activation of pain-sensitive afferent peripheral nerves. This activation may be caused by injury to either somatic (known as somatic pain) or visceral (known as visceral pain) structures. Psychogenic pain is a generic term used to refer to those pains that have sustaining mechanisms related to psychological processes.

2. Why do the definitions of neuropathic pain, nociceptive pain, and psychogenic pain refer to these terms as inferred pathophysiologies?

This classification by pathophysiology is "inferred" because there is no way to prove or disprove that any particular mechanism is operating in the clinical setting to maintain a chronic pain syndrome. The type of pathophysiology that may be involved is conjectured on the basis of the pain description and associated findings on examination and ancillary tests. Because the diagnosis is inferred, there is the potential for imprecision and oversimplification when labeling patients. Indeed, it is likely that patients often have more than one set of pathophysiologies and that each type of pathophysiology actually refers to multiple specific mechanisms. Nonetheless, a pathophysiologic classification has become widely accepted by clinicians, who have observed that it may be useful in defining the type of evaluation that may be needed, selecting appropriate therapies, and determining the prognosis for improvement.

3. What findings on clinical evaluation suggest that a pain is neuropathic?

Neuropathic pain is suggested when patients use terms to describe their pain that are consistent with a dysesthesia, which is defined as an abnormal pain complaint. Pain may be described as burning, electrical-like, or shooting. Patients often say that the pain is unfamiliar, unlike any pain experienced before. The examination may reveal allodynia (pain on light touch), hypalgesia or hyperalgesia (relatively decreased or increased perception of a noxious stimulus, respectively), hypesthesia or hyperesthesia (relatively decreased or increased perception of a nonnoxious stimulus, respectively), or hyperpathia (exaggerated pain response). There may be other focal neurologic deficits, such as weakness or focal autonomic changes. These focal autonomic phenomena may include swelling and vasomotor instability (observed as color changes, livedo reticularis, and focal temperature changes). There may also be trophic changes, including alterations of the skin and subcutaneous tissues or the hair and nails. Ancillary tests, such as electrodiagnostic studies (electromyogram and nerve conduction velocities) can sometimes be helpful in confirming the existence of a neurologic lesion. Tests such as thermography are occasionally useful to confirm autonomic dysregulation.

4. What are some of the challenges inherent in diagnosing neuropathic pain?

When a dysesthesia occurs in the setting of an overt neurologic lesion, the diagnosis of neuropathic pain may be straightforward. Even in this setting, however, it may be difficult to exclude a contribution to the pain of co-existing processes, such as damage to somatic structures sufficient to produce nociceptive pain or psychological processes that exacerbate the pain. Furthermore, neuropathic pain can occur without an overt neurologic deficit (for example, reflex sympathetic dystrophy can follow minor soft-tissue injury and pain may be the first and only manifestation of a small fiber polyneuropathy). Finally, neuropathic pain can be nondysesthetic, such as the deep aching that commonly occurs from nerve or nerve root compression. All of these factors can complicate the diagnosis of neuropathic pain.

5. The clinical diversity of neuropathic pain suggests that the mechanisms responsible are both numerous and complex, presumably involving interactions between the peripheral and central nervous systems. Is there a useful model for conceptualizing these interacting mechanisms?

Three decades of basic research have shown that neuropathic pain may result from any of a variety of mechanisms that interact in complex ways. The normal response of the peripheral nervous system and the central nervous system (CNS) following exposure to a noxious stimulus can become disturbed at multiple levels concurrently, in a process that involves afferent input, efferent activity in the sympathetic nervous system, and pain modulatory processes in both the periphery and CNS. Further research is needed to determine the specific processes that result in these pathologic distortions of normal nociception.

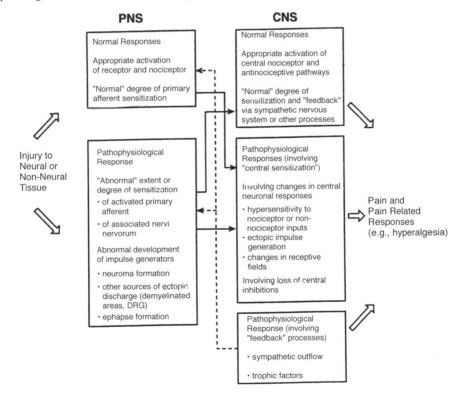

Model demonstrating the complex processes that may be involved in the pathophysiology of neuropathic pain. PNS = peripheral nervous system; CNS = central nervous system; DRG = dorsal root ganglion.

6. From the clinical perspective, what is a useful classification of the heterogeneous population with chronic neuropathic pain?

Although patients with neuropathic pain are traditionally categorized on the basis of diagnosis (e.g., painful diabetic polyneuropathy) or site of the precipitating lesion (e.g., peripheral nerve), it may be most useful to extend the classification based on inferred pathophysiology and to suggest that some patients with neuropathic pain have disorders that are primarily sustained by processes in the CNS while others have disorders sustained by processes in the peripheral nervous system. This distinction is suggested by both clinical and experimental data. For example, a predominant peripheral pathophysiology is suggested by the observation that some patients with neuropathic pain precipitated by nerve injury are cured by a local intervention, such as resection of a neuroma. A predominant central pathophysiology is obvious in those patients whose neuropathic pain is precipitated by stroke.

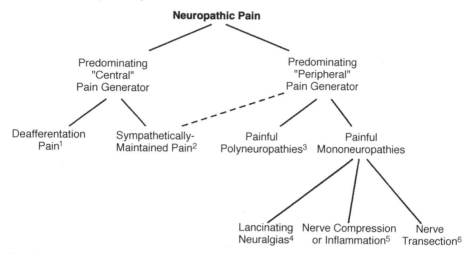

Classification of neuropathic pains by putative predominating mechanism. 1. Response to either peripheral or central nervous system injury. 2. Associated with focal autonomic dysregulation (e.g., edema, vasomotor disturbances), involuntary motor responses, and/or trophic changes that may improve with sympathetic nerve block. 3. Multiple mechanisms probably involved. 4. The patterns of peripheral activity or peripheral and central interaction that yield the lancinating quality of these pains are unknown. 5. Nociceptive nervi nervorum (small afferents that innervate larger nerves) may account for neuropathic pain accompanying nerve compression or inflammation. 6. Injury to axons may be followed by neuroma formation, a source of aberrant activity likely to be involved in pain.

7. What neuropathic pain syndromes are presumably sustained by aberrant somatosensory processing in the CNS?

Neuropathic pains that are inferred to have sustaining mechanisms in the CNS can be broadly divided into a group of disorders known as the deafferentation pains and a disorder known as sympathetically maintained pain. The deafferentation pains include a large number of specific syndromes, such as central pain, pain due to avulsion of a plexus, pain due to spinal cord injury, postherpetic neuralgia, phantom pain, and others. Sympathetically maintained pain, which is believed to be pain sustained by efferent activity in the sympathetic nervous system, is probably a subtype of many syndromes, the most important of which are reflex sympathetic dystrophy and causalgia (now known as complex regional pain syndrome type I and type II, respectively—see question 39).

8. What pain syndromes are presumably sustained by aberrant somatosensory processing in the peripheral nervous system?

Neuropathic pains that are inferred to have sustaining mechanisms in the peripheral nervous system can be divided into a group of painful polyneuropathies and a group of painful mononeuropathies. Each of these groups, in turn, subsumes many specific syndromes.

9. What specific mechanisms in the CNS may be involved in the various types of deafferentation pain?

Studies in experimental models and humans suggest that a state of "central sensitization" may be relevant to all deafferentation syndromes. Although peripheral input may be important in some syndromes (as suggested by the transitory relief of deafferentation pain that is commonly observed following interruption of proximal somatosensory pathways), the sustaining pathophysiology presumably relates to changes in the response characteristics of central neurons that are at least partly independent of this input.

Central sensitization may involve functional and structural changes in CNS pathways involved in nociception (see figure with question 5 and table below). Each of these changes presumably occurs as a consequence of specific mechanisms, which have only begun to be elucidated. Recent studies, for example, have indicated the importance of an interaction between excitatory amino acids (specifically glutamate) and the N-methyl-D-aspartate receptor in producing sensitization of nociceptive neurons in the dorsal horn of the spinal cord. Although the relationship of these functional and structural changes to chronic pain in humans is conjectural, the range of phenomena underscores the plasticity of central connections and suggest a focus for future research targeted at the prevention or treatment of neuropathic pain.

Changes That May Be Involved in Neuropathic Pains Sustained by Aberrant Processes in the Central Nervous System

Functional Changes	Structural Changes
Lowered threshold for activation	Transsynaptic degeneration
Exaggerated activation	Transganglionic degeneration
Ectopic discharges	Collateral sprouting
Enlarging receptive fields	
Loss of normal inhibition	

10. Phantom pain is commonly considered to be a type of deafferentation pain. What is phantom pain?

Although the prototype phantom pain follows limb amputation, the term is applied to pain following amputation of any body part. For example, surveys have described phantom pain following mastectomy and tooth extraction. Some authors also use the term to describe pain in regions of the body that are completely denervated (rendered anesthetic) but not amputated, such as the area below a transected spinal cord or the area supplied by a severely injured peripheral nerve. This may be confusing, however, and it would be preferable to use the term "central pain," or one of its subtypes (see question 28), to describe a pain that occurs in an area denervated as a result of a CNS lesion, and to use either the generic term "deafferentation pain," or the older term "anesthesia dolorosa," to describe a pain that is inferred to have a central mechanism induced by a severe peripheral nerve injury.

11. What is known about the specific mechanisms that may result in phantom pain?

The specific mechanisms that cause phantom pain are not known. One conceptualization suggests that phantom pain is a somatosensory "memory" that does not reside in a specific region of the CNS but may instead involve complex interactions of neural networks in the brain.

12. What is the epidemiology of phantom pain?

Epidemiologic surveys of phantom pain must distinguish this phenomenon from both nonpainful phantom sensations and stump pain. Failure to be precise may be the cause of variation in older surveys, which have reported transitory or occasional discomfort in the phantoms of 25–98% of amputees. A survey of patients undergoing medical amputation identified phantom limb pain in 72%, 65%, and 59% of patients at eight days, six months, and two years, respectively.

Several studies have attempted to define predisposing factors for the development of phantom pain. Phantom limb is rare in congenital amputees or children who lose a limb before the age of six. This observation suggests that some degree of CNS maturation is required before phantom pain can occur. The experience of pain in the limb prior to amputation has been noted to predispose to the development of phantom pain in some, but not all, surveys. A recent study observed that 57% of patients who experienced pain immediately before amputation developed phantom pain that resembled the pre-existing pain in quality and location. A strong association between stump pain and phantom pain has also been reported. Other surveys have suggested that older age, proximal amputations, upper limb lesions, sudden amputations, and pre-existing psychological disturbances may increase the likelihood of phantom pain, but these factors have not been confirmed in more recent studies.

13. What is the natural history of phantom pain?

Although most patients develop phantom sensations and phantom pain soon after the nerve injury, symptoms may develop at any time after denervation. Most surveys observe that the pain substantially declines over time in approximately one-half of patients.

14. How is phantom pain different from phantom sensation?

Phantom pain is one element among many phantom sensations. Pain has been termed an exteroceptive sensation, a description that has also been applied to the perception of touch, temperature, pressure, itch, and other sensations. Kinesthetic sensation, which involves the perception of posture, length, and volume, and kinetic sensations, including the perceptions of willed movements and spontaneous movements, also occur. Among the more common kinesthetic sensations are unusual or bizarre postures, foreshortening of a limb ("telescoping"), or distortions in the size of body parts (usually reduction in proximal regions and expansion of distal regions). All these sensations are usually most vivid immediately after amputation. Over time, the size of the phantom often shrinks, and the intensity of all sensation gradually fades.

15. How is phantom pain different from stump pain?

In contrast to phantom pain, in which the inferred "generator" of the pain is in the CNS, stump pain is a peripheral neuropathic pain presumably related to the development of a neuroma at the end of a severed nerve. Patients usually report some combination of aching, squeezing, throbbing, stabbing, and electrical discomfort localized to the distal stump. The onset of the pain is usually delayed for months, and the incidence is lower than that in phantom pain. Following limb amputation, many patients have both stump pain and phantom pain.

16. Can phantom pain be prevented?

Phantom pain may be difficult to treat, and prevention would clearly be favorable. The possibility of prevention has been highlighted by a small trial that demonstrated the efficacy of a 72-hour preoperative epidural infusion of local anesthetic and/or morphine in reducing postoperative phantom pain among patients with preamputation limb pain. Although the data are too limited to recommend regional anesthesia prior to all amputations, this approach should be considered in a selected group of patients who have intense pre-existing pain.

17. What management strategies are used for phantom pain?

Patients with established phantom pain should be evaluated for the existence of potentially treatable factors that may be exacerbating the pain, such as stump neuroma or depression. Management of these factors may improve outcome. Although there is no compelling evidence that the use of a prosthesis or physical therapy yields analgesic effects in patients with phantom pain, such rehabilitative therapies can have salutary effects on function and should be considered on this basis alone. For the phantom pain itself, a large number of potentially analgesic treatments can be tried in an effort to improve comfort and facilitate functional gains.

There have been very few analgesic clinical trials in patients with phantom pain, and, generally, trials of adjuvant analgesic drugs are offered in a manner identical to that in other types of neuropathic pain (see Chapter 33). A placebo-controlled trial suggested that salmon calcitonin (200 IU via brief intravenous infusion) may be effective, at least in patients with relatively short-lived phantom pain, and a trial of this drug by intranasal or subcutaneous administration should be considered early. The long-term use of opioids can sometimes be effective in phantom pain.

Although sympathetic nerve blocks usually produce minimal or transitory benefit, rare patients appear to do well, and this small potential for long-term favorable effects warrants a trial of sympathetic blockade in selected patients with refractory pain. Prolonged relief from blockade of sensory nerves appears to be even more rare than benefit from sympathetic blocks, and cases have been described in which sensory blockade paradoxically increased the pain. Chemical or surgical neurolysis of proximal somatosensory pathways has more risk than temporary nerve blocks, including the potential to worsen pain, and these procedures are not used to manage phantom pain. The dorsal root entry zone lesion has had promising results in a specific type of deafferentation pain syndromes, plexus avulsion (see question 28), but results have not been favorable in phantom pain. Local injection into the stump, which may be useful for stump pain, also has very limited efficacy in the management of phantom pain.

Neurostimulatory approaches are safer than neurodestructive procedures and have been used in the management of phantom pain. Although the results are usually disappointing with transcutaneous electrical nerve stimulation (TENS), its inherent safety warrants a trial in most patients. A large experience with invasive neurostimulatory procedures, including dorsal column stimulation and deep brain stimulation, has yielded mixed results. These approaches should not be considered until conservative treatments have failed and the patient has undergone a comprehensive evaluation by experienced clinicians.

The value of psychological interventions as part of a multimodality approach to phantom pain deserves emphasis. In the case of phantom pain, disfigurement and physical impairments may compound the distress related to pain and augment the importance of psychological interventions.

18. Postherpetic neuralgia (PHN) is another common deafferentation pain syndrome. What is the definition of PHN?

Although it is axiomatic that PHN is defined solely by the experience of prolonged pain following acute herpes zoster infection, the specific time criterion used to diagnose this condition is a matter of debate. In the medical literature, various reports have defined PHN as pain that persists beyond the crusting of lesions, or pain that continues beyond 1, 1.5, 8, or 24 weeks following resolution of the rash. For research purposes, it is probably most reasonable to require a criterion of four months from onset of the lesion (one month for healing of the lesion followed by three months of pain). This criterion is used to define an early period, during which therapies for acute herpes zoster are appropriate, and an open-ended period that follows, during which treatments appropriate for PHN should be implemented.

19. What is known about the mechanisms that result in PHN?

Following resolution of a systemic varicella infection, which usually occurs in childhood, the virus maintains a dormant phase in dorsal root ganglia. Herpes zoster is the segmental recrudescence of the varicella virus, the appearance of which presumably involves some type of breakdown in immune surveillance.

Herpes zoster produces diffuse inflammation of peripheral nerve, dorsal root ganglion, and, in some cases, the spinal cord. Long after the acute infection resolves, the pathology reveals chronic inflammatory changes in the periphery, neuronal loss in the dorsal root ganglion, and a reduction of both axons and myelin in affected nerve. The relationship between this pathology and the functional changes believed to be involved in the deafferentation pains (see table with question 9) is unknown. One provocative finding is the relatively selective loss of large peripheral nerve fibers in several cases, which suggests that reduced peripheral inhibitory processes mediated by these fibers may be one contributing process.

20. What is the epidemiology of herpes zoster and PHN?

The incidence of herpes zoster, which overall is approximately 1.3 to 4.8 cases per 1000 person-years, increases in the elderly and the immunocompromised (e.g., patients with cancer or AIDS). Some reports have suggested that the incidence may also be influenced by various systemic insults, such as surgery, toxic exposures and infections, and focal pathologic processes affecting the spine or roots.

Although only 10% of all those with acute herpes experience pain for more than one month, the incidence rises steeply with age. In one survey, the prevalence of pain one year after the eruption was 4.2% in patients younger than 20 years old and 47% in those older than 70.

21. What is the natural history of PHN?

PHN gradually improves in most patients, and clinical experience suggests that the best predictor of future improvement is the course during the recent past. Given this natural history, the interpretation of uncontrolled therapeutic trials must be very cautious, particularly if the treatment was administered to patients relatively soon after the acute herpes zoster infection. Many ineffective treatments for PHN have been introduced on the basis of "favorable" effects observed during uncontrolled trials. Clinical studies of treatments for PHN should be controlled, if possible, and include a stringent time criterion, such as four months from onset of the lesion.

22. What are the important clinical features of PHN?

Herpes zoster erupts in the thoracic dermatomes in more than 50% of patients. The trigeminal distribution (usually V^1) is next most common. Lumbar and cervical zoster each occurs in 10 to 20% of patients. Regardless of location, the pain of PHN is usually complex, described as some combination of deep aching, superficial burning, and paroxysmal pain. Itch is also commonly reported. Allodynia or hyperpathia is variable; in some patients, the sensitivity to touch is the most distressing component.

23. Can PHN be prevented?

With the advent of the varicella vaccine, primary prevention of PHN is now feasible. If this vaccine does not itself cause zoster (yet to be determined), a true reduction in the incidence of this lesion will be observed many years after its use becomes widespread.

Early studies of interferon, vidarabine, and acyclovir demonstrated that the administration of antiviral drugs during the acute phase of herpes zoster could produce short-term analgesia and could improve healing of the eruption. More recent trials of the newer oral antiviral agents valacyclovir and famciclovir suggest that these drugs can shorten the zoster episode reliably enough to reduce the incidence of prolonged pain for the study sample overall. These data suggest, therefore, that early treatment with a specific antiviral drug can indeed reduce the incidence of PHN. Additional experience with these drugs will be needed to determine their true efficacy as preventive agents.

There is no good evidence that any of the other currently available therapies for acute herpes zoster prevents PHN. Corticosteroids and early sympathetic nerve block can have valuable analgesic effects during acute zoster, but do not prevent PHN. A recent survey suggests that the use of low-dose amitriptyline during acute zoster reduces PHN, but this finding requires confirmation.

24. What is an appropriate management strategy for acute zoster?

The use of antiviral therapy is the first question to address when developing a strategy for the treatment of acute herpes zoster. Antiviral therapy should be used if patients are at significant risk for tissue injury from the virus itself. Patients who are immunocompromised and those who have overt or imminent injury to the cornea or evidence of damage to motor nerves or nerves supplying viscera (such as the bladder) are in this category. Patients at high risk of PHN, including older patients (> 60 years), those with very intense cutaneous eruptions, and those with very severe pain are also candidates for antiviral therapy. In all patients, the pain should be aggressively managed with some combination of local measures and analgesic drugs (nonsteroidal anti-inflammatory drugs or opioids). The immunocompetent patient with severe pain that has not responded to analgesics and an antiviral should also be considered for a trial of corticosteroid and/or sympathetic blockade.

25. Both topical and systemic analgesic drugs are commonly used in the treatment of PHN. What are the topical therapies for this condition?

Both topical and systemic analgesics are used in the treatment of established PHN. Studies have established that some patients benefit from application of the eutectic mixture of lidocaine and prilocaine (EMLA) or from 10% lidocaine gel. EMLA is commercially available, and patients who are able to apply it should be considered for a trial. Some patients benefit from applications that do not produce dense cutaneous anesthesia, and therapy in such cases usually involves a thin application several times per day. Other patients experience analgesia only if cutaneous anesthesia is produced. This usually requires a thick application of the cream for at least one hour under an occlusive dressing. This may not be feasible if the painful area is very large or situated in areas that cannot be covered.

Some data support the use of topical anti-inflammatory drugs, such as aspirin in chloroform. Clinical experience with this approach has not been very favorable, and it is seldom used.

Another topical therapy, capsaicin cream, has been advocated on the basis of uncontrolled observations. Capsaicin is a naturally occurring compound that selectively depletes peptide neurotransmitters (such as substance P) from small-diameter primary afferent neurons. Current experience suggests that an adequate trial of this drug, which is generally believed to require three to four applications daily for approximately four weeks, will identify a small proportion of patients who report substantial pain relief. Some patients develop local burning and are unable to proceed with a trial.

26. What systemic analgesic therapies have been used for PHN?

Systemic drug therapy for PHN follows the same general approach recommended for other types of neuropathic pain (see Chapter 33). The usual first-line approach comprises one or more adjuvant analgesics. The adjuvant analgesics that have been specifically evaluated for PHN include the antidepressants, amitriptyline, desipramine and maprotiline; the anticonvulsant, carbamazepine; and the alpha-adrenergic agonist, clonidine. Sequential trials with these and other drugs in this category (such as other antidepressants and anticonvulsants, oral local anesthetics, and others) are the major approach to the pharmacotherapy of PHN. Occasional patients benefit from a nonsteroidal anti-inflammatory drug or long-term opioid therapy.

27. What is the status of nonpharmacologic therapy for PHN?

Similar to other types of chronic pain, PHN is best approached using a strategy that addresses the dual goals of comfort and improved function and considers multimodality treatments in every case. For the pain specifically, a variety of nonpharmacologic interventions are sometimes considered.

The anesthetic approaches that have been specifically advocated for PHN include skin infiltration with local anesthetic or local anesthetic and steroids, intravenous local anesthetic, temporary or permanent blocks of peripheral nerves or nerve roots, sympathetic blocks, epidural steroid administration, and application of a cryoprobe to painful scars. With the exception of intravenous lidocaine, all the clinical reports of these procedures describe anecdotal experience. Patients with severe refractory pain are often offered empirical trials of intravenous lidocaine (e.g., 2 to 4 mg/kg over 30 minutes), temporary nerve blocks with local anesthetic (including sympathetic nerve blocks), or techniques that involve subcutaneous instillation of local anesthetic or local anesthetic plus a corticosteroid. Neurolysis is not considered except in the most extreme situations because of the uncertain nature of the results and concern about the possible adverse effects of increased denervation.

In a similarly empirical manner, a trial of a noninvasive neurostimulatory approach, usually TENS, or a trial of acupuncture is often attempted in cases of refractory neuralgia. The use of noninvasive neurostimulatory therapies, specifically dorsal column stimulation, is supported by a small number of favorable case reports, and such an approach is sometimes suggested for patients with severe pain refractory to conservative approaches. Although patients with PHN have been reported to benefit from a very diverse group of surgical procedures, including neurectomy, rhizotomy, sympathectomy, cordotomy, trigeminal tractotomy, mesencephalotomy, mesencephalothalamotomy, and thalamotomy, the accumulated clinical experience with these techniques has been disappointing and none is recommended routinely.

Physiatric and psychological approaches are often recommended to patients with refractory PHN in an effort to improve function and, in some cases, alleviate pain. These techniques should be particularly considered for those patients whose pain leads to immobilization of a limb, general inactivity, or maladaptive behaviors.

28. The existence of central pain syndromes provides strong evidence for the concept that changes in the CNS can result in chronic neuropathic pain. What is central pain?

The term "central pain" generically describes the large number of deafferentation pain syndromes that can occur following injury to the central nervous system. These syndromes are variably named by the location of the lesion (e.g., thalamic pain), the inciting injury (e.g., poststroke pain), or the underlying disorder (e.g., pain due to multiple sclerosis). Syndromes associated with uncommon lesions (e.g., syringobulbia) or common lesions that rarely produce pain (e.g., brain tumors) are usually simply described generically as central pain.

29. What is known about the specific mechanisms that may result in central pain?

Although it is assumed that any of the changes that may be associated with "central sensitization" (see figure with question 5 and table with question 9) could be involved in the development of central pain, little is known of the specific processes involved. Clinical observations suggest that damage to spinothalamocortical pathways is a fundamental element in the development of central pain following a lesion at any level of the neuraxis. Possibly, deafferentation or disinhibition of central nociceptive neurons in the thalamus can follow such a lesion and result in the pathophysiologic changes that underlie the phenomenology of central pain.

30. Central pain following damage to the spinal cord has been best characterized in patients with traumatic or demyelinating lesions. What is the epidemiology of pain following spinal cord injury?

Following acute spinal cord injury, 10 to 49% of patients develop chronic pain. A variety of syndromes have been described, including a deafferentation, or central, pain syndrome. The epidemiology of this specific subtype of pain due to spinal cord injury is unknown.

31. What characteristics suggest the diagnosis of central pain due to spinal cord injury?

Central pain due to spinal cord injury is inferred to exist when dysesthesias occur in a non-segmental distribution below injury to the spinal cord itself. The clinical features are highly variable. Spontaneous and evoked dysesthesias may be associated with uncomfortable paresthesias described as tingling, numbness, or squeezing. These sensations can be experienced in any region below the injury. Painful areas may be small or large, unilateral or bilateral, and stable or fluctuating in size and location. Pain may increase spontaneously or in response to changes in climate, stress, smoking, or other factors. Flexor or extensor spasms, which may be spontaneous or precipitated by movement or by distension of the bladder or bowel, can contribute significantly to the pain. Ill-defined visceral pains, which are usually experienced in the lower abdomen or pelvis, are occasionally reported.

Because the spinal cord ends at the L1 vertebral body, central pain can be diagnosed only if an injury is rostral to this level. If chronic neuropathic pain occurs following a spinal injury below L1, the classification is more complicated. In some cases, the pain is segmental or multisegmental, and the pathophysiology is believed to be sustained by peripheral processes. In other cases, the pain is believed to be sustained by processes in the CNS that are induced by injury to the peripheral nerve. As discussed previously, this type of pain can be labeled a deafferentation syndrome fundamentally similar to phantom pain.

32. Can central pain due to demyelinating lesions of the spinal cord usually occur in the setting of established multiple sclerosis? What are the characteristics of this pain?

Chronic pain occurs in 23% to 80% of patients with multiple sclerosis. Central pain, which is the most prevalent type, usually occurs in patients with disease of long duration. The pain is usually described as continuous burning. It is sometimes associated with other types of dysesthesias or lancinating pains and may fluctuate in intensity spontaneously or in response to activity, stress, or change in weather. The location of the pain is most often the distal legs and feet, but occasional patients present with pain of similar quality in a dermatomal distribution or asymmetric nondermatomal region of the trunk or extremity.

33. What other types of spinal cord pathology have been associated with central pain?

Central pain has been described in association with vascular lesions of the spinal cord, syringomyelia, intramedullary and extramedullary neoplasms, cervical spondylosis, inflammatory lesions (e.g., syphilitic myelitis), subacute combined degeneration, and a toxic myelopathy. Central pain can also be iatrogenic, occasionally complicating spinal surgery or cordotomy.

34. Central pain can also result from lesions in the brain stem. The prototype syndrome is thalamic pain following ischemic or hemorrhagic vascular lesions. What are the characteristics of thalamic pain?

Thalamic pain usually occurs months to years after the injury. The pain is usually dysesthetic (continuous burning, often with intermittent stabbing) and may be associated with uncomfortable paresthesias (e.g., squeezing, gnawing, crawling, or tingling). Allodynia is common, and some patients experience dramatic hyperpathia, with diffuse radiation, duration far in excess of the stimulus, and extreme distress. The pain can be experienced in the entire hemibody or be localized to a small region. Occasional patients have a pseudoradicular distribution or a so-called cheiro-oral distribution (perioral region and ipsilateral hand).

The psychological and neurologic deficits associated with thalamic pain are diverse. Patients often become withdrawn, inactive, and profoundly depressed. The examination usually demonstrates an obvious sensory disturbance in some part of the affected hemibody. A deficit in pain and temperature sensation appears to be a constant. Patients may or may not have associated hemiparesis or choreoathetoid movements. Occasional patients demonstrate unilateral dysmetria or a Horner's syndrome.

35. Can central pain occur following injury to the cerebrum?

Central pain may complicate trauma, vascular lesions, or neoplasm in the cerebral hemisphere. This observation provides evidence that the cerebral cortex is important in the experience of pain. Other evidence includes the observation of disturbed pain perception from suprathalamic lesions, the identification of nociceptive cortical neurons in primates, the description of occasional patients who report pain following stimulation of parietal regions during cortical mapping experiments, and the rare occurrence of central pain in association with epileptiform cortical activity.

36. What management strategies are used for central pain?

The management of central pain is challenging. Like other chronic neuropathic pains, central pain is often best managed using a multimodality approach that focuses on both comfort and function. A controlled trial of amitriptyline and carbamazepine demonstrated clear analgesic effects from the former drug and equivocal effects from the latter in patients with central poststroke pain. Anecdotal reports have described the use of other tricyclic antidepressants, anticonvulsants (including carbamazepine), naloxone (administered as a brief infusion), mexiletine and other local anesthetics, diphenhydramine, propranolol, anticholinesterase inhibitors, chlorpromazine, L-dopa, and 5-hydroxytryptophan. Some patients respond favorably to opioid drugs, and selected patients may be considered for this therapy as well.

Occasional patients with central pain benefit from peripheral stimulation, usually TENS. Invasive neurostimulatory techniques, particularly deep brain stimulation, are considered if pain is refractory to systemic analgesic therapy.

Other invasive approaches play a very limited role in the management of central pain. Temporary somatic or sympathetic nerve blocks with local anesthetic may provide short-lived relief of central pain. These procedures are rarely used. Although the use of surgical neurolytic techniques for the treatment of central pain has been supported in case reports and small series, the likelihood of sustained benefit appears to be extremely low, and these procedures cannot be recommended. The only possible exception to this is the use of the dorsal root entry zone (DREZ) lesion for so-called "end zone" pain in patients with spinal cord injury.

37. Another deafferentation pain syndrome, avulsion of nerve plexus, is a rare but potentially devastating complication of limb trauma. What are the characteristics of this syndrome?

Although severe pain can complicate avulsion of a nerve root at any level of the nervous system, the most important clinical entity follows plexus avulsion injuries, which usually affect the brachial plexus and are commonly followed by severe pain in the insensate limb. Chronic pain, usually continuous burning dysesthesias with superimposed paroxysms, has been reported to complicate brachial plexus avulsions in 26 to 91% of patients. The onset of the pain can be immediate or delayed for months. In one series, approximately one-third had severe unrelenting pain more than two years after the injury. Stress, intercurrent illness, and changes in the weather have been reported to increase the pain; discomfort is sometimes reduced by distraction or stereotyped maneuvers, such as gripping or swinging the arm, or massaging the neck or shoulder. The limb, or portions of it, are anesthetic; most patients do not experience allodynia or hyperpathia, but paresthesias and other phantom-like phenomena may be experienced.

38. What management strategies are used for painful plexus avulsion?

Proper management requires accurate neurologic diagnosis. The distinction between injury to the nerve root itself and avulsion of the root is critical, because the former lesion may be amenable to nerve grafting. Diagnosis usually depends on a combination of clinical findings, electrodiagnostic studies, and imaging procedures (the most important of which is magnetic resonance imaging, which may demonstrate a pseudomeningocele in cases of root avulsion).

Like other chronic neuropathic pains, a multimodality approach to the treatment of painful avulsion should strive to improve both comfort and function. A specific surgical procedure, the DREZ, plays a special role in this disorder. Although there is a small possibility of major morbidity from this procedure, a very favorable clinical experience with this operation suggests that it should be considered only when pain is severe. Other surgical procedures are generally regarded to be ineffective. The favorable outcome associated with the DREZ lesion suggests that the pathophysiology of the pain associated with avulsion resides in the dorsal horn of the spinal cord.

There are no controlled trials of drug therapy in the treatment of pain associated with avulsion injuries. Empirical trials of adjuvant analgesics and opioids should be considered. Other therapies that have been used include sympathetic nerve block, TENS and dorsal column stimulation, trigger point injections into associated regions of myofascial pain, and a variety of psychological and rehabilitative therapies. Splinting of the paralyzed arm and intensive physical therapy to retain residual strength and prevent contractures and joint ankylosis are usually important interventions.

39. A disorder known as sympathetically maintained pain is also inferred to have a predominating CNS pathophysiology. What is sympathetically maintained pain?

Sympathetically maintained pain (SMP) is a subtype of neuropathic pain that appears to be sustained by efferent activity in the sympathetic nervous system. The specific mechanisms involved are unknown and somewhat controversial, and there has been considerable confusion about the classification of pain syndromes that may be included in this category. Historically,

SMP has been viewed as equivalent to the diagnoses of reflex sympathetic dystrophy and causalgia, or, at least, a major subtype of these disorders. The distinguishing features of reflex sympathetic dystrophy and causalgia have been poorly understood, however, and the actual relationship with SMP has been obscure. This has created confusion about all these diagnoses.

In an effort to clarify the nomenclature, the International Association for the Study of Pain has adopted the term "complex regional pain syndrome (CRPS) type I and II" to refer to disorders that have the clinical characteristics of reflex sympathetic dystrophy and causalgia, respectively. Patients with CRPS are assumed to have a neuropathic pain, which is presumably produced by some constellation of mechanisms that may or may not involve the sympathetic nervous system. Patients with CRPS, therefore, may or may not have SMP. Although there is a clear association between CRPS and SMP, such that the clinical findings indicative of CRPS should immediately suggest the potential value of interventions directed to the sympathetic nervous system, the two disorders are considered independent. Some patients who do not meet criteria for CRPS also respond favorably to sympathetic nerve block and, by definition, also have SMP.

40. What is known about the mechanisms of CRPS and SMP?

The specific mechanisms responsible for the unique characteristics of CRPS are unknown. Various mechanisms, which may involve processes in the peripheral nervous system or in the CNS, have been proposed to explain SMP, but no one mechanism, or group of mechanisms, has been confirmed. Based on clinical observations (such as the usual failure of peripheral denervation as a treatment for SMP), there is strong suspicion that the essential pathophysiology involves a process in the CNS. The specifics are unknown, however, and there continues to be controversy about the nature of both SMP and CRPS. Indeed, some authors even question whether SMP actually reflects a relationship between pain and sympathetic efferent function. An alternative hypothesis suggests that SMP is actually related to the transmission of nociceptive information in visceral afferents that travel with the sympathetics.

Mechanisms That May Be Involved in the Development
of Sympathetically Maintained Pain

Peripheral Processes
    Activity in nociceptive visceral afferents that travel with sympathetic efferent fibers
    Processes involving sympathetic-somatic link
        Sympathetic hyperactivity changes peripheral tissues in a way that activates nociceptors
        ("vicious circle")
        Damaged nociceptors have increased sensitivity to catecholamines released by
        sympathetic nerves
        Prostaglandins released by sympathetic nerves may sensitize nociceptors
        Sympathetic-nociceptor ephapses may form

Central Processes
    Sympathetically driven activity in nonnociceptive afferents could increase firing of
        sensitized wide dynamic range neuron in the spinal cord

---

41. What is the epidemiology of the disorders now known as CRPS?

Reflex sympathetic dystrophy (CRPS type I) can complicate injury to soft tissue, joint, or bone at any site, including head and trunk. Orthopedic injury to an extremity appears to be the most common predisposing factor. The precipitating injury can range from mild to severe, and some cases develop without any prior event. Although systematic epidemiologic studies are lacking, the incidence following even severe injury appears to be extremely small.

The classic lesion that predisposes to the development of causalgia (CRPS type II) is a high-speed missile injury that causes stretch, but not interruption, of a peripheral nerve. Surveys of veterans suggest that causalgia can complicate 1 to 5% of such injuries. The vulnerability to causalgia varies with the location of the injury: 90% of cases have damage above the knee or elbow, and the order of nerve involvement is sciatic (40%), median (35%), medial cord of the brachial plexus (12%), and other nerves (13%). The cause of this selective vulnerability is unknown.

There is a variable interval between injury and the onset of dysesthesia and the other clinical findings indicative of a CRPS. Many patients report that the syndrome began immediately or within hours of the event; others state that the onset was delayed by months.

42. What are the clinical characteristics of the complex regional pain syndrome?

CRPS type I and type II are distinguished solely by the history of major nerve injury that characterizes the latter disorder. The diagnosis of either type should be made when chronic pain, which typically has a prominent burning component, is accompanied by autonomic dysregulation in the region of the pain. Autonomic dysregulation may be characterized by swelling, vasomotor instability (e.g., color change or livedo reticularis), or abnormal sweating. Some patients also develop so-called trophic changes and abnormal motor activity. Trophic changes may include skin that becomes thin and shiny, increase or decrease in the growth of hair or nails, focal atrophy of subcutaneous tissue or muscle, or focal osteoporosis. Abnormal motor function may include tremor, other dyskinesias such as myoclonus or chorea, or dystonia. Other findings on the neurologic examination are similarly variable and may include raised thresholds for sensory stimuli (hypesthesia or hypalgesia), exaggerated responses to suprathreshold events (hyperesthesia, hyperalgesia, allodynia, or hyperpathia), or, paradoxically, a combination of these phenomena.

Occasionally, a patient with chronic neuropathic pain is suspected of having a CRPS, but the clinical manifestations of autonomic dysregulation or trophic changes are so subtle that the diagnosis cannot be made. If it is important to establish the diagnosis, ancillary tests may be useful to identify subtle autonomic or trophic phenomena. Autonomic changes in the painful region may be indicated by thermographic demonstration of asymmetric skin temperatures or by testing of sudomotor function. Trophic changes may be indicated by patchy demineralization on plain radiography or abnormal radionuclide uptake on a bone scintigram. A three-phase bone scintigram is preferred by some clinicians, who believe that it may be a more sensitive indicator of the abnormalities associated with CRPS. None of these tests have been evaluated in terms of sensitivity, specificity, or predictive value.

Although some authors have described the progression of reflex sympathetic dystrophy (CRPS type I) in three well-defined stages characterized by specific constellations of symptoms and signs, large surveys have not confirmed these patterns in most patients. Rather, there is great individual variation in both clinical findings and long-term outcomes. There are many reports of remission following early and intensive therapy, and some patients appear to remit spontaneously. Others remit and relapse or have a course characterized by persistent or worsening pain.

43. The diagnosis of CRPS is usually followed by a procedure to block sympathetic innervation to the painful site. If this procedure relieves pain, it may be both diagnostic (establishing the existence of SMP) and therapeutic. How is sympathetic block performed, and how should the response be interpreted?

The traditional method to block sympathetic efferent functions is via neural blockade. A variety of procedures can be used. Pain in the head and upper extremity is usually approached by injection of local anesthetic into the region of the cervical sympathetic chain (the so-called stellate ganglion block), and pain in the lower extremities is typically approached by injection of anesthetic into the region of the lumbar sympathetic chain.

Sympathetic blockade in a limb can also be accomplished using a regional intravenous technique, in which a drug that depletes adrenergic transmitters from sympathetic nerve endings, such as guanethidine or bretylium, is injected into a vein while the venous outflow from the extremity is interrupted with a compression cuff. Although the sympathetic block produced by this procedure can be prolonged, there have been no clinical trials confirming the efficacy of the procedure. A recent meta-analysis of published data failed to demonstrate any benefit whatsoever. Nonetheless, a regional intravenous infusion is still considered for those patients with suspected SMP who are unable or unwilling to undergo neural blockade.

The final approach to sympathetic blockade is via the intravenous injection of the alpha-adrenergic blocking agent phentolamine. This so-called phentolamine test has become widely used as a diagnostic test, and, occasionally, repeated procedures are used therapeutically. Notwithstanding, there have been few studies of the technique, and it is still uncertain that it can fully substitute for sympathetic nerve block.

Most patients undergo a trial period during which at least several sympathetic blocks are performed before the diagnosis of SMP is rejected. The standard approach varies from clinician to clinician. Some recommend the procedure daily, whereas others perform it weekly or less often during this initial period. In some severe cases, continuous sympathetic blockade using local anesthetic infusion is attempted.

The interpretation of a patient's response to sympathetic block can be complicated by technical problems (e.g., how effectively sympathetic outflow was interrupted), the placebo response, and the limitations in the scientific literature about this procedure. Clinical reports of sympathetic nerve block, for example, usually do not apply placebo controls, identical techniques, or standardized criteria for a favorable outcome. Neither these reports nor studies of the phentolamine test provide sufficient information to clearly establish criteria for a positive outcome, or determine the long-term implications of an outcome that appears positive at the time of the test. Most provide no clear indication of the degree or acceptability of pain relief, response of associated phenomena, overall improvement in the functional capacity of the patient, or the ability of the procedure to predict long-term outcome.

Despite these difficulties, clinicians still hold to the view that a diagnosis of CRPS should generally be followed by a trial of sympathetic block to determine whether an SMP also exists. The patient's response is usually considered positive if substantial relief is experienced for a period that exceeds the duration of the local anesthetic by many hours or days.

44. What management strategies are used for patients who have a favorable response to diagnostic sympathetic block?

Patients with CRPS who have a favorable response to a diagnostic sympathetic block and, therefore, are considered to have a co-existing SMP) are usually offered a therapeutic strategy that incorporates repeated or ongoing interruption of sympathetic outflow to the painful area. The approach varies among clinicians and may involve any of the aforementioned procedures on a rigid schedule or on a schedule based on the clinical course of the patient. A variety of responses are observed:

1. Transitory relief after each block that outlasts the duration of local anesthetic effect and lengthens with each block
2. Transitory relief that outlasts the duration of the local anesthetic effect but does increment with subsequent blocks
3. Transitory relief that gradually diminishes with each block, until the block is ineffective
4. A prolonged favorable response after one or a few blocks.

The size of each of these groups relative to the entire population with SMP is unknown.

The small minority of patients who develop a pattern of response to sympathetic blockade characterized by repeated short-lived periods of analgesia have traditionally been considered for permanent sympathetic interruption via chemical or surgical sympathectomy. Reported response rates for these procedures vary greatly, ranging from less than 15% to more than 90%.

Occasionally, systemic pharmacotherapy for a suspected or established SMP is desirable. As mentioned, this is sometimes accomplished using repeated intravenous phentolamine infusions. Orally administered drugs have also been used empirically, including sympatholytic (clonidine, prazosin, and various beta adrenergic blockers, such as propranolol) and nonsympatholytic drugs (calcitonin, nifedipine, and corticosteroids). The medical literature that describes the use of these drugs is very limited. Calcitonin is the only drug studied in a controlled trial, but the population in which it was effective had reflex sympathetic dystrophy, and the value of the drug in those with or without SMP is not known. Clonidine is a nonspecific analgesic and would presumably be effective in some patients with CRPS, irrespective of the co-existence of SMP. The information about the other drugs is limited to anecdotes or small surveys.

Clinicians generally agree that an effort to normalize the function of the painful part using intensive physical therapy is an essential aspect of the therapeutic approach to SMP. Patients with SMP who attain pain relief with sympathetic block should capitalize on periods of increased comfort by focusing on these function-oriented therapies. Rehabilitative approaches also can potentially prevent dysfunction in joints and muscles produced by disuse and trophic changes, optimize function at any given level of impairment, and improve psychological well-being.

45. What management strategies are used for patients with CRPS?

Patients with CRPS who do not have a co-existing SMP are usually managed like other patients with chronic neuropathic pain. All patients require a comprehensive assessment that identifies adverse psychological and behavioral phenomena and the extent of disability associated with the pain. A multimodality therapeutic plan that attempts to optimize both comfort and function ban be developed from this assessment. The most common approach combines sequential trials of analgesic drugs (nonopioid, opioid, and adjuvant analgesics) (see Chapters 31–33) with intensive rehabilitative and psychological interventions. Noninvasive neurostimulatory approaches, such as TENS, are also used.

There is a very limited role for invasive analgesic therapies in CRPS. Experience in the use of invasive neurostimulatory procedures, including acupuncture, percutaneous electrical nerve stimulation, dorsal column stimulation, and deep brain stimulation, is anecdotal. Procedures to isolate the painful part from the central nervous system, either temporarily using somatic nerve blocks or more permanently using chemical or surgical neurolysis, have yielded disappointing results and are not accepted. Similarly, clinical experience with amputation of the painful part has been unfavorable, and this should not be performed for analgesic purposes.

46. Although it is evident that profound changes in CNS occur following peripheral nerve injury, some types of neuropathic pain are inferred to have a sustaining peripheral pathogenesis. What mechanisms may be involved in pain syndromes that are presumably sustained by aberrant somatosensory processing in the peripheral nervous system?

On theoretical grounds, the varied processes that could lead to peripheral neuropathic pains may be broadly divided into those characterized by activation of normal nociceptors and those characterized by pathologic processes precipitated by axonal injury and attempts at regeneration. The inciting events that lead to these various mechanisms and the linkages between such mechanisms and clinical phenomena are largely unknown. The ability to infer a specific mechanism is limited and rarely changes clinical practice. The exception to this may be the development of a neuroma, recognition of which suggests a variety of peripheral therapeutic interventions targeted specifically to this pathology.

Mechanisms That May Be Involved in Neuropathic Pains Sustained by Aberrant Somatosensory Processing in the Peripheral Nervous System

---

Involving activation of nervi nervorum*

Activation of nociceptive nervi nervorum by mechanical or chemical factors
   (e.g., inflammation of nerve)
Sensitization of nociceptive nervi nervorum due to local injury
Disinhibition due to large fiber loss (i.e., loss of segmental inhibition), allowing increased
   transmission of nociceptive information via nervi nervorum
"Backfiring" C fibers, with peripheral release of algogenic substances

Involving aberrant activity from injured nerves[†]

Neuroma formation (severed nerve or incontinuity)
Focal demyelination
Ephapse formation

---

* Nervi nervorum are normal nociceptors that surround large nerves; pain attributed to this activity has been
   termed nerve sheath pain.
[†] Pain attributed to aberrant activity in damaged nerves has been termed dysesthetic pain.

47. What are the characteristics of a neuroma?

Neuromas may form at the end of a cut nerve or develop along the course of a successfully regenerated nerve (so-called neuroma-in-continuity). These regions, which appear pathologically as tufts of regenerating small nerve fibers, generate spontaneous discharges, both locally and at the level of the dorsal root ganglion. Once these regions of aberrant activity are established, ectopic discharges can be evoked by mechanical stimulation and changes in the local environment, including increased concentration of catecholamines, ischemia, and electrolyte disturbances. As illustrated by Tinel's sign, these evoked discharges can be associated with pain.

48. Neuropathic pains inferred to have sustaining mechanisms in the peripheral nervous system can be divided into a group of painful polyneuropathies and a group of painful mononeuropathies. Is anything known about the mechanisms responsible for painful polyneuropathy?

There are many types of painful polyneuropathy, and the variety of etiologies and differences on pathologic examination suggest that the mechanisms responsible for the pain are diverse. Some neuropathies involve predominant injury to the myelin sheath (myelinopathy), and some involve a generalized injury to the neuron itself (axonopathy). Most painful polyneuropathies are axonopathies. Examples include the neuropathies associated with diabetes and nutritional deficiencies.

Many studies have attempted to relate the pain associated with some axonopathies to selective fiber type dysfunction. It has been proposed, for example, that the pain from some polyneuropathies is related to ectopic activity originating from injured small fibers. Studies in patients with painful diabetic neuropathy appear to support this hypothesis. Other studies, however, indicate that all painful polyneuropathies cannot be attributed to this type of mechanism. Some painless neuropathies have selective small fiber loss and some neuropathies that are painful have either no selective damage or damage limited to large fibers. The occurrence of pain in several neuropathies with selective large fiber loss suggests an alternative hypothesis, namely that pain may relate to the loss of peripheral inhibition, which may be mediated by activation of large-diameter peripheral nerves. This hypothesis, however, fails to account for the existence of painless neuropathies with selective large fiber loss. Together, these data suggest that selective fiber type dysfunction may be involved in some painful polyneuropathies, but other mechanisms must be involved as well.

49. What are the characteristics of painful polyneuropathy?

Complaints about pain are relatively uniform among those disorders characterized by a generalized axonopathy. Patients usually report burning or other dysesthesias of the feet and distal legs (and the hands, when the lesion is advanced), paroxysmal lancinating pains that may be spontaneous or provoked, deep aching in the feet and legs, and muscle cramping. Some patients have allodynia or hyperpathia, and many describe accompanying paresthesias. Some patients find these paresthesias, such as tingling, "crawling" sensations, sensations of heat or cold, or a sense of swelling, to be very unpleasant.

Pain associated with myelinopathy, specifically the acute inflammatory polyneuropathy of Guillain-Barré syndrome, is generally aching and occurs in both the back and limbs. Muscle cramps occur as well.

50. Painful polyneuropathies are associated with many types of medical illness. What implications does this have?

The diseases associated with painful polyneuropathy are extremely diverse. Elucidation of those factors that precipitate or sustain the neuropathy may allow specific treatment targeted at the underlying cause of the neuropathy. The ability to prognosticate is also improved by knowledge of the associated illness. These benefits underscore the importance of a detailed medical assessment of all patients with painful polyneuropathy. This assessment complements the evaluation of pain-related morbidity that should be performed in patients with neuropathic pain.

Painful Polyneuropathies

Painful Polyneuropathy Due to Metabolic Disorders
  Diabetes neuropathy
  Neuropathy associated with insulinoma
  Nutritional deficiency
    Alcohol-nutritional neuropathy
    Specific vitamin deficiency (e.g., niacin, B_{12}, or pyridoxine)
  Hypothyroid neuropathy
  Uremic neuropathy
  Amyloid neuropathy
  Neuropathy associated with Fabry's disease
Painful Neuropathy Due to Drugs or Toxins
Painful Polyneuropathy Due to Neoplasm
  Subacute sensory neuronopathy
  Sensorimotor neuropathy associated with carcinoma
  Sensorimotor neuropathy associated with dysproteinemias
Hereditary Painful Polyneuropathy
Painful Polyneuropathies Associated with Guillain-Barré Syndrome

---

* Examples include isoniazid, gold, misonidazole, nitrofurantoin, vincristine, cis-platinum, paclitaxel, arsenic, cyanide, thallium.

51. Where does painful polyneuropathy fit among the heterogeneous peripheral nerve syndromes caused by diabetes?

Diabetes may cause a remarkably varied group of neuropathies. The distal symmetric polyneuropathies are usually distinguished from an autonomic neuropathy and various mononeuropathies, which may be focal or multifocal, and predominantly sensory or predominantly motor. These focal and multifocal mononeuropathies (such as femoral neuropathy and lumbar radiculoplexopathy [diabetic amyotrophy]) can be intensely painful. The distal symmetric polyneuropathies can be divided into distinct groups, each characterized by a predominant disorder either motor or sensory, as well as a mixed group in which all fiber types are affected. Patients who have a polyneuropathy in which sensory fibers are involved can have predominant involvement of large fibers, small fibers, or a mixed syndrome. The pathology associated with painful polyneuropathy is a distal symmetric polyneuropathy with predominant involvement of small-diameter afferent fibers. Studies suggest that the lesion that affects these fibers is both vascular and metabolic.

52. What are the major painful polyneuropathies associated with nutritional deficiency?

Painful polyneuropathy complicates a diverse group of nutritional deficiencies. The major syndromes include alcohol-nutritional deficiency polyneuropathy, thiamine deficiency, niacin deficiency, and pyridoxine deficiency. The pathogenesis of the alcohol-nutritional deficiency polyneuropathy probably involves multiple vitamin deficiencies. With abstinence and vitamin supplementation, symptoms and signs may improve. This neuropathy is indistinguishable from that associated with specific thiamine deficiency. A variety of other neuropsychological (Wernicke-Korsakoff syndrome) and cardiac ("wet" beriberi) manifestations may also develop from a lack of thiamine. Pellagra, the syndrome of niacin deficiency, is also associated with a polyneuropathy clinically similar to that observed in alcoholics. A dermatitis and gastrointestinal disturbances accompany the neuropathy in this condition. The neuropathy associated with pyridoxine (Vitamin B_6) deficiency almost never occurs as a result of inadequate naturally occurring pyridoxine, which is ubiquitous in food; deficiencies are almost always due to ingestion of pyridoxine antagonists, particularly the antituberculous agent, isoniazid.

53. What is the "burning feet" syndrome?

A subgroup of alcoholic patients develop the so-called "burning feet" syndrome, which is an acute syndrome characterized by intense burning pain in the feet associated with erythema and swelling. The syndrome can occur with or without clinical evidence of polyneuropathy, but is presumably neuropathic. Patients with other types of nutritional neuropathy can also develop this syndrome.

54. What metabolic disturbances can result in painful polyneuropathy?

Hypothyroidism and uremia produce well-characterized painful neuropathies. Hypothyroidism can cause a predominantly sensory polyneuropathy, which may be complicated by pain and muscle cramping. On pathologic examination, the neuropathy associated with hypothyroidism is associated with a relative impairment of large nerve fibers. Hypothyroid patients can also develop painful muscle cramping in the absence of a clinical neuropathy and painful mononeuropathies due to entrapment. The most common entrapment neuropathy is due to carpal tunnel syndrome.

A predominantly sensory polyneuropathy, which is often painful, is extremely common among those with chronic renal failure. Occasional patients develop severe dysesthesias, which can mimic the "burning feet" syndrome associated with nutritional deficiencies. Both muscle cramping and "restless legs" (often accompanied by uncomfortable paresthesias) are also common and can occur with or without clinical evidence of polyneuropathy. All these symptoms may improve with dialysis or renal transplantation.

55. Amyloid polyneuropathy is a painful, small fiber polyneuropathy. Which clinical syndrome is associated with this disorder?

Amyloid produces a progressive sensory polyneuropathy, which may occur in both primary and secondary amyloidosis and is usually associated with pain, impaired small fiber function (e.g., loss of pain and thermal sensibility), and signs of autonomic neuropathy (e.g., postural hypotension, impaired sweating, and gastrointestinal dysmotility). On pathologic examination, there is a selective loss of lightly myelinated and unmyelinated axons.

56. Another painful small fiber neuropathy occurs in patients with Fabry's disease. What is this disease, and what clinical syndrome does it produce?

Fabry's disease (also known as angiokeratoma corpus diffusum) is a rare lipid storage disorder with sex-lined genetics that results from a deficiency of the enzyme ceramide trihexosidase. The painful polyneuropathy, which is associated with selective loss of small myelinated and unmyelinated fibers, can cause continuous burning dysesthesias of the distal extremities and intermittent episodes of severe pain, which may be spontaneous or precipitated by activity or other factors. Other features include a maculopapular rash, the so-called angiokeratoma corpuscum, and, in the later phases, dysfunction of the heart, liver, and kidneys.

57. What clinical syndromes caused by exposure to toxins or drugs are associated with painful polyneuropathy?

Although scores of drugs and toxins may damage peripheral nerves, relatively few cause a painful polyneuropathy. Knowledge of these syndromes is important because removal of the drug or toxin usually leads to gradual improvement. The drugs clearly associated with painful polyneuropathy include isoniazid, gold, misonidazole, nitrofurantoin, and the chemotherapeutic agents vincristine, cis-platinum, and paclitaxel. Pain can also be an uncommon accompaniment of other drug-induced neuropathies, but the prevalence of this complication cannot be stated reliably. The toxins associated with dysesthesias include arsenic (acute or chronic exposure), cyanide poisoning (chronic ingestion of sublethal doses), and thallium salts (acute and subacute ingestion).

58. Nerve injury is common in the cancer population and may result from direct compression by tumor, the toxic effects of antineoplastic therapy, associated metabolic disturbances, or poorly understood remote (paraneoplastic) effects. What are the major paraneoplastic painful polyneuropathies?

The painful polyneuropathies associated with cancer include sensorimotor neuropathy associated with carcinoma, sensorimotor neuropathy associated with dysproteinemia, and a specific disorder known as subacute sensory neuropathy. The sensorimotor neuropathy associated with carcinoma is a nonspecific paraneoplastic polyneuropathy that can complicate any tumor type. The clinical features, including the onset and course, are variable. Pain may or may not occur, and the incidence, characteristics, and course of this symptom have not been defined.

The sensorimotor neuropathies associated with the dysproteinemia are somewhat better characterized. A painful polyneuropathy may complicate multiple myeloma, Waldenstrom's macroglobulinemia, solitary plasmacytoma, and osteosclerotic plasmacytoma. Cryoglobulinemia may also result in a pain syndrome, which can be described as acral pain on exposure to cold. In all cases, symptoms and signs often precede the diagnosis of the underlying neoplasm by many months.

Subacute sensory neuronopathy is a well-described subtype of paraneoplastic neuropathy that usually begins with aching pain and dysesthesias and paresthesias in the distal extremities. Small cell carcinoma is the most common associated tumor, but other carcinomas and lymphomas have been reported. Symptoms are progressive and ultimately become associated with severe impairment of sensory functions, particularly those mediated by large fibers. The syndrome often precedes discovery of the tumor by months or years, and the course of the neurologic syndrome is usually independent of the neoplasm. On pathologic examination, this disorder has been associated with degeneration of sensory neurons in the dorsal root ganglia. Although the inciting processes are not known, there is evidence that a humoral immunologic insult mediates this lesion.

59. Are there other painful polyneuropathies?

Aching or lancinating pains may be experienced by patients with hereditary sensory neuropathy type I, a rare dominantly inherited neuropathy that predominantly affects small myelinated and unmyelinated fibers. Other acquired disorders that may be associated with painful polyneuropathy include the Guillain-Barré syndrome, which is an acute myelinopathy, and the chronic myelinopathies, such as the disorder known as chronic inflammatory demyelinating polyneuropathy. Porphyria and any of the autoimmune diseases can also have pain as a prominent symptom in some patients. Rarely will an idiopathic neuropathy be accompanied by disabling pain.

60. What management strategies are used for painful polyneuropathy?

Like patients with other neuropathic pains, patients with painful polyneuropathy must be carefully assessed to develop a multimodality approach that integrates treatments intended to enhance comfort with treatments intended to enhance function. Assessment must include an assiduous search for the underlying etiology of the neuropathy. Primary treatment, such as improved glycemic control for the diabetic or vitamin repletion for those with nutritional neuropathy, can provide some patients with dramatic symptomatic relief and should be implemented whenever appropriate.

The use of analgesic drugs, including nonsteroidal anti-inflammatory drugs, opioids, and many of the so-called adjuvant analgesics, parallels the approaches used for other types of neuropathic pain. A trial of topical capsaicin may also be warranted on the basis of a favorable trial in painful diabetic neuropathy.

Drug therapies directed at the primary disorder and analgesic drugs are usually combined with physiatric and psychological interventions, as appropriate. There is a very limited role for invasive analgesic approaches. There have been favorable anecdotal reports about the use of dorsal column stimulation, but this procedure should be considered only in those patients with refractory disabling dysesthesias who have been evaluated by experienced practitioners. With the exception of trigger point injections, which appear to benefit occasional patients who develop secondary myofascial pains in limbs weakened by the neuropathy, anesthetic approaches are rarely useful. There is no evidence that denervation procedures improve painful neuropathy.

61. In addition to the painful polyneuropathies, neuropathic pains related to aberrant processes in the peripheral nervous system also include mononeuropathies and multiple mononeuropathies. These diverse symptoms have been divided into a few subtypes, including a group of disorders that may be considered "lancinating neuralgias." What are the lancinating neuralgias?

As typically applied, the term "neuralgia" refers to pain caused by damage to a peripheral nerve and is experienced in the distribution of the nerve. This terminology can be confusing given the varying types of painful peripheral mononeuropathies, and it is useful to clarify it by distinguishing a group of disorders related to nerve injury and described as brief paroxysmal pains (i.e., lancinating pains similar to trigeminal neuralgia). These disorders may be called "lancinating neuralgias."

62. What is known about the mechanisms that may be specific to the lancinating neuralgias?

It has been proposed that both a peripheral process and a central process are necessary elements in the pathogenesis of trigeminal neuralgia and, by extrapolation, of the other lancinating neuralgias. In the case of trigeminal neuralgia, the peripheral lesion usually appears to be an arterial loop that chronically injures the trigeminal nerve at a site just outside the brain stem. Presumably, this focus can both produce ectopic impulses and diminish segmental inhibition. Such processes might predispose to paroxysmal discharges of interneurons in the trigeminal nucleus, which, in turn, cause intermittent paroxysmal firing of trigeminothalamic projection neurons that underlie the experience of pain.

63. What are the characteristics of the lancinating neuralgias?

The lancinating neuralgias are characterized by the experience of brief, usually shocklike pains, which may occur in isolation or in runs of variable duration. Some patients also experience a more continuous aching or burning of milder intensity in the region of the neuralgia. The latter pain may occur for a brief period after a severe attack of the lancinating component or more continuously during periods of frequent attacks.

64. What are the common types of lancinating neuralgias?

Trigeminal neuralgia is the best characterized lancinating neuralgia. This syndrome most often affects the mandibular branch of the trigeminal nerve. Pain is usually precipitated by activation of a trigger zone or sometimes by activities such as chewing. The neurologic examination in idiopathic trigeminal neuralgia is normal. When secondary (e.g., related to multiple sclerosis or a tumor in the middle cranial fossa), the examination may demonstrate findings consistent with trigeminal dysfunction. Large surveys have suggested that most patients with idiopathic trigeminal neuralgia have structural pathology, such as an aberrant arterial loop or a fibrous band, that compresses the trigeminal adjacent to the brain stem.

Other neuralgias of the head and neck have been well characterized, including glossopharyngeal neuralgia, occipital neuralgia, geniculate (or nervus intermedius) neuralgia, and superior laryngeal (or vagal) neuralgia. The variety of these syndromes suggests that any focal nerve injury anywhere in the body can result in predominant lancinating dysesthesias. When this occurs, the resulting disorder can be named according to the nerve affected. For example, intercostal neuralgia refers to lancinating chest pains that may follow injury to the intercostal nerves, and ilioinguinal neuralgia is used to describe intense inguinal stabbing pain that can complicate injury to the ilioinguinal nerve.

Uncommon Neuralgias of the Head and Neck

	PAIN SITE	FEATURES	PRECIPITANTS	NERVES
Glossopharyngeal neuralgia	Tonsillar fossa; pharynx	Syncope; cardiac arrhythmias	Swallowing; talking; cough; yawning	Cranial nerve IX
Occipital neuralgia	Suboccipital; occipital	Local tenderness (unilateral)	Head movement	Greater or lesser occipital nerve
Geniculate neuralgia	Deep in ear	Vertigo; tinnitus; herpes zoster (Ramsay-Hunt syndrome	Contact with ear canal; talking; swallowing	Nervus intermedius (Cranial nerve VII)
Superior laryngeal neuralgia	Larynx; throat; angle of the jaw	Hiccups; cough	Coughing; swallowing; talking; yawning	Superior laryngeal nerve (branch of vagus)

* Inference based on location of the pain and potential efficacy of nerve blocks.

65. If a pain syndrome occurs following injury to a peripheral nerve, will it always have a lancinating component?

As noted, injury to any peripheral nerve can result in a syndrome in which lancinating pains predominate. Alternatively, injury can result in a neuropathic pain syndrome largely or exclusively characterized as continuous dysesthesias. Although these differences presumably reflect variation in the underlying pathology or pathophysiology, the nature of this variation is unknown. From the clinical perspective, the difference is important because of the therapeutic implications associated with lancinating neuralgias.

66. What does the diagnosis of a lancinating neuralgia imply for therapy?

The existence of a structural lesion that distorts or compresses the nerve has been identified in a large majority of surgically managed patients with trigeminal neuralgia. Based on this observation, and a smaller surgical experience in patients with glossopharyngeal neuralgia and other syndromes, such structural lesions are assumed to be prevalent among all patients with idiopathic neuralgias of the head. This potential has justified surgical exploration of patients with intractable neuralgia.

Most patients with lancinating neuralgias benefit from drug therapy. The pharmacologic treatment of trigeminal neuralgia is the model for all the lancinating neuralgias. Conventionally, therapy proceeds first with trials of anticonvulsant drugs and a selected group of other drugs, such as baclofen and the oral local anesthetics.

Patients with pain syndromes refractory to drug therapy also may be candidates for invasive measures that destroy the offending nerve. The success of these procedures in some patients illustrates the importance of a peripheral pathophysiology for the pain.

67. Like the lancinating neuralgias, many other types of neuropathic pain can be inferred to have a sustaining peripheral pathogenesis. What are the major similarities and differences among the syndromes that can be classified in this way?

All painful mononeuropathies are associated with a peripheral nerve injury. The injury to the nerve may be traumatic, vascular, neoplastic, or inflammatory. The timing of the injury (acute, subacute, or chronic) may or may not correlate with the temporal characteristics of the pain, and the pain may precede or follow the overt presentation of the injury. The pain may be the only problem associated with the injury, or pain may accompany other neurologic deficits (motor, sensory, or autonomic) referable to the nerve.

The pain is usually experienced, at least partly, in the distribution of the damaged nerve. The descriptors used by patients with painful nerve injury vary. Some use words that are usually applied to nociceptive pains, such as aching, throbbing, or sharp, and others supply terms consistent with dysesthesia, including burning, electrical, or stabbing.

The diversity of these syndromes extends to the findings on examination of the painful area. There may be an area of sensory loss (that is, a raised threshold to response), with or without accompanying areas of hyperesthesia, hyperalgesia, allodynia, or hyperpathia. Focal tenderness is common, and some patients have a highly localized area of exquisite sensitivity along the course of a nerve, which may suggest the site of neuroma formation or entrapment.

The clinical heterogeneity in the population with painful mononeuropathy presumably reflects the varying mechanisms that may be responsible for the pain. As noted previously, these mechanisms may be broadly divided into those that produce pain as a result of axonal transection (resulting in neuroma or related pathology) and those that produce pain without severe damage to axons.

68. What type of pain syndromes are associated with nerve trauma?

The types of painful mononeuropathy that follow nerve trauma exemplify this broad division in the mechanisms that may be responsible for the pain. Trauma that severs axons may be followed by the development of a painful neuroma. The resultant syndromes, which include stump pain, postsurgical pain syndromes, and other traumatic nerve injuries, appear to be fundamentally similar. Nerve compression not severe enough to transect axons also is extremely common, and the pain syndromes that result presumably relate to mechanisms independent of neuroma formation. The latter syndromes, which include cervical or lumbar root compression and entrapment neuropathies, are extremely prevalent.

69. What pain syndromes are associated with other types of nerve pathology?

Severe pain can accompany acute inflammation of a peripheral nerve. This pathogenesis is observed in herpes zoster, idiopathic brachial or lumbar plexopathy (also known as plexitis), and local infection.

Nerve ischemia or infarction due to a vascular insult also can be very painful. The prototype disorder is diabetes mellitus, which is associated with many well-defined painful mononeuropathies related to nerve ischemia, such as femoral neuropathy. These disorders typically present a relatively brief progressive phase characterized by pain and evolving weakness; the pain usually improves gradually and strength slowly returns over months. Pain may also accompany a mononeuritis or mononeuritis multiplex due to vasculitis. Rarely, large vessel occlusion can cause a painful focal neuropathy. The pain in this condition may be due to ischemia of muscle and other soft tissue, as well as injury to the nerve.

Tumors originating from peripheral nerves are usually associated with pain. Whereas benign tumors, such as neurofibroma, typically cause modest pain, malignant neoplasms usually produce severe pain.

70. The diagnosis of a painful peripheral mononeuropathy suggests the potential utility of interventions directed at the site of the lesion. Should invasive approaches be used early in the management of these disorders?

Although invasive approaches intended to ameliorate focal pathology can provide some patients with dramatic analgesia, there are no assurances that such interventions will be helpful, and all carry substantial risks. In one survey, for example, 31 of 48 patients who underwent surgery for pain due to nerve injury were unchanged or made worse by the operation; almost half were made worse. The use of local invasive therapies requires sound clinical judgment informed by recognition of the latter possibility.

71. What noninvasive management strategies should be considered for painful mononeuropathies?

With few exceptions, the pharmacologic approaches to the treatment of painful peripheral mononeuropathies are nonspecific and similar to those applied in the management of other neuropathic pains. Both systemic and epidural corticosteroid therapy have been specifically advocated for painful radiculopathy, but controlled trials have failed to confirm the value of systemic steroids, and the use of epidural steroids remains controversial. Most experienced clinicians will consider the use of epidural steroid injection in selected patients with painful radiculopathy that has not responded to conservative management. A short course of a systemic corticosteroid has been shown to be beneficial in pain due to carpal tunnel syndrome, and it is possible this approach may be helpful in other types of compressive neuropathies.

Given the focal nature of the pain, a trial of a noninvasive neurostimulatory approach, such as TENS, should be considered in most cases. Physiatric and psychological interventions may benefit both pain and disability and should also be considered in all patients with painful peripheral mononeuropathies.

72. What invasive analgesic approaches should be considered for painful mononeuropathies?

Clinical experience indicates that some patients with painful mononeuropathy, particularly a syndrome consistent with neuroma formation, obtain long-term pain relief following repeated temporary nerve blocks or a prolonged block using a local anesthetic infusion technique. These procedures are relatively benign and could be considered earlier than those intended to produce permanent damage to neural tissue.

Neurolysis is sometimes considered for patients who experience transitory relief after each of many repeated nerve blocks. Cryoblock yields a longer lasting interruption of nerve function than local anesthetic instillation and has a lower likelihood of serious complications than chemical neurolysis. Although very limited data are available, the use of cryoblock may be considered an alternative to chemical or surgical neurolysis in carefully selected patients with painful mononeuropathy.

The focal nature of the painful mononeuropathies also suggests the utility of surgical approaches in some patients. As noted, the potential for deterioration exists with all such procedures, and none should be considered until after reasonable conservative measures have been exhausted. Surgery should not be performed unless local anesthetic blocks suggest that the pain could potentially improve if the peripheral focus was eliminated. Unfortunately, pain relief during anesthetic blocks does not predict successful outcomes from surgery.

The surgical approaches applied in the management of peripheral painful mononeuropathies usually address etiologic factors, such as release of entrapment, decompression of a nerve root, or resection of a neuroma. Procedures to denervate the painful part, such as neurectomy or rhizotomy, are rarely considered.

Invasive neurostimulatory approaches, such as dorsal column stimulation, do not damage neural tissue and may be a reasonable step in selected patients with refractory painful mononeuropathy. As with other types of neuropathic pain, the use of invasive neurostimulatory procedures should be considered only by experienced practitioners capable of providing a comprehensive assessment of the patient and expertise in the implementation of the technique.

BIBLIOGRAPHY

1. Asbury AK, Fields HL: Pain due to peripheral nerve damage: An hypothesis. Neurology 34:1587–1590, 1984.
2. Casey KL: Pain and central nervous system disease: A summary and overview. In Casey KL (ed): Pain and Central Nervous System Disease: The Central Pain Syndromes. New York, Raven Press, 1991, pp 1–11.
3. Devor M: The pathophysiology of damaged nerve. In Wall PD, Melzack R (eds): Textbook of Pain, 3rd ed. New York, Churchill Livingstone, 1994, pp 79–100.
4. Elliott KJ: Taxonomy and mechanisms of neuropathic pain. Semin Neurol 14:195–205, 1994.
5. Janig W, Blumberg H, Boas RA, Campbell JN: The reflex sympathetic dystrophy syndrome: Consensus statement and general recommendations for diagnosis and clinical research. In Bond MR, Charlton JE, Woolf CJ (eds): Proceedings of the Sixth World Congress on Pain. Amsterdam, Elsevier, 1991, pp 373–376.
6. Jensen TS, Krebs B, Nielsen J, Rasmussen P: Immediate and long-term phantom limb pain in amputees: Incidence, clinical characteristics and relationship to pre-amputation limb pain. Pain 21:267–278, 1985.
7. Leijon G, Boivie J, Johansson J: Central post-stroke pain—Neurological symptoms and pain characteristics. Pain 36:13–25, 1989.
8. Loeser JD: Cranial neuralgias. In Bonica JJ (ed): The Management of Pain, 2nd ed. Philadelphia, Lea & Febiger, 1990, pp 676–686.
9. Portenoy RK: Neuropathic pain. In Portenoy RK, Kanner RM (eds): Pain Management: Theory and Practice. Philadelphia, F.A. Davis, 1996, pp 83–125.
10. Watson CPN (ed): Herpes Zoster and Postherpetic Neuralgia. Amsterdam, Elsevier, 1993.

V. Psychological Syndromes

28. PSYCHOLOGICAL SYNDROMES

Dennis Thornton, Ph.D.

1. What psychiatric disorders are associated with pain problems?

Pain may be the chief complaint in a number of psychiatric disorders; conversely, pain may lead to many disturbing psychological symptoms. Pain is often the presenting symptom in somatoform disorders. Pain may be the main complaint in "masked depression," and depressive symptoms occur frequently in patients with chronic pain. Pain is rarely the presenting symptom of a delusional disorder. Individuals presenting with chronic pain secondary to accidents, often motor vehicle accidents, may exhibit symptoms of posttraumatic stress disorder. While anxiety is the most common concomitant of chronic pain, depression is the overriding symptom in chronic pain.

2. What is the DSM-IV?

The *Diagnostic and Statistical Manual of Mental Disorders, Fourth Edition*—DSM-IV—is the official manual of the American Psychiatric Association. Its purpose is to provide a framework for classifying disorders and defining diagnostic criteria for the disorders listed. A multiaxial system is employed to foster systematic and comprehensive assessment of the various clinical domains. Five axes are described; the first three relate to clinical diagnoses. Axis I: Clinical disorders and other clinical conditions that may be the focus of clinical attention; Axis II: Personality disorders and mental retardation; Axis III: General medical conditions; Axis IV: Psychosocial and environmental problems; Axis V: Global assessment of functioning. Of note is the fact that the DSM has recently undergone revisions, and some changes are relevant to the field of pain.

DEPRESSIVE DISORDERS

3. Is there an association between chronic pain and depression?

Depression is considered to be the most common emotional response to persistent pain. However, accurate assessment may be difficult. Significant depressive symptoms are present in 30 to 87% of patients with chronic pain, and 8 to 50% of patients meet criteria for a major depressive episode.

4. Name some impediments to the accurate assessment of depression in chronic pain populations.

Several issues lead to underdiagnosis of depressive symptoms. Physicians and patients often view a loss of energy, decreased interest, disrupted sleep pattern, appetite disturbance, and withdrawal as a normal reaction to severe pain and disability. Prolonged duration of these symptoms, however, may be indicative of a depressive syndrome. Patients may become defensive talking about their feelings because of societal stigmas regarding "mental illness" and may be reluctant to portray themselves as weak. Finally, shifting the focus to psychological issues may be threatening for the patient for fear that the examiner may conclude that the pain complaints are secondary to depression and not "organic" in nature.

5. What are the diagnostic criteria for a major depressive disorder?

Over at least a two-week period, and occurring nearly every day, the patient needs to have experienced five of the following: depressed/sad mood, markedly diminished interest or pleasure, significant weight loss or gain, insomnia or hypersomnia, psychomotor agitation or retardation, fatigue, feelings of worthlessness or excessive or inappropriate guilt, diminished cognitive abilities, recurrent thoughts of death, or suicidal ideation. These symptoms should not be better accounted for by another psychiatric disorder, medical illness, or reaction to medication. There is no history of a manic episode. These symptoms should represent a change from the patient's previous affective state.

6. How does the DSM-IV address psychological symptoms in patients with physical illness?

In DSM-III-R the focus was on psychological disturbance and symptoms "clearly due to a physical condition" were not included. This stipulation has been eliminated from the DSM-IV. Therefore, more individuals with chronic pain syndromes may meet criteria for specific psychiatric disorders.

7. What factors may put pain patients at risk for suicide?

Depressive symptoms and suicide are strongly associated. Forty-five to 70% of completed suicides have a history of mood disorder. Chronic illness and pain contribute to depressive symptoms. Physical illness is stated to be a significant contributing factor in 11 to 51% of suicides. Since many pain patients view themselves as disabled by their pain, often with little hope for improvement, they are at risk for affective disorders and suicidal potential. Work status decreases suicidal risk, while the loss of employment increases vulnerability.

8. Do chronic pain patients acknowledge their depression and suicidal feelings?

Willingness of any individual to confide these or other disturbing emotions depends upon a variety of factors. One survey, conducted by a pain self-help organization, found that patients with nonmalignant pain reported that depression was among the most disturbing aspects of the chronic pain experience. Fifty percent of these individuals commented that profound feelings of hopelessness had led them to consider suicide.

9. Are there data on suicide completion within the chronic pain population?

Although it is generally felt that this group is at significant risk, there is a dearth of literature on this subject. White men and women, aged 35–64 years, receiving workers compensation for pain, were shown to be a two to three times greater risk for suicide than the general population. However, this rate was significantly lower than that seen in a psychiatric population. Despite the study limitations, the authors concluded that chronic pain patients are at significant risk for suicide.

10. What depressive symptoms are seen in patients with chronic pain, even without true depression?

Chronic pain patients commonly experience alterations in weight: loss due to an absence of appetite, or gain secondary to a more sedentary lifestyle and/or medications. Sleep disturbances are also quite common, with individuals experiencing difficulty falling asleep or being awakened during the night because of pain. Pain and/or medication may impair concentration and decrease energy. Irritability, frustration, and dysphoria can parallel the level of pain.

11. What is dysthymia?

Dysthymic disorder refers to persistent, low level, depressive feelings. Dysthymia appears to be fairly common among chronic pain patients, individuals for whom the "glass is half-empty, and who describe their mood as "blue" or "down in the dumps" more often than not. There is a long-standing lack of interest, self-esteem is low, and there is a propensity for self-criticism.

Dysthymic patients describe their pessimistic outlook as "normal" for them (ego-syntonic). Major depressive episodes are a marked departure from the patient's normal euthymic mood. Depressed patients describe their pessimistic outlook as abnormal (ego-dystonic).

12. List the diagnostic criteria for dysthymic disorder.
   a. Over at least a two-year period, a depressed mood is present more often than not, i.e., most of the day and most days.
   b. While depressed, two or more of the following:
      (1) Poor appetite or overeating
      (2) Insomnia or hypersomnia
      (3) Low energy or fatigue
      (4) Low self-esteem
      (5) Poor concentration or difficulty making decisions
      (6) Feelings of hopelessness
   c. Over the two-year period, symptoms have not been absent for more than two months.
   d. The syndrome is not better accounted for by a major depressive episode, nor has such an episode occurred during the first two years of the symptoms.
   e. No history of a manic episode.
   f. Symptoms do not occur during the course of a psychotic disorder.
   g. Symptoms are not better accounted for by medication effects or secondary to a general medical condition.
   h. Significant occupational, social, or other impairment results from the symptoms.

13. What are adjustment disorders?
Applies to patients who do not meet criteria for dysthymia or major depressive disorder, but seem to be having significant difficulty coping. The diagnostic criteria are:
   a. Emotional or behavioral disturbance developing in reaction to an identified stressor and occurring within three months of the onset of the stressor.
   b. The syndrome is of clinical significance as noted by either:
      (1) Distress excessive to that expected by exposure to such a stressor
      (2) Impairment in social, occupational, or life sphere functioning
   c. Stress-related disturbance not better accounted for by another Axis I diagnosis or is an exacerbation of a pre-existing disorder.
   d. Symptoms do not represent bereavement.
   e. Upon cessation of the stressor, symptoms resolve within a six-month period.

ANXIETY DISORDERS

14. What is the association between anxiety and pain?
Anxiety is most closely associated with acute injury and pain. Autonomic signs (the "flight-or-fight" response) and emotional distress commonly appear together. Anxiety may also be associated with chronic pain and is often mixed with depressive symptoms.

15. How can anxious and depressive feelings influence the clinical presentation of pain complaints?
The Emergency Department (ED) is a setting in which anxiety symptoms and other disorders play a significant role in the patient's presentation. Thirty-five percent of patients presenting with acute chest pain to an urban ED were identified as displaying significant signs of panic (17.5%) or depression (23.1%). No difference in the prevalence of panic was observed between those with or without acute cardiac ischemia. Both panic and depression increased the likelihood of previous ED visits, and the authors concluded that about one in three patients presenting with acute pain to the ED reports symptoms consistent with a psychiatric disorder.

16. What are the core features of a panic disorder?

The quintessential feature is the unanticipated panic attack, often described as coming "out of the blue." At least two attacks are needed to meet criteria for panic disorder, and they are followed by protracted concern about experiencing additional attacks or the implications of the attacks. The concern continues for at least one month. Patients may seek medical reassurance, request tests, and report that they feel like they are "going crazy." If significant avoidance behaviors develop, the patient may meet criteria for panic disorder with agoraphobia.

17. Is general anxiety disorder (GAD) also associated with the pain experience?

GAD has also been associated with the presentation of somatic complaints, pain in particular. A fairly high incidence of anxiety has been noted within chronic pain inpatient programs. However, little work has been done to assess the prevalence of anxiety disorders among chronic pain patients being treated on an outpatient basis.

18. What are the primary diagnostic criteria for GAD?

Persistent and excessive worry or nervousness. Symptoms continue for six months and are present nearly all the time. The patient is unable, or finds it difficult, to control these concerns. Anxiety must be accompanied by at least three of the following: restlessness; fatigue; difficulty concentrating; irritability; muscle tension; or sleep disturbance. Symptoms are not better ascribed to another Axis I diagnostic category nor a consequence of an underlying medical condition. Distress and any associated physical symptoms result in significant disruption of functioning.

POSTTRAUMATIC STRESS DISORDERS

19. Is there an association between posttraumatic stress disorder (PTSD) and chronic pain syndromes?

PTSD (previously called "shell shock" or "battle fatigue") was a sequela of intense combat and war situations. However, increasing evidence shows that civilians can be subject to symptoms of PTSD, which may follow motor vehicle accidents, work-related injuries, or violent crime. Pain is a common concomitant of the disorder.

20. What are the essential clinical features of DSM-IV diagnostic criteria for PTSD?

    a. Experiencing, being exposed to, or confronted with a traumatic event in which serious harm or the threat of harm was present and the individual experienced an intense emotional reaction of fear, hopelessness, or horror.

    b. The event continues to be re-experienced through intrusive distressing recollections, disturbing dreams, flashbacks, intense emotional and/or physical distress upon re-exposure to symbolic cues.

    c. Persistent avoidance of symbolic stimuli and general psychic numbing manifest in such forms as avoidance of feelings, discussions, exposure to stimuli related to the trauma; amnesia for aspects of the trauma; diminished interest or detachment; restricted affect, and foreshortened future.

    d. Manifest symptoms of increased arousal, e.g., sleep disturbance, irritability, impaired concentration, hypervigilance, and an exaggerated startle response.

    e. Duration of symptoms exceeds one month.

    f. Significant impairment of functioning is present.

21. Do symptoms of PTSD occur commonly among patients with chronic pain?

About one-third of individuals reporting headaches and related pain complaints following a motor vehicle accident meet criteria for PTSD. Compared to those without symptoms of PTSD, those meeting criteria had a greater tendency to suppress their anger, were more depressed, and were more likely to have had a premorbid history of headaches. Individuals who had past anxiety disorders appear more likely to develop driving-related phobias than those without such histories.

22. What are the implications of PTSD in regard to chronic pain?

The early phases of treatment following accidents and injuries are most often focused on the medical and physical aspects, with the assumption that physical healing will allow for full recovery. Psychological trauma may go unnoticed, and functional progress may slow. Closer inquiry may reveal underlying anxieties, painful recollections, and emotional withdrawal. Patients may state that they no longer drive because of physical discomfort, but fail to mention the stress associated with driving. Providing support and informing patients that these psychological sequelae are not uncommon among pain patients will help them convey their fears, so that appropriate support can be provided.

23. Are there specific treatments for pain patients with symptoms of PTSD?

Systematic desensitization is a behavioral technique that has been shown to be quite successful treating phobias and has been successfully applied to pain patients with PTSD. The underlying premise is that you cannot be relaxed and anxious at the same time. The patient is taught relaxation and other coping strategies to foster a state of physical relaxation and inner calm and self-efficacy. The patient is then gradually exposed to the feared object.

24. Does domestic violence place a woman at higher risk for either PTSD or chronic pain syndromes?

Battering is an assault on the entire being. Constant fear, degradation, a lack of control and power, coupled with the physical pain and injury, have a devastating effect on self-esteem and a sense of identity. This continuous state of siege constitutes a unique trauma that can result in a plethora of psychological and somatic syndromes. Depression and posttraumatic stress disorder are commonly observed in this population. Pain complaints, both acute and chronic, may represent a guarded secret of conflict and a sense of helplessness.

25. What approach should the clinician take when domestic violence is suspected?

This is undoubtably a delicate situation where empathy and communication can go a long way. The most practical and effective way to address this problem is to establish the habit of routinely asking all women patients about their home life and violence. This will ease asking the necessary questions, which, in turn, can foster a sense of safety and acceptance, allowing the victim to share her experiences. It is important to avoid insinuations that can only further a sense of guilt.

FACTITIOUS DISORDERS

26. What is Munchausen syndrome?

It is the label given to a subpopulation of individuals diagnosed with a factitious disorder (DSM-IV). The stereotypic portrait is of a life-long history of somatic complaints, attempts to be admitted into hospitals, and requests for tests. Pain complaints often include severe right-lower-quadrant pain associated with nausea and vomiting, dizziness and blacking out, massive hemoptysis, generalized rashes and abscesses, fever of undetermined origin, bleeding secondary to ingestion of anticoagulants, and lupus-like syndromes. Patients often display considerable sophistication in presenting medical facts and treatments. Symptoms may be inconsistent with pathology; additional symptoms may spontaneously emerge during the interview; and symptoms are presented with a dramatic flair. This syndrome is uncommon, and a prevalence of 0.14% has been cited in a series of patients with chronic pain.

27. What are the diagnostic criteria for factitious disorders?

Four types are factitious disorders:
1. With predominantly psychological signs and symptoms.
2. With predominantly physical signs and symptoms.
3. With combined psychological and physical signs and symptoms.
4. Factitious disorder not otherwise specified.

Diagnostic criteria include:
1. The patient intentionally produces or feigns physical or psychological signs or symptoms.
2. The motivation for the behavior is to assume the sick role.
3. External incentives for the behavior (such as receiving economic gain, avoiding legal responsibility, or improving physical well-being, as in malingering) are absent.

28. What is the major distinction of the factitious disorder?
Individuals with factitious disorders intentionally feign either psychological or physical symptoms to assume the "sick role." These acts are voluntary in that the behaviors are purposeful and deliberate. However, they are performed with a degree of compulsivity, denoting the underlying psychopathology and an inability to curb such actions.

29. What is the distinguishing factor between factitious disorders and malingering?
Motivation. While both are intentional behaviors, the malingerer is motivated by external factors rather than an unconscious need to maintain the sick role. This motivational factor also distinguishes malingering from conversion disorder or other somatoform disorders. Because of the conscious and intentional nature of the behaviors, malingering is not considered a psychiatric disorder.

SOMATOFORM DISORDERS

30. What are the somatoform disorders, and what is their relationship with chronic pain syndrome?
Patients in this category express their unconscious conflicts as physical complaints (i.e., they "somatize"). In contrast to malingering, the disorders in this category are considered manifestations of unconscious processes rather than a conscious effort to deceive. These symptoms must be of such severity as to interfere with occupational, social, or interpersonal functioning or prompt the patient to seek and receive medical attention. Of the disorders listed, the most relevant for chronic pain patients are somatization disorder, conversion disorder, pain disorder, and hypochondriasis.

31. What are the DSM-IV diagnostic criteria for somatization disorder?
The somatization disorder was initially based on literature describing Briquet's syndrome. The new criteria are as follows:
a. A history of multiple somatic complaints that began prior to age 30 and have persisted over a number of years. Symptoms have resulted in social or occupational dysfunction and prompted the patient to seek medical treatment.
b. At some point during the course of illness, the patient must report experiencing: four pain symptoms, two gastrointestinal symptoms, one sexual symptom, and one pseudoneurologic symptom.
c. With the benefit of appropriate medical workup, there is either:
(1) No known medical explanation for symptoms or
(2) If a medical condition is identified, the symptoms, complaints, and impairment are excessive to the norm.
d. Symptoms are not feigned as in fictitious disorders or intentionally manufactured as in malingering.

32. What are the essential factors of the somatoform disorder?
Pain is the predominant feature and causes sufficient distress to warrant seeking medical attention and most likely interferes with daily functioning. Considerable time, effort, and money may be expended looking for the physician who will have the "cure," despite the report of negative or minimal findings, failed interventions, or repeated declarations that nothing more can be done to resolve the underlying problem.

33. What are the DSM-IV diagnostic criteria for pain disorder?

a. Pain is the prominent symptom, present in one or more areas of the body and of sufficient severity for the individual to seek medical attention.
b. Impairment of clinical significance is experienced in social and occupational life spheres.
c. Psychological factors are viewed as instrumental in the onset, course, or exacerbation of the pain complaint.
d. Pain is not produced intentionally.
e. The pain symptom is not better accounted for by another mental disorder.

Subtypes and specifics are:

Acute or chronic

1. Pain disorder associated with psychological factors.
2. Pain disorder associated with both psychological factors and a general medical condition.

34. What are the DSM-IV diagnostic criteria for hypochondriasis?

a. Patient is preoccupied with the belief or fear of having a serious illness, which is assumed because of misinterpretation of body sensations.
b. Patient is not dissuaded by appropriate reassurances.
c. Belief is not of delusional intensity.
d. Significant social and occupational impairment occurs in response to the intense distress.
e. Symptoms persist for at least six months.
f. Preoccupation is not better accounted for by another mental disorder.

35. Are pain patients likely to display symptoms of a conversion disorder?

Chronic pain patients may present with nonanatomic sensory symptoms (anesthesias and paresthesias). These symptoms have been noted among individuals said to be suffering from "compensation neurosis" and are cited as the third most frequent symptom following depression and anxiety. These types of nonanatomic sensory abnormalities have been found in anywhere from 24 to 50% of injured workers applying for compensation or Social Security disability. Male and female compensation patients appear equally likely to meet criteria for conversion disorder.

36. What are the DSM-IV criteria for conversion disorder?

a. Symptoms affect voluntary motor or sensory modalities suggesting a neurologic or medical condition.
b. Initiation and/or exacerbation of symptoms is associated with stressors or conflicts implicating psychological influence.
c. Symptoms are not intentionally produced.
d. Symptom pattern is not adequately explained by known medical condition or culturally sanctioned behavior.
e. Symptoms cause significant distress and disruption in function and prompt the patient to seek medical attention.
f. Symptom is not limited to pain or sexual dysfunction and is not better described as part of a somatization or other mental disorder.

37. What makes the somatizing patient difficult to treat?

These patients do not recognize the effect of their emotions. Although the onset of the symptom may have occurred during a stressful period, this connection may have been forgotten or denied by the patient. The symptom may allow the patient to ignore or deny the underlying conflict (primary gain). Individuals with a high degree of conversion are convinced of being ill (disease conviction), show few signs of dysphoria ("la belle indifference"), and tend to deny and/or minimize life problems apart from the physical symptoms.

38. Are chronic pain patients vulnerable to dependency on prescribed medications?

Severe and persistent pain prompts patients to seek virtually any means that will bring relief. Analgesic medications are commonly employed and are appropriate for treating acute pain.

There has been controversy regarding the continued use of analgesic medications, particularly opioids, in individuals presenting with chronic nonmalignant pain syndromes. While a small percentage of pain patients purposefully seek strong analgesics for the euphoric effects, it is not the rule and true addiction is unusual.

39. What determines substance dependence?

Current criteria include a maladaptive use pattern over a 12-month period that results in functional impairment and distress manifested by three or more of the following:

1. Tolerance
   a. Increasing amounts of the substance are needed to achieve the initial effect.
   b. Markedly diminished effect from the same amount.
2. Withdrawal
   a. Characteristic withdrawal symptoms if substance is stopped abruptly.
   b. Withdrawal symptoms are eased or eliminated with re-institution of substance.
3. Substance is used in greater amounts or for a longer duration than originally intended.
4. Persistent desire or unsuccessful efforts to curb or discontinue use.
5. Excessive time is spent in efforts to obtain or recover from the use of the given substance.
6. Occupational, social, and recreational activities are sacrificed because of substance use.
7. Despite acknowledgment of ill effects, substance use is continued.

BIBLIOGRAPHY

1. American Psychiatric Association: Diagnostic and Statistical Manual of Mental Disorders, 4th ed.. Washington, DC, American Psychiatric Association, 1994.
2. Chibnall JT, Duckro PN: Post-traumatic stress disorder in chronic post-traumatic headache patients. Headache 34(6):357–361, 1994.
3. Craig KD: Emotional aspects of pain. In Wall PD, Melzack R (eds): Textbook of Pain, 3rd ed. Edinburgh, Churchill Livingstone, 1994.
4. Dworkin RH, Gitlin MJ: Clinical aspects of depression in chronic pain patients. Clin J Pain 7(2):79–94, 1991.
5. Fishbain DA, Goldberg M, Rosomoff RS, Rosomoff H: Completed suicide in chronic pain. Clin J Pain 7:29–36, 1991.
6. Fishbain DA, Cutler RB, Rosomoff RS, Rosomoff HL: The problem-oriented psychiatric examination of the chronic pain patient and its application to the litigation consultation. Clin J Pain 10:28–51, 1994.
7. Fishbain DA, Goldberg M, Rosomoff RS, Rosomoff HL: More Munchausen with chronic pain. Clin J Pain 7:237–244, 1991.
8. Fishbain DA, Goldberg M, Labbe E, et al: Compensation and non-compensation chronic pain patients compared for DSM-III operational diagnoses. Pain 32(2):197–206, 1988.
9. Hitchcock LS, Ferrell BR, McCaffrey M: The experience of chronic nonmalignant pain. J Pain Symptom Management 9(5):312–318, 1994.
10. Kaplan HI, Sadock BJ: Synopsis of Psychiatry, 6th ed. Baltimore, Williams & Wilkins, 1991.
11. Miller L: Civilian post-traumatic stress disorder: Clinical syndromes and psychotherapeutic strategies. Psychotherapy 31(4):655–664, 1994.
12. Muse M: Stress-related, posttraumatic chronic pain syndrome: Behavioral treatment approach. Pain 25(3):389–394, 1986.
13. Smith GR: The epidemiology and treatment of depression when it coexists with somatoform disorders, somatization, or pain. Gen Hosp Psychiatry 14:265–272, 1992.
14. Smith PH, Gittelman DK: Psychological consequences of battering. Implications for women's health and medical practice. N C Med J 55(9):434–439, 1994.
15. Spence ND, Pilowsky I, Minniti R: The attribution of affect in pain clinic patients: A psychophysiological study of the conversion process. Int J Psychiatry Med 15(1):1–11, 1985–86.
16. Yingling KW, Wilson LR, Arnold LM, Rouan GW: Estimated prevalences of panic disorder and depression among consecutive patients seen in an emergency department with acute chest pain. J Gen Intern Med 8(5):231–235, 1993.

VI. Special Patient Populations

29. PAIN IN CHILDREN

Patricia A. McGrath, Ph.D.

1. What types of pain do children experience?

Like adults, children experience many types of acute, recurrent, and chronic pain. Acute pain is caused by a well-defined noxious or tissue-damaging stimulus (e.g., an injection or superficial skin injury).

Recurrent pain syndromes, such as repeated episodes of headaches, abdominal pains, or limb pains, constitute special pain problems for many otherwise healthy and pain-free children. The recurring pains may not be symptomatic of an underlying disease that requires medical treatment. Instead, the pain syndrome itself is the disorder, and the multiple physical and psychologic factors responsible for the pains must be identified and managed.

Persistent pain is any prolonged pain. The pain may be caused by a disease, such as cancer or arthritis, or may continue beyond the usual period required for healing injuries. In addition, children may experience persistent pain without any clear evidence of injury or tissue damage.

2. What myths have complicated our management of children's pain?

1. Infants have immature nervous systems and do not feel pain in the same way as older infants or children. (They do.)

2. Children do not have the same type of severe pain or chronic pain as adults. (They do.)

3. Health professionals cannot measure pain in children. (They can.)

4. Children are at a higher risk of drug addiction when they receive opioids for pain control. (They are not.)

3. When do infants first perceive pain?

At approximately 26 weeks' gestation, physiologic systems are developed so that a fetus can perceive pain. Thus, at birth, infants have the capacity to perceive pain and should receive appropriate analgesic or anesthetic treatments.

4. What are the primary differences between children's pain and that of adults?

The primary difference may be that the same amount of tissue damage produces stronger pain in children than in adults because of increased plasticity of developing systems. For example, neurodevelopmental research indicates that the endogenous pain inhibitory system is not yet fully developed at birth. Thus, newborn infants may experience greater pain than older infants and children from the same tissue damage.

Also, as children mature, they experience a wider diversity of pains, varying in quality and quantity. Since each new pain is evaluated against the perceptions the child has had to date, moderate tissue damage may evoke strong pain if that tissue damage is the maximum experienced by that child.

5. What is plasticity?

Like adults, children can experience pain without tissue injury or any apparent injury at all. They can also sustain injury without experiencing pain and can experience very different pains from the same type of tissue damage. Children's nociceptive systems are plastic in that they have the capacity to respond differently to the same amount of tissue damage.

We now know that children's perceptions of pain depend on complex neural interactions. Impulses generated by tissue damage are modified both by ascending systems activated by a noxious stimulus (e.g., touch) and by descending pain suppressing systems activated by various situational factors, such as a child's expectations about what he or she will feel.

6. How do you assess the intensity of pain in infants?
Several behavioral scales enable us to measure pain in infants and in children who are unable to communicate verbally about their pain. These scales are based on evaluating either physiologic responses (e.g., heart rate, blood pressure, oxygen level) or overt behaviors (e.g., cries, facial expressions, withdrawal behaviors) throughout a specified period. The greater the number of distress signals, the greater the pain level. Although these distress signals provide an *indirect* assessment of pain, several distress scales have been validated for clinical use.

7. How do you assess the intensity of pain in children?
Toddlers begin to communicate about their pain by pointing to its general location. Gradually, they learn to distinguish different levels, such as a little or a lot. Children under five can use poker chips that represent one to four pieces of hurt to show how much pain they have. Children five years of age and older can use a variety of standardized rating scales, including pain thermometers, visual analogue scales, and colored analogue scales to indicate the strength of their pain.

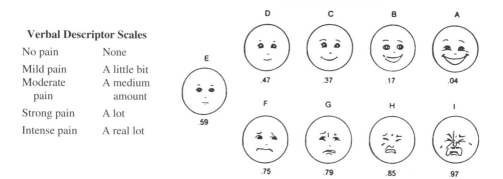

Facial Affective Scale

Verbal Descriptor Scales

No pain	None
Mild pain	A little bit
Moderate pain	A medium amount
Strong pain	A lot
Intense pain	A real lot

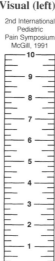

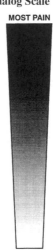

Visual (left) and Shaded Analog Scale

Measures used to assess children's pain: *Above left*, Verbal Descriptor Scales to assess pain intensity for children 7 years of age and older (list on left) and for children younger than 7 years of age (list on right). *Above right*, Facial Affective Scale to assess pain affect. (Reproduced with permission, McGrath, 1990). *Right*, Visual and Shaded Analog Scales to assess pain intensity.

8. Which assessment tool should be incorporated into routine clinical practice?

All clinicians should incorporate a few structured questions into their regular clinical interview to obtain objective information about the pattern, intensity, and quality of children's pain.
Children could be asked to describe their pain according to its similarity to other sensations they
have experienced. In addition, clinicians should use a simple standardized scale such as the visual
analogue scale, colored analogue scale, or pain thermometer (see figure at end of question 7) to
measure the intensity of a child's pain.

9. Is there a basic treatment algorithm that covers pain control in children?

The algorithm shown below provides a brief summary of the steps to controlling pain in children. The first step is to assess the child with pain, evaluating not only the primary sensory characteristics of the pain (its quality, intensity, location, duration, and aversive component) but also
the extent to which situational factors (cognitive, behavioral, and emotional) may be influencing
the child's pain. Appropriate physical and medical examinations should be directed not only at
the primary source of pain but also at secondary sources.

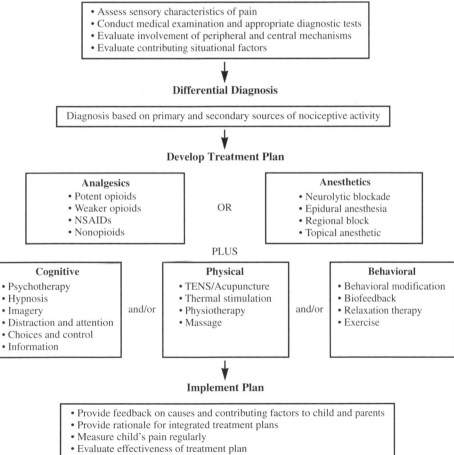

Assessing the Child with Pain

- Assess sensory characteristics of pain
- Conduct medical examination and appropriate diagnostic tests
- Evaluate involvement of peripheral and central mechanisms
- Evaluate contributing situational factors

Differential Diagnosis

Diagnosis based on primary and secondary sources of nociceptive activity

Develop Treatment Plan

Analgesics		**Anesthetics**
• Potent opioids	OR	• Neurolytic blockade
• Weaker opioids		• Epidural anesthesia
• NSAIDs		• Regional block
• Nonopioids		• Topical anesthetic

PLUS

Cognitive		**Physical**		**Behavioral**
• Psychotherapy		• TENS/Acupuncture		• Behavioral modification
• Hypnosis		• Thermal stimulation		• Biofeedback
• Imagery	and/or	• Physiotherapy	and/or	• Relaxation therapy
• Distraction and attention		• Massage		• Exercise
• Choices and control				
• Information				

Implement Plan

- Provide feedback on causes and contributing factors to child and parents
- Provide rationale for integrated treatment plans
- Measure child's pain regularly
- Evaluate effectiveness of treatment plan
- Revise plan as necessary

(From McGrath PA: Pain control in children. In Weiner RS (ed): Innovations in Pain Management. Paul M.
Deutsch Press, 1992, with permission.)

Once a differential diagnosis has been made, the treatment plan for most pains consists of analgesic or anesthetic interventions, plus cognitive, physical, and behavioral interventions, to address all the factors that contribute to the pain.

Children and parents should receive specific feedback on causes and contributing factors as well as the rationale for the treatments selected. Treatment includes measuring children's pain regularly, evaluating the effectiveness of interventions, and revising the plan as necessary. Since the factors that influence a child's pain are dynamic, not static, adjustments must be made to treatment regimens for children who will be experiencing recurrent or long-term pain.

10. What are the basic guidelines for selecting and administering analgesic interventions?

Four simple concepts should be followed when administering analgesics to children: (1) "by the ladder"; (2) "by the clock"; (3) "by the mouth"; (4) "by the child."

11. What is "by the ladder"?

"By the ladder" refers to a three-step approach for selecting progressively stronger analgesic drugs (acetaminophen, codeine, or morphine) based on a child's level of pain (mild, moderate, or strong). If pain persists despite use of the appropriate drug and recommended dosing schedule, the child should receive the next most potent analgesic. Even when children require opioid analgesics, they should continue to receive acetaminophen (or nonsteroidal anti-inflammatory drugs, if appropriate) as supplemental analgesics.

12. What is "by the clock"?

"By the clock" refers to the timing for administering analgesic medications. Analgesics should be administered on a regular schedule, e.g., every 4 or 6 hours, based on the drug's duration of action and the severity of the child's pain, not on an as needed basis, unless a child's episodes of pain are truly intermittent and unpredictable. When PRN dosing is used, children must first experience pain before they can obtain pain relief. These breakthrough episodes of pain can cause serious problems for children who fear that their pain cannot be controlled. As a result, they may become progressively frightened and upset, so that their pain increases. Moreover, the doses of opioids required to relieve existing or breakthrough pain are higher than those required to prevent the recurrence of pain.

13. What is "by the mouth"?

"By the mouth" refers to the route of drug administration. Medication should be administered to children by the simplest effective route, usually by mouth. Since children are afraid of injections, they may deny that they have pain or may not request medication. When possible, children should receive medication through routes that do not cause additional pain. However, attention must be paid to the fact that opioid analgesics are less potent when administered orally, rather than parenterally. (See Chapter 32.)

14. What is "by the child"?

"By the child" refers to the need to base analgesic doses on each child's individual circumstances. No one analgesic dose will reliably relieve pain for all children who have a similar medical condition or similar level of pain. Instead, children vary with respect to how much of a drug or what type of a drug is required to control their pain. It is essential to monitor a child's pain regularly and adjust analgesic doses as necessary.

15. How do parents know which over-the-counter (OTC) products are safe and effective for children?

Parents should be advised that most OTC analgesic medications have not been specifically evaluated and approved for use in children. The labeling on most drugs states that the product is contraindicated for children under 16 years of age. Yet, some of these drugs may be extremely beneficial for children. Thus, it is important to consult with physicians who would know differences between prescription and OTC drugs and are able to provide advice to parents on how to use them. (Note: Both the Food and Drug Administration and the pharmaceutical industry are attending more to the need to develop and evaluate analgesic products specifically for use in infants and children.)

16. Which nondrug methods of treatment should be incorporated routinely into clinical practice?

Nondrug interventions are classified according to whether the interventions modify thoughts and coping abilities (cognitive), the peripheral or central nervous system (physical), or children's behavior (behavioral). Specific cognitive, physical, and behavioral interventions are listed in the figure at the end of question 9. Although each method is listed within a main category, there may be significant overlap. For example, hypnosis is considered primarily a cognitive intervention because children learn to reduce pain by their mental focus through intense concentration, even though a hypnotic induction process often includes a behavioral component of progressive muscle relaxation and may also affect central nervous system function.

Cognitive interventions are the most powerful and versatile nondrug pain therapies for children. When health professionals provide children with age-appropriate information about pain or teach them how to use simple coping strategies, they are administering a basic cognitive intervention. When children receive accurate information about what will happen to them and what they may feel, they can improve their understanding, increase their control, lessen their distress, and reduce their pain.

Distraction and focused attention, as well as guided imagery, are practical tools that health professionals and parents can routinely use when children experience pain. Genuine distraction and attention—when the child's attention is fully absorbed by an activity or topic other than his or her pain—is a very active process that can lessen neuronal responses evoked by tissue damage. Parents and staff members can assist children to concentrate fully on something besides their pain. Music, lights, colored objects, tactile toys, sweet tastes, and other children are effective attention-grabbing stimuli, particularly in young children. Conversation, games, computers, and interesting movies are effective distracters for older children and adolescents.

17. Which behavioral methods should be incorporated routinely into clinical practice?

Behavioral interventions are designed to change either children's own behavior or the behavior of the adults who interact with them. The therapeutic objective is to lessen behaviors that can increase children's pain and distress while increasing behaviors that can reduce pain. Progressive muscle relaxation and simple repetitive physical exercise (depending on children's preference) are convenient methods for most children to use during painful medical treatments. During stressful treatments, many children seem naturally to tense their muscles and hold their breath. Some children can learn to relax by alternately tightening and loosening their fists, by rhythmically moving a leg, or by deep, paced breathing.

General exercise regimens are an important component of pain management for children experiencing recurrent or persistent pain, as well as for children requiring multiple and repeated painful treatments. The objective is to restore as many of children's normal activities as possible to provide them with enjoyment, increase their participation in social events, increase their independent pain management, and help them reduce their stress.

18. What should be done to minimize pain for children experiencing multiple invasive procedures (e.g., bone marrow aspirations, catheter placements, lumbar punctures)?

It is essential to provide them with appropriate analgesic or anesthetic treatments, such as topical anesthetic creams before painful needle insertions and sedatives for aversive procedures. However, health professionals should be aware that many children prefer not to be sedated but to be alert and aware. Children can use simple coping strategies. Pain can be minimized when children have increased control, increased choice, and accurate information about what will happen. Imagery, distraction, and attention-focusing may also be helpful.

19. How do you treat children with recurrent pain syndromes?

Recurrent pain syndromes such as frequent headaches, abdominal pains, chest, or limb pains may affect otherwise healthy children. Many of the children referred to our pain clinic have experienced these pains for periods of years rather than months. In this type of pain, unlike disease-induced pain, the pain itself, rather than an underlying disease, is the problem.

After adequate investigation, it is important for parents and children to understand that there is no single source of tissue damage that can be fixed by a single treatment. Instead there may be multiple causes (see figure below). A cognitive-behavioral approach, which modifies the primary and secondary contributing factors, is most effective.

Regardless of some apparent similarity in a child's pain characteristics (e.g., frequency, intensity), certain factors may be primary causes for one child's pain but almost negligible causes for another child's pain. Thus, treatment emphasis must include a general approach to address the common factors and an individual approach to address the unique relevant factors for each child. The extent to which various cognitive, emotional, behavioral, and familial factors are the primary causes for recurrent pain will determine the particular composition of a multistrategy treatment. Because pharmacologic methods relieve the painfulness of an individual episode but do not generally change the syndrome, an integrated, flexible approach for combining physical, behavioral, and cognitive methods should be used.

Factors Involved in Pain of 10-Year-Old Girl with Recurrent Headaches

Cognitive Factors	Behavioral Factors	Emotional Factors
• Inaccurate understanding of headache syndrome	• Strong secondary gains from temporary stress reduction	• Anxiety related to unrealistic expectations for her academic performance
• Poor independent control	• Withdrawal from social and physical activities	• Anxiety related to unrealistic expectations for her and her friends' behaviors
• Expectations for continuing pain and disability	• Passive approach to pain control	• Parental anxiety regarding the cause of her headaches
• Aversive relevance	• Multiple learned triggers	• High frustration levels
• Few pain control strategies	• Positive family history of headaches	• Anxiety related to her peer relationships
• Failure to identify and resolve stress	• Inappropriate use of analgesics	• Increasing stress because of her failure to resolve stressful issues effectively

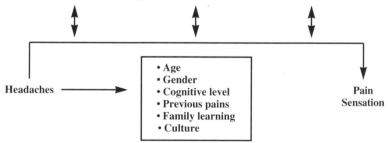

Headaches ⟶

• Age
• Gender
• Cognitive level
• Previous pains
• Family learning
• Culture

Pain Sensation

Treatment Recommendations:

1. Assist child in identifying and resolving stressful situations.
2. Teach child to cope more effectively with routine frustrations.
3. Teach parents and child about pain systems, recurrent pain syndromes, and true vs. learned headache triggers.
4. Reduce secondary gains associated with child's pain by providing consistent and nonmaladaptive responses to her pain complaints.
5. Teach child nonpharmacologic methods of pain control, such as muscle relaxation through biofeedback and nonstressful exercise.

(From McGrath PA, Hillier LM: Controlling children's pain. In Gatchel R, Turk D (eds): Psychological Treatment for Pain. New York, Guilford Press, 1996, with permission.)

20. What is the best approach for treating neuropathic pain in children?

Neuropathic pain differs from nociceptive pain in that the pain is generated not by ongoing tissue damage but by changes in the nervous system as a consequence of injury to it. (See Chapter 27). Pain may follow injury to the peripheral spinal cord or brain.

Chronic neuropathic pain should be managed from a multimodal perspective. Patients may benefit from relaxation training, biofeedback, and structured counseling to learn specific pain-reducing strategies and stress management. Families require supportive therapy to encourage children's functional rehabilitation with return to school and to social and physical activities. In addition, tricyclic antidepressants and anticonvulsants and sympathetic blocks may be useful in patients believed to have sympathetically maintained pain, who fail to progress with a vigorous regimen of physical therapy and cognitive-behavioral treatments.

21. What is pediatric palliative care?

A 16th century aphorism defines the essence of pediatric palliative care: "To cure sometimes, to relieve often, to comfort always." The comprehensive care of children includes curative therapies when available, pain and symptom management, and compassionate support for children and their families. It is essential to focus not only on the medical management of children's diseases but also on the psychosocial and spiritual factors that affect children's pain and suffering.

22. Are there special dosing considerations for neonates and infants?

Neonates and infants require the same three categories of analgesic drugs as older children. However, the difference in pharmacokinetics and pharmacodynamics among neonates, preterm infants, and full-term infants warrants special dosing considerations for infants and close monitoring when they receive opioids. Acetaminophen can be safely administered to neonates and infants without concern for hepatotoxicity when given for short courses at the recommended dose (10 to 15 mg/kg). The starting doses for opioid analgesics in infants under six months of age are $\frac{1}{4}$ to $\frac{1}{2}$ the suggested doses. (See table below). As for children, the dosage and mode of administration of opioids need to be titrated between the degree of analgesia required and a reasonable level of sedation.

Opioid Analgesic Dosing*

DRUG	EQUIANAL-GESIC DOSE	USUAL STARTING DOSE IV/SC:		IV/SC:PO	USUAL STARTING DOSE PO:		BIOLOGIC HALF-LIFE
	PARENTERAL	< 50 kg	≥ 50 kg	RATIO	< 50 kg	≥ 50 kg	HALF-LIFE
Short half-life opioids							
Morphine	10 mg	Bolus dose – 0.1 mg/kg q 2–3 hr Continuous infusion = 0.03–0.05 mg/kg/hr	5–10 mg q 2–4 hr	1:3	0.3 mg/kg q 3–4 hr	30 mg q 3–4 hr	2.5–3 hr
Hydro-morphone	1.5 mg	0.015 mg/kg q 3–4 hr	1–1.5 mg q 3–4 hr	1:5	0.06 mg/kg q 3–4 hr	4–8 mg q 3–4 hr	2–3 hr
Codeine	130 mg				0.5–1 mg/kg q 3–4 hr	60 mg q 3–4 hr	2.5–3 hr
Oxycodone					0.2 mg/kg q 3–4 hr	10 mg q 3–4 hr	1.5 hr
Meperidine*	75 mg	0.75 mg/kg q 2–3 hr	75–100 mg q 3 hr	1:4	1–1.5 mg/kg q 3–4 hr	50–75 mg q 3–4 hr†	3 hr*
Fentanyl	100 mcg	0.5–2 mcg/kg/hr as continuous infusion	25–75 mcg q 1 hr				

(Table continued on following page.)

Opioid Analgesic Dosing* (Cont.)

DRUG	EQUIANAL-GESIC DOSE	USUAL STARTING DOSE IV/SC:		IV/SC:PO	USUAL STARTING DOSE PO:		BIOLOGIC HALF-LIFE
	PARENTERAL	< 50 kg	≥ 50 kg	RATIO	< 50 kg	≥ 50 kg	HALF-LIFE
Long half-life opioids							
Controlled release morphine					0.6 mg/kg q 8 hr or 0.9 mg/kg q 12 hr	30–60 mg q 12 hr	
Methadone	10 mg	0.1 mg/kg q 4–8 hr	5–10 mg q 4–8 hr	1:2	0.2 mg/kg q 4–8 hr	10 mg q 4–8 hr	12–50 hr

Doses are for opioid naive patient. For infants under 6 months, start at ¼ to ⅓ the suggested dose and titrate to effect.

* Meperidine not recommended for chronic use because toxic long half-life metabolite normeperidine may accumulate.

† "Usual" starting doses are often determined empirically, not always dosed according to equianalgesic principles (i.e., starting dose of meperidine IV/PO of 75 mg even though IV:PO ratio is 1:4).

Adapted with permission from WHO monograph, Cancer Pain Relief and Palliative Care in Children (in press).

23. What are the guidelines for opioids in managing pain?

1. Pick an appropriate route. For chronic dosing, oral administration is preferred. Intravenous and subcutaneous administration are essentially equivalent. Avoid intramuscular administration because it hurts. A table of equianalgesic doses by drug and by route is in Chapter 32. Whenever using continuous IV infusion, hourly PRN rescue doses with short-onset opioids should be available. A rescue dose is usually 50–200% of continuous hourly dose. If more than six rescue doses are necessary in a 24-hour period, increase daily infusion total by the total amount of rescues for the previous 24 hours. An alternative is to increase the infusion rate by 50%.

2. Pick an appropriate drug.

3. Pick an appropriate dose. Starting doses are shown in the table at the end of question 22.

4. To change opioids: Because of incomplete cross-tolerance, if changing between short half-life opioids, start the new opioids at 50% of the calculated equianalgesic dose. Titrate to effect. If changing from short to long half-life opioid (i.e., morphine to methadone), start at 25% of equianalgesic dose and titrate to effect.

5. When discontinuing drug or tapering opioids: For anyone receiving opioids for more than one week, the dose should be tapered to avoid withdrawal symptoms. Taper by 50% for two days, then decrease by 25% every two days. In patients weighing less than 50 kg, the target dose before discontinuation is the equivalent of 0.6 mg/kg/day. If the patient weighs more than 50 kg, the largest dose is 30 mg of oral morphine.

Meperidine is not recommended for chronic use because normeperidine may accumulate. Normeperidine is a toxic metabolite with a long serum half-life and can cause myoclonus, hyperreflexia, and seizures. "Usual" starting doses are often determined empirically.

24. Are children at particular risk for addiction?

No. The fear of opioid addiction in children has been greatly exaggerated. While physical dependence—the body's routine and gradual adjustment to the drug so that the body requires the drug on some regular basis—is common, it can be controlled easily by gradual tapering of medication doses. Similarly, tolerance is a pharmacokinetic/pharmacodynamic phenomenon in which progressively higher levels of the drug are required to achieve the same physiologic effect. The terms physical dependence and tolerance are not synonymous with addiction and may occur independently.

Addiction represents a pattern of drug use in which an individual is wholly absorbed in the compulsive use and procurement of a drug and has a tendency to relapse after withdrawal. Drug dosing continues despite harmful effects. There is no empirical evidence that children receiving opioid analgesics for pain control are at risk for addiction. In contrast, children who do not receive appropriate analgesic medications are probably more at risk for pseudoaddiction by becoming excessively concerned about receiving their next medication dose in the hope that they might eventually relieve their suffering.

25. What is the role of adjuvant medication for children with chronic pain?

Adjuvant medications (Chapter 33) play a primary role for children suffering persistent pain or for children receiving palliative care. Drugs, indications, and starting doses are listed below.

Adjuvant Analgesic Drugs

DRUG CATEGORY	DRUG, DOSAGE	INDICATIONS	COMMENTS
Antidepressants	Amitriptyline, 0.2–0.5 mg/kg Escalate by 25% every 2–3 days up to 1–2 mg/kg if needed. Alternatives: doxepin, imipramine, nortriptyline.	Neuropathic pain (i.e., vincristine-induced, radiation plexopathy, tumor invasion). Insomnia.	Usually, improved sleep and pain relief within 3–5 days. Anticholinergic side effects are dose-limiting. Use with caution in children at increased risk for cardiac dysfunction.
Anticonvulsants	Carbamazepine, 2 mg/kg PO q 12 hr Phenytoin, 2.5–2 mg/kg PO q 12 hr Clonazepam, 0.01 mg/kg q 12 hr	Neuropathic pain, especially shooting, stabbing pain.	Monitor for hematologic, hepatic, and allergic reactions. Side effects: GI upset, ataxia, disorientation, somnolence.
Neuroleptics	Chlorpromazine, 0.5 mg/kg IV/PO q 4–6 hr Promethazine, 0.5–1 mg/kg IV/PO q 4–6 hr Haloperidol, 0.01–0.1 mg/kg IV/PO q 8 hr	Nausea, confused child psychosis, acute agitation. Enhancement of opioid analgesia.	Consider concurrent use of antihistamine (e.g., diphenhydramine) to avoid dystonic reaction if high doses or prolonged course is used.
Sedatives, Hypnotics, Anxiolytics	Diazepam, 0.05–0.1 mg/kg IV/PO q 4–6 hr Lorazepam, 0.02–0.04 mg/kg IV/PO q 4–6 hr Midazolam, 0.05 mg/kg IV q 5 min prior to procedure; 0.3–0.5 mg/kg PO q 30–45 min prior to procedure	Acute anxiety, muscle spasm. Premedication for painful procedures.	Sedative effect may limit opioid use. Other side effects include depression and dependence with prolonged use.
Antihistamines	Hydroxyzine, 0.5–1 mg/kg q 4–6 hr Diphenhydramine, 0.5–1 mg/kg q 4–6 hr	Opioid-induced pruritis, anxiety, nausea.	Sedative side effects may be helpful.
Psychostimulants	Dextroamphetamine, Methylphenidate, 0.1–0.2 mg/kg twice a day. Escalate to 0.3–0.5 as needed	Opioid-induced somnolence, potentiation of opioid analgesia.	Side effects include agitation, sleep disturbance, and anorexia. Administer second dose in early afternoon to to avoid sleep disturbances.
Corticosteroids	Prednisone, prenisolone, and dexamethasone dosage depends on clinical situation (e.g., dexamethasone 6–12 mg/m$^{2/d}$)	Headache from raised intracranial pressure, spinal or nerve compression; widespread metastases.	Side effects include edema, dyspeptic symptoms, and occasional gastrointestinal bleeding.

Adapted with permission from WHO monograph, Cancer Pain Relief and Palliative Care in Children (in press).

BIBLIOGRAPHY

1. Anand KJS, McGrath PJ (eds): Pain in Neonates. New York, Elsevier, 1993.
2. Apley J: The Child with Abdominal Pains. Oxford, Blackwell Scientific, 1975.
3. Jacox A, Carr DB, Payne R, et al: Management of Cancer Pain. Clinical Practice Guideline. Rockville, MD, Agency for Health Care Policy and Research, U.S. Department of Health and Human Services, Public Health Service, 1994.
4. McGrath PA: Pain in Children: Nature, Assessment and Treatment. New York, Guilford Press, 1990.
5. McGrath PA: Pain control in paediatric palliative care. In Doyle D, Hanks GW, MacDonald N (eds): Oxford Textbook of Palliative Medicine. Oxford, Oxford University Press (in press).
6. McGrath PA, Hillier LM: Controlling children's pain. In Gatchel R, Turk D (eds): Psychological Treatment for Pain: A Practitioner's Handbook. New York, Guilford Press, 1996, pp 331–370.
7. McGrath PJ, Unruh A: Pain in Children and Adolescents. Amsterdam, Elsevier, 1987.
8. Ross DM, Ross SA: Childhood Pain: Current Issues, Research, and Management. Baltimore, Urban & Schwarzenberg, 1988.
9. Schechter NL, Berde C, Yaster M (eds): Pain Management in Children and Adolescents. Baltimore, Williams & Wilkins, 1992.
10. World Health Organization: Cancer Pain Relief and Palliative Care in Children. Geneva, World Health Organization (in press).

30. PAIN IN THE ELDERLY

Ronald Kanner, M.D.

1. What is meant by elderly?

Of interest, most medical dictionaries do not give a definition for "old" or "elderly." The *International Dictionary of Medicine and Biology, Stedman's Medical Dictionary,* and the *Mosby Medical, Nursing, and Allied Health Dictionary* omit the word "old" and define "elder" as "sambucus" (the elderberry). The most commonly used working definition of elderly is over 65. However, most aging studies that began with people 65 and older now have a large cadre of people over 85. New definitions are emerging rather rapidly. "Old" is now generally taken to mean 75 or older and the "old old" is now 80 or older. Most physicians, however, have in their practice octogenarians who are athletic, fit, and active.

2. Why is it important to address pain in the elderly?

The over 85 population is proportionally the fastest growing segment in American society. As older patients represent an increasingly larger proportion of the population, their health care needs assume a much greater role. Furthermore, the prevalence of pain in the elderly is probably double what it is in younger adults. This number grows even larger in institutionalized elderly patients. Some of the common painful diseases, such as arthritis and cancer, are also more prevalent in the elderly. It is estimated that the British population of over 85 year olds will have increased by almost 90% between 1981 and 2001. Furthermore, relatively few studies address the needs and specific problems of the aged population.

3. What are the impediments to accurate pain assessment in the elderly?

Pain is a truly subjective phenomenon. Its assessment requires appropriate communication between the person suffering the pain and the health care practitioner assessing it. Elderly patients are more likely to underreport pain than are younger patients, possibly because of their desire to be perceived as "good patients." In a study of patients with duodenal ulcer or myocardial infarction, older patients reported milder pain than younger patients. They tend to have more faith in the medical system and more respect for physicians. Cognitive impairment, a fairly common problem in the elderly, may render patients unable to use appropriate descriptors for pain. In such cases, behavioral signs may be used to assess pain, and they are often less accurate than good verbal reports. Although the precise severity of pain may be difficult to assess, even patients with significant cognitive impairment can report the presence of pain. Unfortunately, there are relatively few well-validated scales for the elderly. The verbal and visual analog scales used in younger patients do not have the same degree of validation in the elderly. Impaired hearing and vision also may lead to difficulties with communication.

4. What scales are available for assessment of pain in patients with dementia?

The Discomfort Scale for Patients with Dementia of the Alzheimer Type (DS-DAT) is difficult to validate because it was generated from the impressions of nursing staff caring for demented patients. It lists a series of items that, in the staff's opinion, indicated that the patient was in pain. Examples include noisy breathing, negative vocalization, sad vs. content facial expression, frightened facial expression, frown, tense vs. relaxed body language, and fidgeting. As its name indicates, the DS-DAT is a discomfort scale and may not assess pain directly. It is unclear whether distress, discomfort, or pain is being assessed. Behavioral methods of pain assessment may be valid for the presence or absence of pain, but they do not assess the intensity of pain. Certain facial expressions are common with intense pain, but they are not necessarily graded responses.

5. Are nonsteroidal anti-inflammatory drugs safe in elderly patients?

Advancing age greatly increases the risk of side effects from nonsteroidal anti-inflammatory drugs (NSAIDs). The incidence of gastrointestinal (GI) bleeding from NSAIDs is nearly twice as high in patients over 65 as in young patients. Elderly patients are also at greater risk for adverse renal and cardiac effects. Many adverse effects may owe part of their increased incidence to the fact that such disorders are generally more common in the elderly, even without NSAIDs. The daily dose of NSAIDs is related directly to the risk of GI complications, regardless of age. Unfortunately, because elderly patients commonly see more than one physician, they may receive multiple prescriptions for NSAIDs. Patients exposed to multiple NSAIDs have a higher risk of GI bleeding than patients taking a single drug. Changing the route of administration does not seem to offer much benefit in terms of GI bleeding. One study showed that patients receiving rectal forms were more likely to bleed than patients receiving oral forms. Some of this difference may have been due to the mistaken belief that rectal administration was safer; patients given the drug by the rectal route may already have been at risk for GI bleeding.

6. What pharmacokinetic factors affect drug dosing in the elderly?

All phases of pharmacokinetics are affected in aging, including absorption, distribution, metabolism, and elimination. However, effects are often in opposite directions. In general, the elderly tend to require lower doses of medications than younger patients. Absorption is often irregular in the elderly because of delayed transit time or malabsorption syndromes. The volume of distribution of most drugs is smaller in the elderly than in the young. Elderly patients tend to have a lower lean body mass. Hepatic metabolism and renal clearance are also diminished. Such factors lead to relatively higher levels of drug at a given dose. In many instances, increased effects from medications are due to longer duration of action rather than simply higher peaks of concentration.

7. Are older patients less sensitive to pain than younger patients?

Both clinical and experimental tests offer conflicting data. Some studies have shown that pain threshold is slightly elevated in elderly patients. Others have shown no difference between the old and young. Pain tolerance has similarly been reported as either slightly increased or unchanged in the elderly. In some large epidemiologic studies, pain complaints have been listed as being less frequent in the elderly than in the young. Some of the difference may be a reporting bias. Joint pain, however, is clearly more prevalent in the elderly population. Elderly patients suffering from clinical pain syndromes may be less likely to report pain than their younger counterparts.

8. What are the clinical implications of the pharmacokinetic changes seen in the elderly?

Given diminished volume of distribution, longer half-life, and reduced clearance, it follows that plasma levels will be elevated for a longer period after a given dose. Therefore, drugs with a short serum half-life are generally preferable to longer-lasting drugs. With the opioid analgesics, four or five serum half-lives are required to reach steady-state drug levels, putting patients at greater risk for accumulation. Close monitoring is required after any drug change or increase in dose.

9. What specific problems are seen with tricyclic antidepressants used for pain in the elderly?

Most of the troublesome side effects of the tricyclic antidepressants (TCAs) are due to their anticholinergic effects. In patients with cognitive impairment, anticholinergic activity can lead to increased confusion. (One of the major deficits in Alzheimer's disease is a deficit in cerebral acetylcholine.) Narrow-angle glaucoma, another common problem in the elderly, may be markedly exacerbated by anticholinergic drugs. Elderly patients with benign prostatic hypertrophy are at greater risk for urinary retention because of the anticholinergic effects of TCAs. A mild degree of dysautonomia is often present in the elderly, causing slight dizziness on arising. This orthostatic hypertension may be markedly exacerbated by the anticholinergic side effects. Finally, cardiac conduction blocks can be worsened by TCAs.

10. What are the common side effects of opioid analgesics in the elderly?

Constipation is by far the most common and troublesome side effect of opioids. It is even more prevalent in the elderly, in whom constipation is generally more common. Respiratory depression is unusual, unless appropriate pharmacokinetic guidelines are disregarded. Cheyne-Stokes breathing patterns during sleep are not uncommon in the elderly, and opioids should not be discontinued solely on the basis of observing this respiratory pattern. The situations in which respiratory depression can become a problem are primarily two:

1. When drugs with a long serum half-life are used, many days may pass before a steady state is reached. Thus, with drugs such as levorphanol and methadone, serum levels may rise for over 1 week, despite steady dosing. If elderly patients are not monitored carefully, this may lead to respiratory depression.

2. If patients with severe pain receive escalating doses of opioids, they are usually tolerant to such doses. However, if the underlying pain syndrome is relieved, previously tolerated doses of opioids may produce respiratory depression.

11. What is the most common cause of adverse side effects in the elderly?

Polypharmacy (the use of more than one drug for a specific problem) is a prescription for disaster in the elderly. In a study of falls in the elderly, prescription of multiple drugs was the single most common cause. Patients taking a combination of analgesics, antidepressants, and sedatives are much more likely to suffer confusion than patients taking a single agent.

12. What is the basic rule of thumb for analgesic therapy in the elderly?

Start low, go slow. Initial dosing in the elderly should be started at about half the level that one would use in a younger patient. TCAs should be started at no higher than 10 mg at bedtime. Titration must be gradual and careful. Doses of TCAs should be increased only by the amount at which they were started and only after around 3 or 4 days at each level.

13. What pain syndromes are more common in the elderly than in the young?

Arthritis and other articular complaints leap immediately to mind. However, trigeminal neuralgia and postherpetic neuralgia are more common in the elderly than in the young. Temporal arteritis and polymyalgia rheumatica are also almost exclusively diseases of the elderly. Pure psychogenic pain is seen much less commonly in the elderly than in the young. However, masked depression may present as a pain syndrome in elderly patients. The prevalence of cancer also rises with advancing age, bringing with it all of the pain syndromes associated with malignancy.

14. What are the consequences of poorly controlled pain in the elderly?

Elderly patients with pain tend to have reduced mobility. As they become more and more immobile, depression ensues. Lack of functional ability appears to be more of a determinant of depression than severity of disease. As with younger patients, chronic pain may lead to decreased socialization, sleep disturbances, and possibly even impaired immunity. When pain is poorly controlled, physicians tend to prescribe more medications. Polypharmacy may lead to increased confusion and falls.

Most analgesic studies have been conducted in patients between 18 and 65 years of age. The exclusion of the very young and the very old makes it difficult to make firm statements about the analgesic efficacy of drugs in either age group.

15. What factors lead to the underprescribing of opioid analgesics in elderly patients?

Both factual and fictional ideas lead to the relatively low doses of opioids prescribed for elderly patients. First, elderly patients tend to respond to lower doses than younger patients. However, they are also less likely to complain about pain and to request analgesic medications. There also seems to be a belief in the medical community that elderly people require less analgesia than young patients. Even when left to their own devices (patient-controlled analgesia), elderly patients tend to take lower doses of analgesics than younger patients.

16. What kinds of drugs should be avoided in the elderly?

Within each class of drug used for pain treatment, certain drugs are more likely to produce side effects in the elderly. With nonnarcotic analgesics (NSAIDs), it is generally a good idea to use nonacetylated drugs with a relatively simple metabolism. Indomethacin and piroxicam have relatively long serum half-lives and tend to produce more GI problems than drugs such as salsalate and ibuprofen. This caution applies to their role as analgesics, not as anti-inflammatories. With the opioid analgesics, it is probably best to stay with a pure agonist rather than a mixed agonist-antagonist such as pentazocine or butorphanol. The mixed drugs are more likely to produce psychotomimetic effects in the elderly. In addition, drugs with a long serum half-life, such as methadone and levorphanol, require a greater length of time to reach steady state than drugs with a short serum half-life. Among antidepressant medications, the tertiary amine tricyclics are more likely to produce anticholinergic side effects than the secondary amine drugs.

17. How should the side effects of analgesics be treated in the elderly?

All patients taking opioid analgesics should be put on a bowel regimen before starting the drug. A simple combination of a senna preparation and stool softener is usually sufficient. Nausea, on the other hand, should not be treated prophylactically. Not all elderly patients become nauseated on opioids, and the side effects of the antiemetics may be worse than the problems caused by the opioids.

18. How should analgesics be chosen for elderly patients in pain?

The same three-step ladder that applies to younger patients should apply to the elderly. Mild-to-moderate pain should be treated with nonopioid analgesics. Moderate pain requires minor opioids, possibly in combination with nonnarcotics and adjuvant drugs. Severe pain requires potent opioids. The only difference is that lower doses should generally be used, and combinations of medications may cause more cognitive impairment.

BIBLIOGRAPHY

1. Closs SJ: Pain in elderly patients: A neglected phenomenon? J Adv Nurs 19:1072–1081, 1994.
2. Egbert AM: Help for the hurting elderly. Safe use of drugs to relieve pain. Postgrad Med 89(4):217–222, 225, 228, 1991.
3. Enck RE: Pain control in the ambulatory elderly. Geriatrics 46(3):49–53, 57–58, 60, 1991.
4. Gordon M, Preiksaitis HG: Drugs and the aging brain. Geriatrics 43:69–78, 1988.
5. Parmelee PA, Smith B, Katz IR: Pain complaints and cognitive status among elderly institution residents. J Am Geriatr Soc 41:517–522, 1993.
6. Portenoy RK, Farkash A: Practical management of non-malignant pain in the elderly. Geriatrics 43(5):29–40, 44–47, 1988.
7. Wall RT: Use of analgesics in the elderly. Clin Geriatr Med 6:345–364, 1990.

VII. Pharmacologic Management

31. NONSTEROIDAL ANTI-INFLAMMATORY DRUGS

Robert A. Duarte, M.D.

1. What are the indications for treatment with aspirin or other nonsteroidal anti-inflammatory drugs (NSAIDs)?

Aspirin, acetaminophen, and other NSAIDs are generally the drugs of choice for mild-to-moderate pain. They represent the first step in the analgesic ladder proposed by the World Health Organization. NSAIDs have a primarily peripheral site of action, relatively little in the way of central nervous side effects, and a clear ceiling effect. The ceiling effect refers to the fact that increased dose levels after a certain point cause unacceptable side effects without improving analgesia. NSAIDs have a relatively low abuse potential and are particularly useful for somatic nociceptive pain syndromes, such as bone pain or arthritis.

2. What is the mechanism of action of NSAIDs?

Aspirin and the other NSAIDs decrease the production of prostaglandin (PG), particularly PGE_2, through inhibition of an enzyme called cyclooxygenase. This inhibition reduces inflammatory mediators (e.g., bradykinin) known to sensitize peripheral nociceptors. Although it is intuitive to hypothesize that PG inhibition produces analgesia, this has not been firmly established as the only analgesic mechanism. There may be central effects as well, but the peripheral site of action is believed to be more important.

3. Do the various NSAIDs have similar or different pharmacokinetic characteristics?

All NSAIDs possess similar absorption characteristics. In general, they are rapidly absorbed after oral and rectal administration. They are highly protein-bound and metabolized primarily in the liver. However, durations of action vary markedly. Some drugs, such as ibuprofen, require dosing at least every 4–6 hours, whereas piroxicam can be given once a day and choline magnesium trisalicylate is dosed every 12 hours. Elimination half-lives range from 4 hours for the propionic acid derivatives to nearly 2 days for piroxicam.

4. What is considered the prototypical NSAID?

Aspirin (acetylsalicylic acid) is the standard of a group of medications known as salicylates. It is inexpensive, widely accessible worldwide, and available over the counter. It has demonstrated analgesic efficacy in treating pain secondary to musculoskeletal disorders, dysmenorrhea, arthritis, and headaches.

5. What are the potential adverse side effects of aspirin?

The most frequent limiting side effects from aspirin are primarily gastrointestinal (GI) and include nausea, vomiting, and dyspepsia as well as occult GI bleeding. Aspirin irreversibly acetylates platelet cyclooxygenase and may lead to prolonged bleeding time. In contrast to aspirin, the newer NSAIDs produce a reversible inhibition of platelet cyclooxygenase that lasts only as long as the serum drug concentration is effective. This factor is of major concern in patients with cancer pain who already have a bleeding diathesis due to cancer or chemotherapeutic agents.

Some of the nonacetylated salicylates (e.g., choline magnesium trisalicylate) do not inhibit platelet function. Doses of aspirin greater than 1,000 mg every 4 hours may produce salicylate toxicity, which manifests as tinnitus, hyperventilation, and acid–base disturbances.

6. Is there an association between NSAIDs and renal disease?

Yes. Although aspirin and other NSAIDs do not generally cause renal disease in patients with normal renal function, problems such as nephrotic syndrome, acute interstitial cystitis, and acute renal failure have been observed when aspirin is given to patients with abnormal renal function. The proposed mechanism is decreased availability of renal prostaglandins, which serve a protective role in maintaining adequate renal function.

7. Discuss the major differences between aspirin and acetaminophen.

Acetaminophen appears to be equal to aspirin and other NSAIDs in terms of analgesia but has no appreciable anti-inflammatory effects. Acetaminophen seems to have more central than peripheral prostaglandin-inhibiting effects. One major advantage of acetaminophen is its lack of upper GI tract irritation. Protein binding is significantly lower with acetaminophen than with aspirin, varying from 20–50%.

8. Does acetaminophen inhibit peripheral cyclooxygenase activity like the other NSAIDs?

No. The exact mechanism of action is unclear. Acetaminophen has only weak antiprostaglandin activity in peripheral tissues; it may have some central antiprostaglandin activity. Acetaminophen is equianalgesic with aspirin in single-dose studies of pain due to cancer, postoperative pain, and headache.

9. What is the clinical presentation of acute acetaminophen overdose?

At high doses (200–250 mg/kg), acetaminophen is hepatotoxic. At doses of 400 mg/kg, acetaminophen may be fatal. Symptoms of acetaminophen overdose include vague abdominal pain during the first week followed by signs of hepatic failure.

10. Are there any serum tests to prognosticate hepatic damage?

Yes. Measurement of the plasma half-life of acetaminophen in the first day of intoxication is a better prognosticator of hepatic damage than a single measurement of plasma levels. The longer the half-life, the worse the prognosis of hepatic involvement.

11. What are the risks of combining other NSAIDs with acetaminophen?

The risk of analgesic nephropathy appears to be increased when different NSAIDs are used together or in combination with acetaminophen. This effect is generally seen in long-term use. The primary lesion is papillary necrosis with secondary interstitial nephritis and may be a function of prostaglandin inhibition at the renal tubular level.

12. What contributing factors may increase the risk for renal failure?
- Congestive heart failure
- Hepatic cirrhosis
- Collagen vascular disease
- Intravascular volume depletion
- Atherosclerotic heart disease

13. Describe two different clinical pictures associated with aspirin hypersensitivity.

Some patients with **asthma** and **nasal polyps** may be particularly aspirin-sensitive. Urticaria, angioneurotic edema, hypotension, and shock are possible reactions to aspirin. Hypersensitivity syndromes to aspirin usually develop within minutes to 1 hour of ingestion. Patients who are sensitive to aspirin may also demonstrate hypersensitivity to other NSAIDs.

14. What groups of NSAIDs are available on the market today? Which is most effective?

1. Salicylates (salsalate, diflunisal, and choline magnesium trisalicylate)
2. Propionic acid derivatives (ibuprofen, flurbiprofen, fenoprofen, ketoprofen, and naproxen)
3. Indoles (indomethacin, sulindac, tolmetin, and etodolac)
4. Fenamates (mefenamic acid and meclofenamate)
5. Mixed group (piroxicam, ketorolac, and diclofenac)

No clear evidence indicates that any group has greater analgesic effects than any other group. However, certain pharmacokinetic differences may make one group preferable over another for a given patient. Furthermore, certain idiosyncratic reactions are not directly explicable by the pharmacokinetics of a drug and may have more to do with individual reactions to medications.

15. What are the differences among the various salicylate derivatives?

Aspirin is the prototype of the salicylates, and other members of the group are judged against it. It is an acetylated salicylate that irreversibly inhibits platelet prostaglandin synthetase. This inhibition lasts for the life of the platelet and inhibits adhesion and aggregation. The other drugs in this group, if they inhibit platelet activity at all, do so in a reversible fashion; that is, the inhibition lasts only as long as the drug lasts in serum.

Diflunisal is a salicylate derivative that attains peak concentrations within 2 hours of oral administration. It has a considerably longer half-life than aspirin, ranging from 8–12 hours. It may be given every 12 hours. The incidence of GI side effects seems to be lower with diflunisal than with aspirin.

Choline magnesium trisalicylate is a nonacetylated salicylate derivative. It has no effect on platelet function, and its effects on the gastric mucosa are significantly less important than those of aspirin. As with diflunisal, it may be given every 12 hours and has a serum half-life of 9–17 hours. It is also available in a liquid form that may be useful for patients who have difficulty with swallowing pills.

Salsalate (salicylsalicylic acid) also has fewer GI side effects than aspirin.

16. Do salicylates follow linear or nonlinear kinetics?

Salicylates follow nonlinear or dose-dependent kinetics. For example, if one doubles the dose of a particular salicylate, plasma levels will more than double. In addition, the elimination half-life at the low dose will significantly increase at a high dose.

17. What particular drug interactions occur with the salicylates?

Salicylates add to the analgesic efficacy of opioid agents. They decrease the rate of absorption of fenoprofen and indomethacin. When taken with oral anticoagulants, they significantly increase the risk of bleeding. Salicylates also displace naproxen, phenylbutazone, and phenytoin from their plasma binding proteins, resulting in a higher free fraction of these agents and a fall in salicylate concentration.

18. Give examples of the pyrrole-acetic acid group.

Indomethacin, an indoleacetic acid derivative, is highly effective in the management of pain. It is specifically effective in certain headache syndromes, such as paroxysmal hemicrania. GI side effects are common. It has a half-life of 5–10 hours and is usually dosed every 6–8 hours. Indomethacin is also available as a time-released capsule.

Sulindac, a pyrrole-acetic acid derivative, was synthesized in search of a compound less toxic than but equally effective as indomethacin. Some evidence suggests that sulindac can be used safely in patients with renal disease in comparison to the other NSAIDs, but caution is still warranted.

Ketorolac, a pyrrole-acetic acid derivative, is available as an intramuscular (IM) as well as an oral preparation. Studies have shown that 30 mg of IM ketorolac are equally effective as 6–12 mg of IM morphine in postoperative pain.

19. How is sulindac (Clinoril) different pharmacokinetically from the other NSAIDs?

The parent drug (sulfoxide) is inactive. It is reduced to a sulfide, the active metabolite, and then oxidized to a sulfone (inactive metabolite). The active metabolite is eliminated slowly from plasma, resulting in a relatively longer half-life (16 hr).

20. What are the characteristics of the propionic group?

The aromatic propionic derivatives, also known as the profens, are the largest single class of NSAIDs. The prototype of this class is ibuprofen; its major analogs include naproxen, fenoprofen, ketoprofen, and flurbiprofen. Naproxen tends to be less toxic, but its anti-inflammatory action is equal to that of aspirin and indomethacin. The pharmacokinetics of naproxen allow it to be given on a twice-daily basis, which may improve patient compliance.

21. What is the primary difference between naproxen sodium and naproxen?

The sodium moiety attached to naproxen sodium allows quicker absorption. Naproxen sodium may be helpful in patients who need quicker relief; for example, as an abortive agent in the management of headaches.

22. If a patient fails to obtain sufficient analgesia from one class of NSAID, what should the next step be?

If an adequate trial of one class of NSAIDs fails to provide analgesia, the clinician should switch to an alternative class. For example, if aspirin is effective but produces intolerable side effects, a trial of another salicylate (e.g., diflunisal) is recommended. However, if aspirin was not effective in producing analgesia despite an adequate trial, one should switch to another class, such as the propionic group.

23. What is considered an adequate trial of NSAIDs?

An analgesic should not be considered a failure unless it has been pushed to the maximal tolerated dose. For benign pain, 2 weeks of a maximal scheduled dose constitute an adequate trial. For malignant pain, 1 week is sufficient.

24. Do NSAIDs cause an increase in duodenal ulceration?

No. Duodenal ulceration is probably not increased by NSAIDs, but the complications of duodenal ulceration are greater with NSAIDs. NSAIDs are associated with a 5-fold increase in gastric ulceration.

25. What are the potential risk factors for NSAID-associated GI toxicity?

• Advancing age
• Concomitant administration of corticosteroids
• History of either ulcer disease or prior GI complications from NSAIDs

26. Is dyspepsia a reliable predictor of ulceration?

No. Although nausea and vomiting can be produced by NSAIDs, dyspepsia is in fact a poor predictor for perforation.

27. What is the role of protective therapies in association with administration of NSAIDs?

The role has not been established. To date, only misoprostol has been proved to reduce the risk for serious GI toxicity. Misoprostol diminishes the incidence of endoscopically detectable lesions. However, no evidence has confirmed that misoprostol diminishes the risk of complications from these lesions when they occur. Protective agents may be indicated in patients over 60 years of age and patients with a predisposition to GI problems.

28. What central nervous system side effects are seen with NSAIDs?

All NSAIDs have the potential to produce central nervous system side effects, including sedation, dizziness, and headaches. Headaches occur in about 10% of patients taking indomethacin.

Central side effects are usually mild and transient, except in the elderly. When they occur, lower doses should be used.

29. What electrolyte disturbances are associated with NSAIDs?

NSAIDs can cause hyponatremia and hyperkalemia as a result of altered renal function. In addition, the action of antidiuretic hormone may be increased, exacerbating congestive heart failure. Such potential problems should be of concern in elderly or medically compromised patients.

30. Which NSAID is the agent of choice for pain control?

No conclusive evidence supports one NSAID over another for analgesia. It is recommended to begin with an NSAID with which the physician is familiar and which has a low incidence of side effects. In addition, patient compliance should be considered. For example, if you know that the patient will remember to take a medication only once a day, do not begin with an NSAID that requires a twice-daily regimen.

BIBLIOGRAPHY

1. American Pain Society: Principles of Analgesic Use in the Treatment of Acute and Chronic Cancer Pain: A Concise Guide to Medical Practice, 2nd ed. American Pain Society, 1989.
2. Beaver WT: Nonsteroidal antiinflammatory analgesics in cancer pain. Adv Pain Res Ther 16:109–131, 1990.
3. Bloom BS: Risk and cost of gastrointestinal side effects associated with nonsteroidal anti-inflammatory drugs. Arch Intern Med 149:1019–1022, 1989.
4. Brune K, Lanz R: Non-opioid analgesics. In Kuhar M, Pasternak G (eds): Analgesics: Neurochemical, Behavioral, and Clinical Perspectives. New York, Raven Press, 1984, pp 149–173.
5. Denson DD, Katz JA: Nonsteroidal anti-inflammatory agents. In Raj PP (ed): Practical Management of Pain, 2nd ed. St. Louis, Mosby, 1992, pp 614–615.
6. Edelson JT, Tosteson AN, Sax P: Cost-effectiveness of misoprostol for prophylaxis against nonsteroidal anti-inflammatory drug-induced gastrointestinal tract bleeding. JAMA 264:83–84, 1990.
7. Johnson AG, Seideman P, Day RO: Adverse drug interactions with nonsteroidal anti-inflammatory drugs (NSAIDs). Recognition, management and avoidance. Drug Saf 8(2).99–127, 1993.
8. Portenoy RK: Principles of treatment with nonopioid analgesics and adjuvant drugs: Post-graduate course. In Current Concepts in Acute, Chronic and Cancer Pain Management, 1993.
9. Sunshine A, Olson N: Nonnarcotic analgesics. In Wall PD, Melzack R (eds): Textbook of Pain. London, Churchill-Livingstone, 1989, pp 670–685.
10. Verbeeck RK, Blackburn JL, Looewen GR: Clinical pharmacokinetics of nonsteroidal anti-inflammatory drugs. Clin Pharmacokinet 8:297–331, 1983.
11. Weinblatt ME: Nonsteroidal anti-inflammatory drug toxicity: Increased risk in the elderly. Scand J Rheumatol 91(Suppl):9–17, 1991.
12. World Health Organization: Cancer Pain Relief. Geneva, World Health Organization, 1986.

32. OPIOID ANALGESICS

Ronald Kanner, M.D.

1. What is an opioid?

Opioid is the term used to refer to a group of analgesics which have the properties of morphine. This includes the naturally occurring opiates, semisynthetic opiates, and the endogenous opioids. The term opiate was initially used to denote any derivative of the poppy plant. In poetic terminology, an opiate is anything that assuages suffering. As synthetic and semisynthetic products became available, it became clear that the term opiate had to be modified. This was furthered by the discovery of peptides in the brain and spinal cord mimicking the action of morphine.

2. What is a narcotic?

Narcotic is now a term that has more legal implications than it does pharmacologic ones. It was initially used to denote any drug capable of producing sleep (narcosis). It was generally applied to the opiates. However, it is now used to denote drugs of abuse that are controlled by government agencies. The old terminology for one of the agencies was The Bureau of Narcotics and Dangerous Drugs (DNDD). The main regulatory agency on a national level is the Drug Enforcement Agency (DEA).

3. What are the two main naturally occurring opioid alkaloids, and what are their properties?

Morphine and codeine are two of the most widely used naturally occurring opioid alkaloids. Morphine is the prototype of the opioid drug. It binds primarily to mu receptors, producing analgesia and respiratory depression.

4. What is the mechanism of opioid analgesia?

Opioid analgesia is thought to be mediated through a direct interaction with an opioid receptor. These receptors are found mainly in the spinal cord and brain stem. However, there are some sites that are far removed from these, and their exact function is unknown.

5. What subtypes of opioid receptor are important in analgesia?

The three main opioid subtypes are the mu, kappa, and delta receptors. From the standpoint of analgesia, the mu receptor seems to be the most important. There may be subtypes of these receptors, with different drugs having different affinities for given receptor subtypes. There may be analgesic activity at the delta and kappa sites as well.

6. What is meant by a mixed agonist/antagonist drug?

When a drug combines with a receptor site to produce the action of that receptor it is considered an agonist. A drug that binds with a receptor and inhibits activity is considered an antagonist. Semisynthetic and synthetic products have been produced that are both agonist and antagonist. The hope in producing these drugs was that they would be agonist for analgesic affects and antagonist for the respiratory depression and sedative effects of the opioids. Examples include pentazocine, butorphanol, buprenorphine. Naloxone is a pure antagonist drug.

7. What are the endogenous opioids?

The first endogenous opioids to be discovered were endorphins and the enkephalins. These are polypeptides that are synthesized in the brain and spinal cord. They bind with opioid receptors and produce analgesia. Since the discovery of endorphins and enkephalins in the early 1970s, a number of other peptide products have been described.

8. How do agonist/antagonist drugs differ from pure agonist analgesics?

Clinically, the most important concept is that these drugs have a "ceiling effect." That is, with increasing doses, side-effects supervene and further analgesia cannot be achieved. With pure agonist drugs, as tolerance develops drug doses can be increased to obtain further analgesia. In patients who are opioid tolerant, administration of a mixed agonist/antagonist may precipitate withdrawal.

9. What is the difference between efficacy and potency?

Efficacy refers to the ability of the drug to produce a given response in an appropriate clinical setting. Potency refers either to the number of milligrams required to produce an effect or to the affinity with which a drug binds to a receptor. Thus, a drug may be very potent (able to produce a response at a very low dose) but not have great efficacy (because of intolerable side effects).

10. What is meant by an equi-analgesic dose?

Most studies done to determine the clinical potency of the opioid analgesics were done against a standard dose of 10 mg of intramuscular morphine. Thus, the number of milligrams of a given drug required to produce the same degree of analgesia as 10 mg of morphine is referred to as the "equi-analgesic dose." Most opioids are far more potent when given parenterally than orally. To achieve a dose equi-analgesic to 10 mg of intramuscular morphine, anywhere from 20 to 60 mg would have to be administered orally. This is because of a "first pass effect" in the liver. Anywhere from 50 to 80% of an opioid is inactivated by hepatic metabolism after oral administration. The extent of this first pass effect varies from drug to drug. Hydromorphone, for example, is five times as potent on a milligram basis after intramuscular injection than it is after oral administration. Methadone, on the other hand, has only a 2:1 ratio.

11. By the intramuscular route, what are the equi-analgesic doses of hydromorphone, methadone, demerol, and levorphanol that would equate with 10 mg of intramuscular morphine?

At this dose level, one would require 1.5 mg of hydromorphone, 10 mg of methadone, 75 mg of meperidine, and 2 mg of levorphanol.

12. What are the major differences among the opioid analgesics?

The first major difference is between agonists and mixed agonist/antagonist drugs. The relatively pure opioid agonists include drugs such as morphine, codeine, oxycodone, levorphanol, meperidine, fentanyl, and methadone. The mixed agonist/antagonist drugs that are in popular use are pentazocine, butorphanol, and buprenorphine.

The next major differentiation is between long serum half-life and short serum half-life. Methadone and levorphanol are two of the most commonly used long serum half-life drugs, having a half-life of anywhere from 12 to over 50 hours. (With prolonged use, half-life extends markedly.) Morphine and hydromorphone are prototypes of the short serum half-life drugs.

13. What are appropriate dosing intervals for the opioid analgesics?

When used as immediate release products, morphine and hydromorphine should generally be dosed anywhere from every 2 to every 4 hours. If a sustained- or controlled-release product is used, morphine can be dosed every 8 to 12 hours. The long serum half-life drugs may have a greater duration of efficacy and can often be dosed every 4 to 6 hours. Despite the long serum half-life, analgesic efficacy does not directly parallel the serum half-life.

14. What routes of administration are available for the opioids?

Opioids can be successfully delivered by virtually any route. In general, the most convenient route is orally. However, allowances must be made for the first pass effect in the liver. When given by the intramuscular route, opioids are anywhere from two to five times as potent on a milligram basis than when given orally. They are also readily absorbed after subcutaneous injection and can be administered intravenously. Rectal and sublingual preparations are also available for some opioids. Fentanyl is available as a transdermal patch.

15. What are the benefits and drawbacks of transdermal fentanyl?

Fentanyl is a relatively potent opioid analgesic. The application of a transcutaneous patch allows for relatively stable serum levels of fentanyl over 48 to 72 hours. This cuts down the need for repeated dosing and for the pain of parenteral administration. However, after application of the first patch, there is a delay of 12 to 24 hours in achieving adequate analgesia. During this time, rescue doses must be given. Furthermore, if side effects ensue, removal of the patch will not immediately eliminate them because a subcutaneous reservoir of drug has been formed. The dose of drug is directly related to the surface area of the patch. It is available as 25, 50, 75, and 100 micrograms per hour. Direct equi-analgesic studies with morphine have not been published, but 100 micrograms per hour is approximately equi-analgesic to 2 mg per hour of morphine.

16. What are the most common side effects of the opioids?

Constipation is the most common and bothersome clinical side effect of the opioids. While respiratory depression, tolerance, dependence, and addiction get the lion's share of the adverse press, constipation is the problem with which the clinician most often has to deal. It is also a complication to which tolerance does not usually develop. Any patient being started on opioid analgesics should be given a bowel regimen. In general, a combination of the senna alkaloids and a stool softener is sufficient. However, care should be taken not to allow constipation to progress too far. Once the patient has missed more than a few days of bowel movements, disimpaction may be necessary.

17. Under what circumstances is respiratory depression a serious worry in patients treated with opioids?

If opioids are used carefully, in gradually increasing doses, respiratory depression usually is not a problem. However, there are two circumstances in which respiratory depression may occur unexpectedly. First, when using long serum half-life drugs, it must be kept in mind that five serum half-lives are required to reach steady state. Thus, when using a drug such as methadone or levorphanol, it may require more than a week to achieve steady state. During this titration period, great care must be taken because serum levels may be escalating despite stable dosing.

The second circumstance occurs in patients who undergo a pain-relieving procedure after they have been on large doses of opioids. Patients may tolerate large doses while they are in pain. However, if they undergo radiation therapy, cordotomy, or some other procedure directed at the pain syndrome itself, they may no longer be as tolerant to the opioids. Patients should be monitored carefully for a number of days following these procedures. If respiratory rate decreases or they become overly somnolent, doses should be cut back.

18. How should opioid overdose be treated?

This depends directly on the situation in which the overdose has occurred and the severity of side effects. If there is only somnolence, without respiratory depression, simply cutting back on the dose or holding a few doses is usually enough to reverse the side effects. If there is severe respiratory depression, more urgent measures are required. In these cases, naloxone may be administered intravenously. However, if it is given as a bolus, patients who have been taking opioids chronically may experience withdrawal. Therefore, naloxone should be diluted in 10 ml of saline and administered slowly. Keep in mind that opioids primarily depress respiratory rate. Therefore, simply counting respirations as they increase is enough to judge efficacy of opioid reversal. Naloxone, however, has a much shorter serum half-life than do most opioids. Repeated doses may be required.

19. What is meant by tolerance and what are its clinical manifestations?

Tolerance refers to a situation in which decreased effects are noticed despite stable doses of a drug, or increasing doses of a drug are required to maintain a given effect. In experimental models, this can develop quite rapidly. Clinically, however, many patients with stable pain syndromes can be maintained on steady doses of opioids for prolonged periods of time. As pain increases (as with advancing cancer), progressively higher doses of drug may be used to control pain. In these cases, increasing analgesia may occur without significant respiratory depression or somnolence.

20. What is meant by physical dependence?

Physical dependence is a state in which rapid discontinuation of a drug or administration of an antagonist produces an abstinence syndrome. With the opioids, an abstinence syndrome is characterized by abdominal discomfort, borborygmus, goose flesh, nausea, and yawning. In addicted subjects, there is marked drug craving. In nonaddicted subjects, there is simply severe discomfort.

21. What is meant by opioid addiction?

Addiction is a state in which there is psychological dependence on a drug, preoccupation with securing its supply, use despite harm, use for nonmedical purposes, and a high incidence of recidivism. This is actually quite rare in patients treated appropriately with opioids for pain. Even in patients with pain of nonmalignant origin, opioid addiction is quite uncommon.

22. What is patient controlled analgesia (PCA)?

As generally used today, PCA refers to a setup in which patients are able to administer their own drugs on a set basis. Usually, this is by the intravenous route. Intravenous access is established, and a system is attached in which the patient may bolus small amounts of opioid every few minutes. A "lockout period" is also established to avoid overdosing. This may be done with or without a continuous infusion.

BIBLIOGRAPHY

1. Acute Pain Management Guideline Panel: Acute Pain Management. Clinical Practice Guideline. ACHPR Pub No 92-0032. Agency for Health Care Policy and Research, Public Health Service, U.S. Department of Health and Human Services, Rockville, MD, February 1992.
2. Kanner RM, Foley KM: Patterns of narcotic drug use in a cancer pain clinic. Ann N Y Acad Sci 362:161–172, 1981.
3. Portenoy RK: Chronic opioid therapy for nonmalignant pain: From models to practice. APS J 1:285–288, 1992.
4. Portenoy RK: Opioid analgesics. In Portenoy RK, Kanner RM (eds): Pain Management: Theory and Practice. Philadelphia, FA Davis, 1996, pp 248–276.
5. Porter J, Jick H: Addiction rare in patients treated with narcotics. N Engl J Med 302:123, 1980.

33. ADJUVANT ANALGESICS

Brian Thiessen, M.D., and Russell K. Portenoy, M.D.

1. What are "adjuvant analgesics"?

"Adjuvant analgesics" are drugs that have primary indications other than pain, but are analgesic in some painful conditions. This definition distinguishes a very diverse group of drugs from the traditional analgesics, which comprise the nonopioid analgesics (acetaminophen and the nonsteroidal anti-inflammatory drugs) and the opioid analgesics.

Adjuvant Analgesics: Major Classes

Multipurpose Analgesics	Analgesic Agents for Neuropathic Pain Syndromes	Analgesic Agents for Musculo-skeletal Pain Syndromes
Antidepressants	Antidepressants	Muscle relaxants
Alpha-2 adrenergic agonists	Anticonvulsants	Benzodiazepines
Neuroleptics	GABA agonists	Analgesic Agents for Bone Pain
Corticosteroids	Oral local anesthetics	Corticosteroids
Topical anesthetics	Topical anesthetics	Osteoclast inhibitors
	Sympatholytics	Radiopharmaceuticals
	NMDA receptor blockers	
	Calcitonin	

GABA = gamma-aminobutyric acid; NMDA = N-methyl-D-aspartic acid.

As suggested by the label adjuvant, these analgesics are often co-administered with the traditional analgesics. In some patient populations, particularly those with cancer pain, the conventional approach involves the addition of an adjuvant analgesic drug only after the dose of a traditional analgesic (usually an opioid) has been optimized. In these populations, the adjuvant analgesics are administered to (a) manage pain that is refractory to the traditional analgesics, (b) allow reduction in dose of the traditional analgesic for the purpose of lessening side effects, or (c) concurrently treat a symptom other than pain.

In some clinical settings, adjuvant analgesics have become so well accepted that they are administered as the first-line drug. This is particularly true for chronic neuropathic pain syndromes unrelated to cancer, such as postherpetic neuralgia, trigeminal neuralgia, or painful polyneuropathy. In these situations, the term adjuvant is a misnomer.

2. What factors should be considered prior to prescribing an adjuvant analgesic?

To select and administer an adjuvant analgesic properly, the physician must be aware of the drug's clinical pharmacology and its particular use in patients with pain. The following information about the analgesic is necessary: (a) approved indications; (b) unapproved indications widely accepted in medical practice; (c) common side effects and uncommon, but potentially serious, adverse effects: (d) important pharmacokinetic features, including half-life, usual time-action relationships, extent of interindividual variability, and factors that may alter disposition (e.g., age or interactions with other drugs); and (e) specific dosing guidelines for pain.

3. What are the special considerations for the elderly?

In the medically frail and the elderly population, a cautious approach to the use of the adjuvant analgesics is warranted. It is prudent to select a drug with a good safety profile and begin therapy at a relatively low dose. Gradual escalation of the dose is the safest technique for confirming an effective regimen or determining that the drug is ineffective.

4. Are responses to the adjuvants uniform?

There is considerable interindividual and intraindividual variation in the response to adjuvant analgesics. This variation underscores the potential utility of sequential drug trials, which may be needed to identify a drug with a favorable benefit:risk ratio. Moreover, most trials benefit from the use of gradual dose escalation to identify the most optimal dose. The use of gradual dose escalation and the potential need for multiple trials should be explained to patients who are about to begin therapy with an adjuvant analgesic. This information helps the patient maintain appropriate expectations and reduces frustration during a period of ineffective dosing.

5. Which classes of adjuvant analgesics may be considered multipurpose, nonspecific analgesics?

Adjuvant analgesics that have been demonstrated to be effective in diverse pain syndromes can be designated multipurpose analgesics. The best characterized of these drugs are the tricyclic antidepressants. Other classes that may be considered multipurpose include the alpha-2 adrenergic agonists (e.g., clonidine), the neuroleptics, and the corticosteroids. Although there is some evidence that would support the labeling of local anesthetic drugs in this way, conventional practice now limits the use of this class to patients with neuropathic pain syndromes (see next question).

6. What is the evidence that antidepressant drugs are multipurpose analgesics?

Antidepressant drugs, especially the tricyclic antidepressants, have been extensively evaluated in many different pain syndromes, including neuropathic pain, low back pain, headache, fibromyalgia, arthritis, cancer pain, and others. A trial of an analgesic antidepressant is warranted in most patients with chronic pain.

7. Which antidepressants are commonly used for chronic pain?

The tertiary amine compound, amitriptyline, has been best studied, but there is evidence supporting the analgesic efficacy of other tertiary amine tricyclic drugs as well, including imipramine, clomipramine, and doxepin. Of the secondary amine tricyclic compounds, which are generally better tolerated than the tertiary amine drugs, desipramine has been most carefully studied and nortriptyline is also probably analgesic. Compared with the tertiary amine drugs, these secondary amine compounds are less likely to produce sedative, anticholinergic, or hypotensive side effects.

Among the newer classes of antidepressants, analgesic effects have been suggested for trazodone, maprotiline, and the selective serotonin reuptake inhibitor (SSRI), paroxetine. Of these newer classes, the SSRIs have the most favorable safety profile. They are usually better tolerated than the tricyclic antidepressants.

8. What is the relative efficacy of the various classes?

There have been few studies directly comparing the analgesic efficacy of the various antidepressant drugs. From the very limited data available, an analgesic response is most likely to be produced by the tertiary tricyclic drugs; amitriptyline is preferred because of the extensive data available for this drug. The secondary amine tricyclic drugs, such as desipramine, are probably less analgesic than the tertiary amine drugs, but are more likely to be effective than the SSRIs. But SSRIs have fewer side effects than either secondary or tertiary amines. Based on this information, the clinician should attempt to select the drug most likely to provide benefit and be tolerated by the patient.

Monoamine oxidase inhibitors (MAOIs), such as phenelzine and tranylcypromine, have been evaluated as analgesics in relatively few clinical settings. In a controlled trial, phenelzine was analgesic in patients with atypical facial pain, and a few uncontrolled trials suggested analgesic properties in other types of chronic pain. Despite these findings, use of MAOIs as analgesics has been limited because of the risk of hypertensive crises and the need for significant dietary restrictions.

Comparison of Antidepressant Side Effects

DRUG EFFECTS	CARDIOTOXICITY	SEDATION	ANTICHOLINERGIC
Tertiary amines			
Amitriptyline	++	+++	+++
Secondary amines			
Nortriptyline	+	++	+
Desipramine	+	+	+
SSRIs			
Paroxetine	–	+/–	–

SSRI = Serotinin selective reuptake inhibitors

9. What mechanisms may be responsible for antidepressant analgesia?

Relief of depression is not required for the analgesia produced by antidepressant drugs, although improvement in mood no doubt plays a role in some patients. The analgesia produced by the tricyclic antidepressants occurs at a dose significantly lower than that required to treat depression and usually appears within one week after this dose is reached—much sooner than the antidepressant effects typically appear.

The primary pharmacologic action of the antidepressants is to block reuptake of monoaminergic neurotransmitters (e.g. serotonin and norephinephrine) in the central nervous system. Descending pain modulatory pathways that use serotonin and norepinephrine as neurotransmitters have been well-characterized, and altered activity in these pathways could be the mechanism by which these drugs yield analgesic effects. The tricyclic antidepressants also interact with many other receptors, some of which have been implicated in other pain-modulating systems.

10. What are the common adverse effects of the antidepressants?

The secondary amine tricyclic antidepressants are less toxic than the tertiary amine compounds, and the SSRIs are less toxic than either tricyclic subclass (see table at question 8). At doses commonly used for pain control, the tricyclic compounds have few serious adverse effects. Cardiovascular toxicity, including hypotension and cardiac arrhythmia, is the most serious concern. Significant heart disease, including conduction disturbances, arrythmias, or failure, is a relative contraindication to treatment. Secondary amine compounds and SSRIs have a lower incidence of cardiotoxicity and are preferred if cardiac disease is present.

The more common side effects of the tricyclic antidepressants are less serious. Anticholinergic effects include dry mouth, urinary retention, blurred vision, and constipation. Somnolence and mental clouding are often transient but are a particular problem in the elderly.

Nausea is usually the most common side effect of the SSRIs. Some patients report tremulousness or insomnia, and some experience somnolence. Sexual dysfunction can be a problem for others.

11. Do any particular characteristics among patients suggest a trial of an antidepressant analgesic?

A trial of an antidepressant analgesic is potentially appropriate for any type of chronic pain. The presence of a psychiatric disorder that may also respond to these drugs, such as major depression or panic disorder, suggests an early trial. Insomnia may justify an early trial of an antidepressant analgesic, such as amitriptyline, which has sedating properties.

When the antidepressants are used to treat chronic neuropathic pain, they are often considered first-line drugs for the management of pain characterized by continuous dysethesias. These dysesthesias are often described by patients as burning, electrical, or painful numbness. Although lancinating (stabbing) neuropathic pain can respond, antidepressants are not usually considered first-line drugs for pain of this type.

In the management of cancer pain, the usual indication for a trial of an antidepressant is chronic neuropathic pain that has not responded adequately to opioid analgesics. In this setting, these drugs are used as adjuncts to an optimized opioid regimen.

12. A healthy 70-year-old man is beginning therapy with amitriptyline for painful neuropathy. What is an appropriate starting dose and dosing schedule?

The starting dose of any tricyclic agent should be low, especially in the elderly. With one of the tricyclic antidepressants, such as amitriptyline, the recommended initial dose is 10 mg/day in the elderly and 25 mg/day in younger patients. The dosage can be gradually increased every 2 to 3 days until an effective dose is reached. For amitriptyline and desipramine, this is usually in the range of 50 to 150 mg/day. Blood levels may help guide therapy. The tricyclic drugs are usually administered as a single night-time dose, thereby allowing sedative effects to occur while the patient is asleep. Some patients, however, experience morning "hangover" effect and respond better to divided doses.

The inability to tolerate a trial of amitriptyline or the existence of relative contraindications to this drug (such as pre-existing cognitive impairment, prostatism, constipation, or dry mouth) might be addressed by a trial of a secondary amine tricyclic, such as desipramine. If the risks associated with a tricyclic antidepressant are too high, a trial of an SSRI, such as paroxetine, should be considered.

13. What role does clonidine have as an adjuvant analgesic?

There is abundant evidence that alpha-2 adrenergic agonists are multipurpose, nonspecific analgesics. Clonidine is the only drug of this class available in the United States. Although one study suggests that only a small proportion of patients with chronic pain respond to this drug, responders may attain excellent analgesia. Clonidine has been shown to be analgesic in chronic headache, chronic neuropathic and nonneuropathic nonmalignant pain syndromes, and cancer-related neuropathic pain. Given the limited experience with the use of clonidine as an analgesic, however, it is not generally considered a first-line drug, but it can be considered for a trial in any refractory case of chronic pain.

The major side effects of clonidine are dry mouth and sedation. Hypotension can occur, and the drug must be used cautiously in patients predisposed to this effect.

14. What is the mechanism of analgesia produced by alpha-2 adrenergic agonists?

The mechanism or mechanisms that produce clonidine analgesia are unknown. Noradrenergic pain-modulating systems exist in the central nervous system, and it is possible that the alpha-2 adrenergic receptor is involved in the functioning of this pathway. Central sympathetic inhibition may be the analgesic mechanism involved in those pain syndromes sustained, at least in part, by sympathetic efferent activity (so-called sympathetically maintained pain).

15. What is the role of neuroleptic drugs in the treatment of pain?

Their role is limited. Methotrimeprazine is a phenothiazine neuroleptic that has been demonstrated to be a multipurpose analgesic. This drug, which is available in the United States only as a parenteral formulation, is highly sedating and can produce hypotension. It is used only in the cancer population, generally for bedridden patients at the end of life. For these patients, it can be a very effective therapy for pain associated with agitation, insomnia, or nausea. In controlled studies of this drug, the analgesic potency of 10 to 20 mg intramuscularly (IM) approximated that of morphine 10 mg IM in opioid-naive patients.

Although the experience with methotrimeprazine suggests that neuroleptic drugs can be nonspecific analgesics, there is actually very little evidence that other drugs in this class have analgesic effects. In one controlled trial, chlorpromazine was not analgesic, and other controlled trials are lacking. Anecdotal reports have suggested that drugs such as haloperidol or fluphenazine may be analgesic in neuropathic pain, and on this basis, a therapeutic trial of one of these drugs is sometimes administered in cases of neuropathic pain that has been refractory to other therapies.

16. Describe the extrapyramidal side effects of neuroleptics.

The extrapyramidal effects of neuroleptics can be divided into two groups: those that occur early in the course of treatment and those that are delayed in onset. The early effects include acute dystonic reactions (such as torticollis) parkinsonism, akathisia, and neuroleptic malignant syndrome. The late effects include tardive dyskinesia and other tardive movement disorders.

Other side effects include sedation, orthostatic hypotension, and anticholinergic effects such as dry mouth, blurred vision, and urinary hesitancy. Mental clouding and confusion are relatively common in the elderly and medically ill. Rarely, neuroleptics may cause idiosyncratic side effects such as skin rashes, blood dyscrasias, and hepatic damage.

17. List some of the common pain syndromes for which corticosteroids have shown benefit.

In the nonmalignant pain population, short courses of corticosteroids are often given to provide symptomatic relief of acute herpetic neuralgia, carpal tunnel syndrome, and reflex sympathetic dystrophy. Long-term therapy is avoided because of the risk of toxicity. In the cancer population, the use of these drugs is far more extensive. Controlled trials and clinical series have shown that corticosteroids can be beneficial in many types of cancer pain, including malignant epidural spinal cord compression, bone pain, pain due to increased intracranial pressure, neuropathic pain from compression or infiltration of peripheral neural structures, and pain from expansion of visceral capsules or obstruction of a hollow viscus.

18. How do corticosteroids produce analgesia?

It is likely that corticosteroids have a variety of analgesic mechanisms. Corticosteroids have direct anti-inflammatory effects, reducing the tissue concentrations of inflammatory mediators that activate nociceptors. These drugs also reduce the aberrant firing that can originate from sites of nerve injury. Pain related to malignant compression may lessen because of steroid-induced reduction of peritumoral edema and, in cases of steroid-responsive neoplasms, reduction of tumor bulk.

19. List the common side effects associated with corticosteroid use.

Acute treatment with corticosteroids is usually well tolerated. Potential toxicities include hyperglycemia, fluid retention (which may cause hypertension or cardiac failure in predisposed patients), dyspepsia, peptic ulcer disease, insomnia, and neuropsychological effects (ranging from frank delirium to isolated mood or cognitive or perceptual disturbances). Chronic administration of corticosteroids can cause the following adverse effects: cushingoid habitus, weight gain, hypertension, osteoporosis, myopathy, increased risk of infection, hyperglycemia, and peptic ulcer disease. Rarely, chronic treatment results in aseptic necrosis of the femoral or humeral head.

20. What dosing regimens are commonly used when corticosteroids are administered for pain?

Dexamethasone has been the preferred corticosteroid in the cancer population. Use has been justified by the low mineralocorticoid effects produced by this drug. Dosing regimens have traditionally been divided into low and high-dose schemes. A high-dose regimen (most commonly 100 mg loading dose followed by 24 mg every 6 hours) is often initiated in the setting of very severe, often rapidly escalating pain ("crescendo pain") that has not responded promptly to an opioid. Severe bone pain and worsening malignant plexopathy are examples of such pain syndromes. In addition, oncologic emergencies that are steroid-responsive, such as superior vena cava syndrome and malignant epidural spinal cord compression, are commonly managed with high-dose steroid regimens.

Low-dose dexamethasone regimens vary from 4 mg every 6 hours to 1 to 2 mg twice daily. They are commonly used in the setting of advanced medical illness with pain refractory to opioids and other adjuvant agents. Given the side effects of these agents, the patient must be continually assessed for efficacy and toxicity during long-term therapy. In all cases, the lowest dose that achieves the desired analgesic benefit should be sought.

Other corticosteroids have also been used as analgesics, including prednisone and methylprednisone. There have been no comparative trials of the various drugs, and the doses that have been administered have varied.

21. Neuropathic pain describes a diverse set of pain syndromes in which the sustaining mechanism is believed to involve aberrant somatosensory processing in the peripheral or central nervous system. The term includes syndromes such as painful polyneuropathy, trigeminal neuralgia, central pain, postherpetic neuralgia, and phantom pain. What is the role of the adjuvant analgesics in the treatment of chronic neuropathic pain?

Neuropathic pain syndromes are often refractory to traditional analgesics. The adjuvant analgesics are extremely valuable for these diverse disorders. Although data from clinical trials are inadequate to guide the selection of specific drugs, some general guidelines can be recommended on the basis of clinical experience. For example, patients with neuropathic pain characterized by continuous dysesthesias (often described as constant burning or electrical sensations) are usually offered an antidepressant analgesic early. Orally administered local anesthetics are also commonly used, and other multipurpose analgesics (such as clonidine or a neuroleptic) may be considered in refractory cases. Patients with lancinating (stabbing) pain or neuropathic pain characterized by a paroxysmal onset and longer duration are usually offered trials of anticonvulsants or baclofen, a gamma-aminobutyric acid, first; trials with the drugs used for continuous neuropathic pain usually follow. Finally, patients suspected of having neuropathic pain sustained by efferent activity in the sympathetic nervous system (sympathetically maintained pain) are sometimes treated with adjuvant analgesics that may modulate sympathetic function.

Adjuvant Analgesics Typically Selected for Neuropathic Pain
with Predominating Continuous Dysesthesias

	Examples
First Line	
Tricyclic antidepressants	Amitriptyline, desipramine
"Newer" antidepressants	Paroxetine
Oral local anesthetics	Mexiletine, tocainide, flecainide
For Refractory Cases	
Alpha-2 adrenergic agonists	Clonidine
Anticonvulsants	Carbamazepine, phenytoin, valproate, clonazepam
Topical agents	Capsaicin, local anesthetics
Neuroleptics	Prochlorperazine, haloperidol
NMDA receptor antagonists	Dextromethorphan, ketamine
Calcitonin	
Baclofen	

NMDA = N-methyl-D-aspartic acid

Adjuvant Analgesics Typically Selected for Neuropathic Pain
with Predominating Lancinating or Paroxysmal Dysesthesias

	Examples
First Line	
Anticonvulsants	Carbamazepine, phenytoin, valproate, clonazepam
Baclofen	
For Refractory Cases	
Oral local anesthetics	Mexiletine, tocainide, flecainide
Tricyclic antidepressants	Amitriptyline, desipramine
"Newer antidepressants	Paroxetine
Neuroleptics	Pimozide
Alpha-2 adrenergic agonists	Clonidine
Topical agents	Capsaicin, local anesthetics
NMDA receptor antagonists	Dextromethorphan, ketamine
Calcitonin	

NMDA = N-methyl-D-aspartic acid.

22. How are anticonvulsants used in the management of neuropathic pain?

Abundant survey data and controlled studies have established the efficacy of anticonvulsant drugs for neuropathic pain characterized by lancinating dysesthesias or dysesthesias that have a paroxysmal onset but may be more prolonged (see second table at question 21). Carbamazepine is most widely used for this indication, but other anticonvulsants, including phenytoin, valproate, and clonazepam, have been used for many years.

More recently, newer anticonvulsants have been tried for neuropathic pain. In a recent series, gabapentin was shown to benefit some patients with reflex sympathetic dystrophy. Lamotrigine reduced hyperalgesia in an animal pain model, but its efficacy has yet to be described in humans. Anecdotal experience suggested that felbamate might be analgesic but, given the recent reports of aplastic anemia associated with felbamate therapy, the utility of this drug is limited. Gabapentin appears to have a favorable safety profile, and preliminary clinical experience supports its use as an analgesic for neuropathic pain.

23. List some painful conditions with prominent lancinating or paroxysmal symptoms for which the anticonvulsant agents have shown benefit.

Trigeminal neuralgia was the first painful condition for which the analgesic benefit of carbamazepine was described. Other anticonvulsants have also been used to treat this condition. Studies have also demonstrated the efficacy of these drugs in the treatment of lancinating pain associated with postherpetic neuralgia and painful diabetic neuropathy. Other reports suggest benefit in glossopharyngeal neuralgia, tabetic lightning pains, paroxysmal symptoms of multiple sclerosis, stabbing pain following laminectomy, lancinating pain due to cancer, and posttraumatic mononeuropathy.

24. Can anticonvulsants be used for continuous dysesthesias?

Clinical observation suggests that some patients with continuous dysesthesias, such as the constant burning reported by many patients with painful polyneuropathy, do experience relief from anticonvulsant drugs. These agents should be considered second-line therapy for neuropathic pain of this type (see first table at question 21).

25. Of all the analgesic anticonvulsants, carbamazepine has been most widely used. What are the adverse effects associated with this drug?

Carbamazepine commonly causes sedation, dizziness, diplopia, unsteadiness, and nausea. These effects can be minimized by starting with low initial doses (100 mg, 2 or 3 times/day) and increasing the dose gradually (by 100 mg every other day). The effective analgesic dose is variable, and dosing should be increased until pain is relieved, side effects occur, or the plasma concentrations exceed the therapeutic range for seizure control.

Carbamazepine often lowers white blood cell counts, but clinically significant leukopenia or thrombocytopenia occurs rarely. A complete blood count should be obtained prior to therapy, several weeks later, then two or three months after that. Therapy should be discontinued if a serious decline in blood count (e.g., a leukocyte count below 3000/cm^3) occurs. Hepatotoxicity is also rare with carbamazepine, but the possibility dictates periodic monitoring of liver function tests. Hyponatremia due to inappropriate secretion of antidiuretic hormone is an uncommon and usually asymptomatic adverse effect. Hypersensitivity reactions, usually rash, occur rarely, and cases of Stevens-Johnson syndrome have been reported.

26. Is there much individual variation in the response to drugs used for the management of lancinating or paroxysmal dysesthesias?

Patients with lancinating or paroxysmal dysesthesias may respond to one anticonvulsant but not to others, or they may not respond to any of the anticonvulsants but may do well with one of the other drugs used to treat pain of this type (see next question). For this reason, it is appropriate to undertake sequential trials of anticonvulsant drugs in patients with refractory pain.

27. What other drugs are used in the management of lancinating or paroxysmal dysesthesias?

Baclofen, a gamma-aminobutyric acid-B receptor agonist, is generally considered the best alternative to the anticonvulsants in the treatment of lancinating or paroxysmal dysesthesias, including trigeminal neuralgia. Treatment is usually started at 5 mg 3 times/day and slowly increased to the range of 30 to 90 mg/day. Baclofen must not be withdrawn abruptly, as this can precipitate a withdrawal syndrome characterized by restlessness, delirium, and seizures.

Many other drugs have also been used to treat refractory lancinating neuropathic pain (see second table at question 21). Orally administered local anesthetics are often selected if an anticonvulsant and baclofen have failed. A butyrophenone neuroleptic, pimozide, has been shown to be effective for trigeminal neuralgia and has been used for similar pains. This drug has a high side-effect profile, however, and is often poorly tolerated. Other drugs, including antidepressants (e.g., amitriptyline) and other agents usually selected for neuropathic pains of other types, are also used in this setting.

28. What is the role of systemically administered local anesthetics in the treatment of neuropathic pain?

Systemically delivered local anesthetics have been used to treat both acute and chronic pain for many years. Brief intravenous infusions of lidocaine or procaine can potentially relieve diverse types of pain, including those not categorized as neuropathic. The need for careful monitoring during this therapy and uncertainty about the optimal dosing guidelines and durability of effects have limited its utility.

Treatment with systemic local anesthetics has become commonplace with the advent of oral local anesthetic drugs, such as mexiletine, tocainide, and flecainide. The use of these drugs has focused on neuropathic pain because of evidence of efficacy from several controlled trials in painful polyneuropathy and painful traumatic mononeuropathy. A trial of an oral local anesthetic is usually recommenced in patients without medical contraindications who have continuous dyesthesias that have been refractory to antidepressant treatment and those with lancinating neuropathic pain that have not responded to anticonvulsants or baclofen (see tables at question 21 and next question). In the United States, mexiletine is the preferred drug for this indication.

29. Cardiovascular toxicity is a major concern with oral local anesthetic agents. What are the relative contraindications to the use of these drugs, and how should the potential for this toxicity be monitored?

Toxic concentrations of systemically delivered local anesthetics can produce cardiac conduction disturbances and myocardial depression. Patients with a history of cardiac failure or arrhythmia and those at risk for these problems (e.g., patients with known coronary artery disease) should not receive these drugs without an appropriate evaluation. Referral to a cardiologist may be required.

Most patients older than 50 and all those with known heart disease should be monitored with repeated electrocardiograms (ECG) during dose escalation. Younger patients with no known cardiac disease should also undergo an ECG if relatively high doses are reached. The first sign of local anesthetic toxicity is prolongation of the PR interval and QRS duration. With higher concentrations, bradycardia and arrythmias occur.

Additional toxicities include dizziness, perioral numbness, encephalopathy and seizures. Nausea and vomiting is common with mexiletine. Liver damage and blood dyscrasias are rare complications.

30. What is the role of topical drugs in the treatment of pain?

Three types of topical drugs have been used in the management of chronic pain: local anesthetics, capsaicin, and nonsteroidal anti-inflammatory drugs. Although these drugs are most often used in the treatment of neuropathic pains, they are sometimes used in other syndromes as well.

A trial of a topical local anesthetic is often considered for neuropathic pain syndromes characterized by a predominant peripheral mechanism and continuous dysesthesias and nonneuropathic pain syndromes attributable to a focus of cutaneous or subcutaneous tissue injury. Of the topical local anesthetics, only one commercially available formulation can produce dense cutaneous anesthesia: a 1:1 mixture of lidocaine and prilocaine known as a eutectic mixture of local anesthetics (EMLA). This drug, which is approved for the prevention of pain due to needle punctures, was shown to be beneficial in a limited study of patients with postherpetic neuralgia and has been used to treat a variety of chronic pain syndromes. Cutaneous anesthesia is produced if the cream is applied in a thick layer and covered with an occlusive dressing for at least one hour. The need for cutaneous anesthesia for pain relief has not been established in all syndromes, however, and it is possible that some patients will respond to a thin application of EMLA without a dressing, or to other commercially available topical anesthetic preparations that do not produce cutaneous anesthesia. Therefore, patients who are offered a trial with EMLA should be encouraged to try different modes of application. If an occlusive dressing is needed and a large area of skin must be covered, ordinary plastic wrap often suffices.

31. How is topical capsaicin used in the treatment of chronic pain?

Capsaicin, the active ingredient in hot peppers, is known to deplete small peptides in primary afferent neurons, including those involved in pain transmission. For example, this compound releases and then depletes the peptide known as substance P, which mediates pain transmission at the first central synapse in the dorsal horn of the spinal cord. The evidence suggests that some patients with neuropathic pain will benefit from the topical application of this drug to the painful site. Several controlled trials also indicate that patients with painful arthritic small joints can also benefit from the topical application of this drug.

32. Discuss the method of application of capsaicin.

Capsaicin cream is commercially available in 0.025% and 0.075% concentrations. The higher concentration has been tested most often in clinical trials and in most instances should be tried first. The cream is applied locally to the painful region 3 to 4 times/day. A minimum 4-week trial is necessary to obtain maximal benefit. The major adverse effect is local burning, which can be intense and necessitate discontinuation of the cream. Initial burning may diminish with repeated applications. Alternatively, applying a topical local anesthetic or ingesting an analgesic prior to application of the capsaicin may allow continuation of the therapy.

33. Are topical nonsteroidal anti-inflammatory drugs effective?

The evidence that topical anti-inflammatory drugs can reduce pain is equivocal. Such a formulation is sometimes administered for arthritis or postherpetic neuralgia.

34. Which adjuvant agents are useful for the treatment of sympathetically maintained pains?

Sympathetically maintained pain is a form of neuropathic pain in which the pain is believed to be sustained through efferent sympathetic activity. This diagnosis is usually suspected when patients fulfill criteria for reflex sympathetic dystrophy or causalgia. The latter two syndromes, which have recently been renamed by the International Association for the Study of Pain as complex regional pain syndrome (CRPS) types I and II, are characterized by the association of pain and local autonomic dysregulation and/or trophic changes. This constellation of findings raises the possibility of sympathetically maintained pain, which could potentially be ameliorated by interruption of sympathetic outflow to the painful site. Sympathetic interruption is usually accomplished by sympathetic nerve blocks. This procedure can be both diagnostic and therapeutic. (See Chapter 27).

Drug therapy is usually considered for patients with CRPS type I or II who are not candidates for sympathetic nerve blocks or who have had blocks but experienced declining efficacy. Anecdotal reports have described the use of virtually all of the multipurpose analgesics and the adjuvant analgesics for neuropathic pain. Although the mechanism of action is unknown, a trial of intranasal calcitonin is often administered on the basis of a successful controlled trial. Several drugs modulate the activity of the sympathetic nervous system and have also been used anecdotally for the diagnosis or treatment of sympathetically maintained pain. Intravenous phentolamine, an alpha-1 adrenergic antagonist has been touted as a diagnostic test for sympathetically maintained pain, and anecdotal reports have suggested the efficacy of other adrenergic drugs.

35. Do benzodiazepine medications have a role to play as adjuvant analgesics?

As previously mentioned, the anticonvulsant benzodiazepine, clonazepam, is used as an adjuvant analgesic, typically in the treatment of lancinating or paroxysmal neuropathic pain syndromes. Apart from this drug, however, the evidence for benzodiazepine analgesia is limited and often contradictory. Although a survey suggested that alprazolam, a benzodiazepine with antidepressant activity, is efficacious for chronic neuropathic pain in the cancer population, other benzodiazepines have not shown similar analgesic properties.

Despite the limited supporting data, the benzodiazepines may have a role in the management of some pain syndromes. Patients with pain associated with anxiety disorders may report less discomfort if the anxious mood can be improved. In addition, benzodiazepines such as diazepam and lorazepam have been used to lessen muscle spasm and may be helpful in patients whose pain is related to spasm or spasticity.

36. What is the role of the so-called muscle-relaxant drugs?

Musculoskeletal pain syndromes are among the most common ailments in medical practice. Many of these conditions can be managed with nonpharmacological approaches. Muscle relaxants represent a diverse group, which includes antihistamines (e.g., orphenadrine), chemicals similar in structure to tricyclic compounds (e.g., cyclobenzaprine), and drugs of other structures (e.g., methocarbamol, carisoprodol, chlorzoxazone). Although each of these drugs has been demonstrated in controlled trials to offer analgesic effects in musculoskeletal pain, there is no evidence that they actually relax skeletal muscle. Nonetheless, these drugs are analgesic and are generally well tolerated. Sedation is the major side effect. They are usually used on a short-term basis and, like the benzodiazepines and opioids, should not be prescribed over a long period unless patients are carefully monitored by experienced clinicians.

37. Which adjuvant analgesics are used in the management of cancer pain?

As noted, patients with neuropathic cancer pain are offered trials of the same adjuvant analgesics used to manage nonmalignant neuropathic pain syndromes. Other adjuvant analgesics may be useful in other cancer pain syndromes. The most important of these are adjuvant analgesics for the treatment of malignant bone pain or pain caused by bowel obstruction.

38. Discuss the analgesic potential of calcitonin.

The effects on bone produced by calcitonin may yield analgesia in malignant bone pain and other painful conditions of bone, such as osteoporosis. This drug also has analgesic potential beyond these indications. Clinical trials have shown efficacy in the treatment of sympathetically maintained pain and phantom limb pain, suggesting a possible role for this agent in patients with diverse types of refractory neuropathic pain syndromes (see tables at question 21). The mechanisms that account for analgesia in the latter conditions are unknown.

39. How are radiopharmaceuticals used in the treatment of bone pain?

Radiopharmaceuticals are radionuclide compounds that have preferential uptake into bone and thereby deliver a concentrated dose of radiation to bony metastases. Phosphorus-32 orthophosphate was the initial compound used in treating pain from bony metastases. Although it relieved bone pain in up to 80% of patients, it had a tendency to produce significant bone-marrow suppression. Of the newly developed radiopharmaceuticals, strontium-89 is commercially available in the United States. Other radiopharmaceuticals with similar bone-seeking properties are being developed. Some degree of pain relief occurs in approximately 80% of patients receiving strontium-89; 10% achieve complete relief. Onset of action takes from 7 to 21 days postinjection and the duration of action is typically from 3 to 6 months. Bone marrow suppression is the major toxicity, occurring in some 30% of patients.

BIBLIOGRAPHY

1. Backonja M: Local anesthetics as adjuvant analgesics. J Pain Symptom Manage 9:491–499, 1994.
2. Cherny NI, Portenoy RK: Cancer pain: Principles of assessment and syndromes. In Wall PD, Melzack R, (eds): Textbook of Pain, 3rd ed. Edinburgh, Churchill Livingstone, 1994, pp 787–823.
3. Fromm GH: Baclofen as an adjuvant analgesic. J Pain Symptom Manage 9:500–509, 1994.
4. Hegarty A, Portenoy RK: Pharmacotherapy of neuropathic pain. Semin Neurol 14:213–224, 1994.
5. Holmes RA: Radiopharmaceuticals in clinical trials. Semin Oncol 20:22–26, 1993.
6. Monks R: Psychotropic drugs. In Wall PD, Melzack R, (eds): Textbook of Pain, 3rd ed. Edinburgh, Churchill Livingstone, 1994, pp 963–990.
7. Onghena P, Van Houdenhove B: Antidepressant-induced analgesia in chronic nonmalignant pain: A meta-analysis of 39 placebo-controlled studies. Pain 49:205–219, 1992.
8. Patt RB, Proper G, Reddy S: The neuroleptics as adjuvant analgesics. J Pain Symptom Manage 9:446–453, 1994.
9. Payne R: Pharmacologic management of bone pain in the cancer patient. Clin J Pain 5:S43–S50, 1989.
10. Rowbotham MC: Topical analgesic agents. In Fields HL, Liebeskind JC (eds): Pharmacological Approaches to the Treatment of Chronic Pain. Seattle, IASP Press, 1994, pp 211–229.
11. Swerdlow M: Anticonvulsant drugs and chronic pain. Clin Neuropharmacol 7:51–82, 1984.
12. Watanabe S, Bruera E: Corticosteroids as adjuvant analgesics. J Pain Symptom Manage 9:442–445, 1994.

VIII. Nonpharmacologic Management

34. TEMPORARY NEURAL BLOCKADE

Michael Hanania, M.D., and Martin R. Boorin, D.M.D.

1. What is the role of temporary nerve blocks in pain management?

Nerve blocks can help in the diagnosis and treatment of pain. Peripheral and central nerve blocks help to localize the origin of the specific pain problem. When pain seems to cover multiple dermatomes, a selective peripheral nerve block helps to diagnose which nerve or dermatome is primarily responsible for the pain. Temporary nerve blocks are also necessary before more permanent neurolytic procedures can be attempted. When a permanent neurolytic procedure is contemplated, a temporary nerve block should produce complete pain relief before the longer-lasting block is instituted.

For unclear reasons, a temporary nerve block sometimes results in prolonged pain relief, outlasting the duration of the local anesthetic. In cases of somatic pain, such as mechanical low back pain, temporary nerve blocks may break the pain cycle and allow increased function. This helps to facilitate physical therapy and rehabilitation, thereby preventing disuse muscle atrophy and joint dysfunction.

In some syndromes (such as nerve injury) it is unclear whether the primary pain generator is peripheral (at the site of nerve injury) or central (within the spinal cord). If peripheral nerve block produces complete pain relief, it is inferred that the generator is peripheral.

2. What is the mechanism of action of local anesthesia? What are the implications for differential blockade?

Local anesthetics are weak bases that reversibly block sodium channels and impair the propagation of an action potential along a nerve fiber. In general, thinner fibers are more sensitive to anesthetic blockade than thicker, myelinated fibers. Sympathetic fibers are very thin. Nociceptors (which are responsible for the perception of noxious stimuli) are A-delta and C-fibers (also quite thin, although somewhat thicker than the sympathetic nerves). Fibers subserving proprioception and light touch are relatively thick; motor fibers are the thickest. Thus, when progressively increasing concentrations of an anesthetic are used, sympathetic fibers are blocked first, followed by nociceptors, proprioceptors, and motor fibers. Function returns in the opposite order as anesthetics wear off.

3. Which are the ester and amide local anesthetics? Discuss their fundamental differences.

The **ester local anesthetics** have an ester linkage between the aromatic moiety and amine group and are metabolized by plasma cholinesterases. Their half-lives in the circulation are short. A product of their metabolism is p-aminobenzoic acid, which is sometimes associated with hypersensitivity reactions. Procaine, cocaine, chloroprocaine, and tetracaine are ester anesthetics. The **amide local anesthetics** have an amide linkage and undergo primarily hepatic metabolism. The amide local anesthetics include lidocaine, mepivacaine, bupivacaine, ropivacaine, and etidocaine.

4. What are the differences in duration of action among the commonly used local anesthetics?

Typical durations of sensory anesthesia for peripheral nerve blocks are about 30–90 min for procaine and chloroprocaine, 2–4 hr for lidocaine, 3–5 hr for mepivacaine, and 6–12 hr for bupivacaine. Durations vary depending on size of the nerve and proximity of the needle to the nerve. The addition of epinephrine to anesthetic solution also prolongs duration of action because of local vasoconstriction.

5. List the toxic dose limits for peripheral nerve blockade for chloroprocaine, procaine, lidocaine, mepivacaine, bupivacaine, and tetracaine.

Local Anesthetic	Toxic Dose (mg/kg)	Local Anesthetic	Toxic Dose (mg/kg)
Chloroprocaine	11	Mepivacaine	5 (7 if epinephrine added)
Procaine	6	Bupivacaine	2.5
Lidocaine	5 (7 if epinephrine added)	Tetracaine	1.5

Overdoses usually produce symptoms indicative of central nervous system dysfunction (dizziness, tinnitus, metallic taste, slurred speech, and seizures). These are often followed by cardiovascular symptoms, such as hypotension, tachy- or bradyarrhythmias, ventricular fibrillation, and, in extreme cases, electrical standstill.

6. What is the role of neuraxial block in pain management?

Epidural or spinal blocks provide temporary block of neural function at a spinal cord level. They help to differentiate a peripheral from a central origin of pain. If a peripheral nerve or root block has failed, but a spinal block relieves pain, it may be inferred that the origin of the pain is more central (within the spinal cord). Epidural blockade also offers the option of leaving the catheter in place for prolonged treatment. Thus, epidural analgesia or anesthesia can be provided on an ongoing basis or through intermittent boluses. This procedure may facilitate rehabilitation.

7. What are the common complications of epidural or intrathecal anesthetic blockade?

Epidural blockade involves the risk of inadvertent dural puncture. When this occurs, cerebrospinal fluid (CSF) may leak and a postlumbar puncture (low-pressure) headache may develop. This complication is described in greater detail in the chapter on headaches. Rarely, the needle used for puncture may injure a nerve root. Even less common are the formation of epidural abscesses, epidural hematoma, or injury to the cauda equina. Local anesthetics also may induce temporary neuritis. Cephalad migration of the anesthetic agent may produce an anesthetic level much higher than the level anticipated. In cervical blocks, cephalad migration may lead to respiratory arrest. Transient hypotension is fairly common as a result of vasodilatation. If methylprednisolone is injected into the subarachnoid space, chronic arachnoiditis is an uncommon but serious late complication.

8. What are the indications and contraindications for epidural steroid injections?

The efficacy of epidural steroid injections for chronic low back pain is still highly controversial. In acute exacerbations of radicular nerve pain, injections may be of some benefit. Radicular pain is more likely than mechanical low back pain to respond to steroid injections. Recovery from an acutely herniated lumbar or cervical disc may be hastened by epidural steroid injections. With acute low back pain, most clinicians use 2–3 weeks of conservative management before attempting epidural steroid injections. Epidural steroids seem to be least helpful in spinal stenosis, mechanical low back pain, or long-standing chronic low back pain. Contraindications include coagulopathy, local infection, or progressive weakness that may require surgical decompression.

9. What is the appropriate timing of epidural steroid injections?

A steroid formulation such as methylprednisolone or triamcinolone is usually injected in doses of 40–80 mg every 2–4 weeks to a maximum of 3 injections in 6 months. Evidence suggests that more than 3 injections offer no added benefit and may increase the risk of side effects. Adrenal suppression with decreased cortisol levels has been shown to occur for 3–5 weeks after a typical epidural steroid injection. Multiple injections may produce ligamentous laxity.

10. What are the various brachial plexus blocks? For what pain conditions are they useful?

The brachial plexus can be blocked proximally at the level of the nerve roots and trunks by the interscalene approach; at the level of the divisions and cords by the supra- or infraclavicular approach; and distally at the level of the terminal branches or nerves by the axillary approach. A brachial plexus block can be performed by single injection or continuous catheter technique for repeated injections or infusion. It may be useful for painful conditions such as complex regional pain syndrome (CRPS), shoulder-hand syndrome after stroke, acute or postherpetic neuralgia involving dermatomes within C5–T1, vascular insufficiency of Raynaud's disease, and phantom limb pain. Brachial plexus block also facilitates range-of-motion exercises in cases of frozen shoulder, elbow, or wrist. Because the thoracocervical sympathetic nerves travel in close relation to the somatic nerves of the brachial plexus, brachial plexus block results in sympathetic blockade as well. It also may be used for postoperative pain management and prevention of phantom limb pain after amputation.

11. What are the possible side effects and complications of the various brachial plexus blocks?
Hematoma, neuropathy, and unintentional intravascular injection are possible with any of these blocks. Interscalene block may be associated with unintentional injection of local anesthetic into the epidural or subarachnoid space; recurrent laryngeal nerve block, which causes hoarseness; phrenic nerve block; and ipsilateral Horner's syndrome. Pneumothorax, although rare, is most often associated with the supraclavicular block.

12. What is the sensory innervation of the lower extremities?
The sciatic nerve divides at the level of the knee into the tibial and common peroneal nerves. The sural nerve, which forms from the tibial and common peroneal nerves, provides sensory innervation to the lateral aspect of the lower leg and foot. Anteriorly, the femoral nerve eventually becomes the saphenous nerve and provides sensory innervation to the medial aspect of the lower leg and foot. The lateral femoral cutaneous nerve and obturator nerve provide sensory innervation to the lateral and medial thigh, respectively.

13. What painful conditions are treated with intercostal nerve blocks?
Intercostal nerve blocks are useful in acute herpetic neuralgia involving the thoracic dermatomes. Early sympathetic or neural blockade may reduce the incidence of postherpetic neuralgia. The sympathetic fibers travel with the intercostal nerves and can be blocked easily at the posterior midclavicular line, along the inferior aspect of the rib. Intercostal nerve blocks can be used to differentiate between pain originating in the chest or abdominal wall and pain with a visceral origin because the intercostal nerves innervate only the outer structures. Intercostal neuralgia and scar neuromas after thoracotomy and some cases of postherpetic neuralgia may be treated by intercostal blocks. Neurolysis by cryoanalgesia or radiofrequency lesioning may be considered if satisfactory temporary relief is obtained after local anesthetic block.

14. What is the role of facet blockade in back pain?
Facet joints may be the source of significant mechanical back and neck pain. Pain is usually deep in the paravertebral regions of the back or neck and associated with with areas of referred pain. Pain due to facet disease increases with extension, rotation, or lateral flexion of the spine. The facet joint is innervated by the medial branch of the posterior primary ramus from the level involved and the level above. Hypertrophic arthropathy and eventually osteophytic degeneration and arthritic changes in these joints are postulated to cause the pain. Local anesthetic block of the medial branch nerve helps to make the diagnosis, although false-positive results are possible. Intraarticular or periarticular steroid injections may provide prolonged relief. Cryo or radiofrequency neurolysis of the medial branch nerve is an option if local anesthetic block gives good but temporary pain relief.

15. What are the indications for a suprascapular nerve block?
The suprascapular nerve not only supplies the supraspinatus muscle but also provides sensory fibers to the shoulder joint. Therefore, suprascapular nerve block can temporarily relieve shoulder joint pain and allow the patient to perform active range-of-motion exercises. Frozen shoulder syndrome as a result of immobilization may be prevented. When suprascapular nerve entrapment is suspected as the cause of shoulder pain, steroids also may be injected into the suprascapular notch at the superior border of the scapula.

16. When is a lateral femoral cutaneous nerve block used in chronic pain management?

A lateral femoral cutaneous nerve block is sometimes useful for treatment of meralgia pares-thetica, a syndrome of pain and dysesthetic cutaneous sensation in the anterolateral thigh sec-ondary to entrapment of the lateral femoral cutaneous nerve as it passes posterior to the inguinal ligament. It is commonly associated with obesity, diabetes, or tight belts.

17. Describe the primary CNS center for nociceptive input from the upper cervical and craniofacial regions. Why is the diagnosis of orofacial pain often so difficult?

Pain impulses from the orofacial region are carried by primary afferent fibers that pass through the trigeminal ganglion to the trigeminal brainstem sensory nuclear complex, where they synapse with second-order neurons. This orofacial sensory relay center, which extends from the pons into the upper cervical cord, can be divided into the main trigeminal sensory nucleus and the trigeminal spinal tract nucleus. The main relay for pain information occurs in the subnucleus caudalis, the most caudal section of the trigeminal spinal tract nucleus. Second-order neurons in the cervical spinal dorsal horn and in the nucleus caudalis cross to the contralateral side and ascend to the thalamus via spinothalamic and trigeminothalamic pathways. The final signals sent to the thalamus by these two relay centers are influenced through the convergence of several af-ferent inputs from the skin, oral mucosa, dental pulp, temporomandibular joint, masticatory mus-cles, and cervical region into one neural path. This convergence on the second-order neuron may explain the often perplexing pain-referral patterns observed in the head, face, and neck.

Excitatory areas also may arise centrally, with pain perceived at a peripheral site. In such cases, treatment directed at the painful site rather than the central source is ineffective. Clinical examination and local anesthetic blockade may help to identify the true source of the pain.

Cranial nerves IX and X, as well as upper cervical nerves (C1–C3) carrying nociceptive input from the cervical spine, converge on the nucleus caudalis with the trigeminal afferent neu-rons. The convergence of impulses from both areas is the basis for referral of pain from the cervi-cal spine to the face and head.

18. Describe the use of diagnostic anesthetic blocks to identify referral of pain to the face and teeth by muscles of mastication.

In both myofascial pain syndrome and acute single muscle myofascial disorders, pain is be-lieved to be derived from trigger points (TPs) within the myofascial tissues. TPs are characterized by localized, deep tenderness in a taut band of skeletal muscle, tendon, or ligament that has the ability to refer pain to a specific anatomic distribution. The area of perceived pain referred by the irritable TP is known as the **zone of reference** and may be located in a distant location. Systematic palpation of the musculature may identify a zone of referral through a consistent and repro-ducible altered pain sensation in the area of complaint. Multiple TPs may have overlapping areas of referred pain. The symptoms of myofascial pain may outlast the initiating events and set up cyclical muscle pain. This cycle may be sustained by numerous perpetuating physical and psy-chosocial factors. Patterns of pain referral from the muscles of mastication frequently involve re-gions of the face and mouth and complicate proper diagnosis and treatment. Injection of small volumes of local anesthetic solution directly into the muscle may be diagnostic.

The temporalis muscle has three muscle fiber regions that may refer pain to the maxillary teeth and/or ipsilateral mid-face, sometimes mimicking sinus disease. Diagnostic injection of the temporalis muscle requires caution to avoid intravascular injection into the superficial temporal artery. The masseter muscle may contain TPs in several regions and is readily accessible for diag-nostic block. The superficial body of the masseter commonly refers to regions involving the pos-terior maxillary and mandibular teeth, whereas the deep body may refer to the posterior mandible, styloid region, and ipsilateral ear. The lateral pterygoid muscle, although not readily palpated, is associated with pain deep into the temporomandibular joint and maxillary sinus region. Spasm of this muscle leads to acute interference with mandibular movement. The medial pterygoid muscle may refer pain to the back of the mouth and pharynx, temporomandibular joint, and ear. Diagnostic blockade may be approached via intraoral and transcutaneous injections.

Pterygoid muscle blocks may be complicated by temporary facial paresthesia and intravascular injection into the maxillary artery.

Fricton JR, Gross SG: Muscle disorders. In Pertes RA, Gross SG (eds): Clinical Management of Temporomandibular Disorders and Orofacial Pain. Chicago, Quintessence Publishing Co., 1995, pp 94–99.

Phero JC, McDonald JS, Green DB, et al: Orofacial pain and other related syndromes. In Raj PP: Practical Management of Pain. St. Louis, Mosby, 1992, pp 228–229.

19. How may local anesthetic blocks be used for the management of headache?

Although most types of headaches are treated with a combination of medications, some causes of headache or head pain are readily managed with nerve blocks. Head pains may arise from myofascial pain syndromes. However, other diseases and neoplasms involving the sensory distribution of cranial nerves V, IX, and X and cervical plexus nerve roots must be considered. Myofascial pain syndromes, which may include head pain, are characterized by steady aching muscle pain at multiple sites and are often associated with poor sleep, morning stiffness, chronic fatigue, depression, and TPs. TPs may lead to secondary central excitatory effects such as hyperalgesia, protective muscle spasm, or even autonomic responses. The superficial sternal and deep clavicular divisions of the sternocleidomastoid muscle may have referral patterns that lead to occipital and frontal headaches. The upper trapezius and occipitofrontalis muscles also may produce recurring, tension-type headache, which is often described as beginning in the occipital region and radiating over the parietal and frontal areas of the skull. These TP sources sometimes may be inactivated by noninvasive measures (pharmacotherapy, spray-and-stretch therapy) or dry needling of the TP and injection of local anesthetic with or without steroid. Results of these interventions may include analgesia, relaxation of muscle fiber shortening, increases in local muscle blood flow, and, if a corticosteroid is used, an anti-inflammatory effect. Complications are rare but may involve local hematoma, local anesthetic toxicity, and pneumothorax when the trapezius muscle is treated.

De Sio JM, Warfield CA, Kahn C: Benign pain. In Brown D (ed): Regional anesthesia and analgesia. Philadelphia, W.B. Saunders, 1996, p 688.

Okeson JP: Bell's orofacial pains. Chicago, Quintessence Publishing Co., 1995, pp 273–277.

Phero JC, McDonald JS, Green DB, et al: Orofacial pain and other related syndromes. In Raj PP: Practical Management of Pain. St. Louis, Mosby, 1992, pp 238–239.

20. What are the indications for cervical epidural injections in pain management?

Neck pain may result from nerve root irritation, myofascial dysfunction, arthritic cervical spine changes, trauma, or cancer of the head and neck. Cervical epidural injections of steroids are indicated primarily for neck pain secondary to cervical disc disease. Pain secondary to spinal stenosis, which leads to a narrowed intervertebral foramen, or a preexisting arthritic disorder may be treatable with cervical epidural steroid injections, but results are not as satisfactory. Complications may include spinal headache from dural puncture and, less often, epidural abscess, hematoma, and meningitis. It is often not possible to restrict an epidural block with local anesthetic to the cervical segments. Cephalad spread may produce respiratory depression or extended blockade. Long-acting local anesthetics are best avoided to prevent respiratory compromise secondary to phrenic nerve blockade and cardiac effects, such as reduced inotropicity and total peripheral resistance secondary to unintentional sympathetic blockade.

21. Discuss the role of superficial and deep cervical blocks in the management of acute and chronic pain and the relative risk with each block.

Cervical plexus blocks, which may be used in numerous surgical procedures involving the neck and shoulder, are occasionally used for the diagnosis of vague neck discomfort in the superior cervical dermatomes (C2–C4). More definitive diagnostic or therapeutic procedures are usually performed on peripheral nerve extensions, such as the occipital nerve block. The superficial cervical plexus block, located in the posterior triangle of the neck at the midpoint of the posterior border of the sternocleidomastoid, leads to complete blockade of the cutaneous nerve supply to the neck. The deep cervical plexus block is a paravertebral block that also blocks posterior primary rami for additional analgesia over the back of the neck. The proximity of the vertebral artery leads to the potential for an intravascular injection. In even small doses, local anesthetic injected intravascularly may lead to rapid development of CNS toxicity and seizures. The risk of unintentional intrathecal or epidural injection as a result of needle placement also exists. Phrenic nerve paresis may result from blockade of the motor innervation of the diaphragm.

22. When is an occipital nerve block indicated? What complications may occur?

Occipital nerve block is indicated for the diagnosis and treatment of headaches resulting from occipital neuralgia. Occipital neuralgia often results from compression or trauma to the greater occipital nerve (sensory branch of C2) along its course through the semispinalis capitis and the occipital attachment of the upper trapezius muscle. Compression of this nerve induces paroxysmal dysesthesia or paresthesia of the occiput, radiating upward to the vertex. Diagnostic TP blocks within adjacent muscles may be used to differentiate neuralgia from myofascial pain. Management of neuralgia, if anticonvulsants are unsuccessful, usually involves one or a series of nerve blocks with local anesthetic and long-acting corticosteroid. Complications consist of inadvertent subarachnoid administration, intravascular injection, and hematoma.

De Sio JM, Warfield CA, Kahn C: Benign pain. In Brown D (ed): Regional anesthesia and analgesia. Philadelphia, W.B. Saunders, 1996, p 689.

Dunn JJ, Mannheimer JS: The cervical spine. In Pertes RA, Gross SG (eds): Clinical Management of Temporomandibular Disorders and Orofacial Pain. Chicago, Quintessence Publishing Co., 1995, pp 17–18.

Graff-Radford SB: orofacial pain of neurogenous origin. In Pertes RA, Gross SG (eds): Clinical Management of Temporomandibular Disorders and Orofacial Pain. Chicago, Quintessence Publishing Co., 1995, p 336.

23. What is the gasserian ganglion? What are the indications for blockade?

The gasserian ganglion contains the cell bodies for the sensory neurons of the trigeminal (fifth cranial) nerve. It is located in Meckel's cave, an indentation in the petrous pyramid. It may be blocked with glycerol in cases of intractable trigeminal neuralgia.

24. How is the gasserian ganglion block performed? What side effects and complications may be experienced?

The trigeminal ganglion is partly contained within the dura mater, and the posterior two-thirds is bathed by cerebrospinal fluid. The ganglion is bordered medially by the cavernous sinus and internal carotid artery and superiorly by the temporal lobe of the brain. The transcutaneous gasserian ganglion block is directed, often under fluoroscopic guidance, into the foramen ovale, through which the mandibular division exits the skull base. Paresthesia or dysesthesia is usually elicited along one of the trigeminal nerve divisions. When indicated, a sensory change in the specific division affected is sought by needle repositioning. When adequate pain relief is obtained from local anesthetic placed into the ganglion, successful long-term pain reduction may be obtained with either a chemical or radiofrequency gangliolytic block. When the neurolytic block is performed, an increase in pain, masseteric weakness, and paresthesia may persist for weeks to months. Significant complications include bleeding, infection, facial dysesthesia, corneal hypesthesia, and anesthesia dolorosa. Acute complications, such as unconsciousness and paralysis, may result from injection into the cerebrospinal fluid.

25. What are the branches and functions of the first division of the trigeminal nerve?

The first division of the trigeminal nerve—the ophthalmic nerve (designated cranial nerve V1)—is distributed primarily to the forehead and nose. The ophthalmic nerve leaves the superior aspect of the trigeminal ganglion, lies in the lateral wall of the cavernous sinus, and enters the orbit through the superior orbital fissure, where it divides into three separate nerves: the lacrimal, frontal, and nasociliary nerves. The ophthalmic nerve provides sensory innervation to the bulb and conjunctiva of the eye, lacrimal gland, and skin over the forehead, eyes, and nose. Intraorbital branches of the nasociliary nerve are blocked by retrobulbar block. The largest branch, the frontal nerve, divides shortly after entering the superior aspect of the orbit into the supratrochlear and supraorbital nerves, which are accessible for cutaneous blockade. The supratrochlear nerve provides sensory innervation to the conjunctiva and skin of the medial aspect of the eye and the skin over the forehead. The supraorbital nerve, passing through the supraorbital notch, innervates the frontal sinus and then the upper lid, forehead, and scalp as far as the lambdoidal suture.

26. What role do supraorbital and supratrochlear nerve blocks play in the management of herpes zoster?

Repeated sympathetic nerve blocks, in combination with subcutaneous infiltration with a local anesthetic–steroid mixture for supraorbital and supratrochlear nerve blocks, have been shown to reduce the severity of pain associated with acute herpes zoster. The injections should be given during acute illness rather than delayed until postherpetic pain is experienced. Pain may be eliminated for periods greatly exceeding the length of the anesthetic block.

27. What are the major nerve branches of the maxillary division of the trigeminal nerve? How are nerve blocks of the maxillary division used in pain management?

The maxillary nerve (designated as cranial nerve V2) is purely sensory, providing innervation of the nose, cheek, eyelids, mid-face, maxillary sinus, and associated structures of the upper jaw. Mucosal sensory innervation includes part of the nasopharynx, tonsil, palate, and maxillary gingiva as well as maxillary teeth. The maxillary nerve exits the middle cranial fossa via the foramen rotundum, traverses the pterygopalatine fossa medial to the lateral pterygoid plate, and enters the orbit through the inferior orbital fissure. Major nerve branches arise in the cranial vault, pterygopalatine fossa, and orbit as well as on the face. Blockade of the maxillary nerve provides pain relief in some cases of local disease of the mid-face region. The major nerve trunk may be blocked via an extraoral approach under the zygomatic arch as well as an intraoral approach. Intravascular injection and hematoma may result from the vascular nature of the pterygopalatine fossa and presence of the maxillary artery medial to the pterygoid plates. Wide dispersal of local anesthetic may lead to temporary anesthesia of the ocular muscles or optic nerve and loss of the corneal reflex.

28. How is the sphenopalatine ganglion block used for the management of pain conditions of the head?

The sphenopalatine ganglion is a parasympathetic ganglion of the facial nerve. Postsynaptic fibers leave the ganglion and distribute with branches of the maxillary division of the trigeminal nerve. These fibers provide parasympathetic innervation to the lacrimal and mucosal glands of the nasal fossa, palate, and pharynx. In a similar fashion, the maxillary nerve carries sympathetic nerve efferents from the superior cervical ganglion to target structures. The sphenopalatine ganglion block has been associated with alleviation of the frequency and intensity of headache, specifically cluster headache and migraine, that are poorly controlled with conventional drugs such as beta blockers. The block is carried out on a daily basis for 5–7 days, using topical application of local anesthetic to the nasopharynx posterior to the inferior and lower middle turbinate. Adverse effects include bleeding, orthostatic hypotension, and local anesthetic systemic toxicity. Excessive pressure with the anesthetic applicator against the cribriform plate may increase the risk of a high spinal block with respiratory embarrassment. Further controlled trials are needed to define the indications and efficacy of this procedure.

BIBLIOGRAPHY

1. Hanania MM, Brietstein D: Postherpetic neuralgia: A review. Cancer Invest 15(2):165–176, 1997.
2. Hanania MM: A new technique for piriformis muscle injection using a nerve stimulator. Reg Anesth 22(2), 1997.
3. Haddox JD: Lumbar and cervical epidural steroid therapy. Anesthesiol Clin North Am 10:179–203, 1992.
4. Katz J: Somatic nerve blocks. In Raj PP: Practical Management of Pain, 2nd ed. St. Louis, Mosby, 1992, pp 713–753.
5. Winnie AP, Collins VJ: The pain clinic I: Differential neural blockade in pain syndromes of the questionable etiology. Med Clin North Am 52:123–129, 1968.
6. Winnie AP, Hartwell PW: Relationship between time of treatment of acute herpes zoster with sympathetic blockade and prevention of post-herpetic neuralgia: Clinical support for a new theory of the mechanism by which sympathetic blockade provides therapeutic benefit. Reg Anesth 18:277–282, 1993.

35. PERMANENT NEURAL BLOCKADE AND CHEMICAL ABLATION

Michael Hanania, M.D.

1. What is neurolysis?
The application of a chemical or physical destructive agent to a nerve to create a long-lasting or permanent interruption of neural transmission.

2. What types of agents are commonly used?
Chemical agents include alcohol, phenol, glycerol, ammonium compounds, chlorocresol, and aminoglycosides. Hypotonic or hypertonic solutions may also be used. The most commonly used physical agents are cold (cryotherapy) and heat (radiofrequency lesions or laser).

3. What are the indications for neurolysis?
The use of neurolytic agents is almost exclusively reserved for the treatment of intractable cancer pain. Rarely, some forms of nonmalignant pain can be treated this way (for example, intractable postherpetic neuralgia and chronic pancreatitis). Several requisites must be met before neuroloysis is performed. In most cases, successful pain relief should be demonstrated with temporary blockade. The painful area must be sufficiently limited to be served by a readily accessible nerve or plexus. A thorough knowledge of the relevant anatomy and the mechanism by which the agent destroys nerve tissue are essential. Neurolysis should be regarded as an irreversible and potentially permanent procedure whose use is usually considered only when other treatment modalities have failed.

4. What are the potential side effects or complications of neurolysis?
Extravasation or malplacement of the solution, resulting in injury to nerves other than the target nerve, can produce unwanted sensory and motor block. Anesthesia dolorosa, or pain in the deafferented area, may occur. Systemic effects, such as hypotension, may be severe enough to require resuscitation.

5. How do commonly used neurolytics, such as alcohol and phenol, work?
Alcohol and phenol cause protein coagulation and necrosis of the axon without disruption of the Schwann cell tube. Thus, axonal regeneration can occur. Recovery is faster with phenol than with alcohol. However, if cell bodies are destroyed along with axons, as is more likely with alcohol, regeneration is not possible, and permanent blockade will result.

6. What are the indications for celiac plexus neurolysis?
This is a commonly performed neurolytic procedure that is useful in reducing visceral pain from structures that have sensory fibers passing through the celiac plexus. The structures innervated through the celiac plexus include the lower esophagus, stomach, small intestine, large intestine to the midtransverse colon, liver, pancreas, adrenals, and kidneys. Pancreatic cancer pain is most commonly treated with this block.

7. Under what circumstances is celiac plexus neurolysis preferred over systemic opioids for the management of pain from pancreatic cancer?
Most patients do well with systemic opioids and require no further intervention for controlling pain from pancreatic cancer. In fact, analgesia after celiac neurolysis may not be superior to that after treatment with systemic opioids. However, patients who develop severe side effects from systemic opioids benefit most from celiac neurolysis. Following celiac neurolysis,

a decreased need for opioids is observed as well as fewer associated side effects, such as sedation, confusion, nausea, and constipation.

8. Where is the celiac plexus, and what are the approaches and techniques for celiac plexus blockade?

The celiac plexus is the largest plexus of the sympathetic nervous system. It lies near the aorta, just anterior to the body of the first lumbar vertebra. Guidance by fluoroscopy or CT scan must be used when injecting neurolytic solution to ensure correct needle placement. One technique is a posterior percutaneous approach using a needle to pass transaortic or anterior to the crura of the diaphragm at the level of L1 where the celiac plexus is situated. Variations of this approach exist, including using two needles for bilateral injection in the retrocrural region. Recently, an anterior percutaneous approach was described.

9. What must be done prior to actual neurolysis of the celiac plexus?

A celiac plexus block using local anesthetic must be performed first to determine if significant pain relief is likely with celiac neurolysis. The patient should therefore reduce opioid consumption the day of the procedure so that pain relief can be assessed.

10. What is the success rate with celiac plexus neurolysis for pancreatic cancer pain?

A success rate of 85 to 94% of good to excellent pain relief has been obtained in several large series of patients undergoing neurolytic celiac plexus block for pain from pancreatic cancer. In a series of 136 patients, analgesia was present until the time of death in 75% of cases. Repetition of the block is required in some patients. The earlier in the disease process the block is performed, the better the results. This may be due to better spread of neurolytic solution around the celiac plexus when tumor infiltration is minimal.

11. What are the potential complications of celiac neurolysis?

Reported complications include pneumothorax, chylothorax, pleural effusion, convulsions, and paraplegia. Postural hypotension and diarrhea occur frequently secondary to the sympathetic blockade, but are usually self-limited.

12. What is intrathecal neurolysis, and when is it used?

Intrathecal neurolysis is a form of chemical rhizotomy in which a neurolytic agent is introduced into the cerebrospinal fluid which is used for blockade of specific dermatomes. This can be performed at any spinal level up to the midcervical region. At higher levels, there is risk of spread of neurolytic agent to the medullary centers. Indications for intrathecal neurolysis include any peripheral pain within a specific dermatomal distribution.

13. How is intrathecal neurolysis performed using phenol or alcohol?

Studies have demonstrated that all nerve fibers are affected indiscriminately by both phenol and alcohol. The concentration and quantity of agent used determines the extent of nerve fiber destruction and, therefore, the degree and extent of sensory loss. Phenol is hyperbaric relative to cerebrospinal fluid, and therefore, the patient would need to be positioned so that the sensory nerve roots are down with gravity (i.e., semisupine). Alcohol is hypobaric, so the nerve roots involved need to be in the up position or against gravity (i.e., semiprone). Positioning of the patient and use of small incremental doses of neurolytic solution are critical for obtaining the proper block. Average duration of analgesia is three to four months, with a wide range of distribution.

14. What are typical concentrations and volumes for intrathecal neurolysis with phenol or alcohol?

Recent reports suggest a higher success rate of analgesia is obtained with intrathecal phenol in preparations of 10 and 15% solution versus a 7.5% solution for treating pain due to a variety of neoplasms. Absolute alcohol may be used in increments of 0.1 ml until pain relief is obtained (usually a total of 0.7 ml is required).

15. What are the complications associated with intrathecal neurolysis?

If this is performed at the lumbar level, bowel and bladder dysfunction are among the most feared complications, although the actual incidence and severity are low, regardless of the agent used. At the thoracic level, solution is introduced distant from the major limb plexuses and nerve subserving bladder and bowel function; however, intercostal muscle paresis can occur. Chemical rhizolysis at the cervical level has to be carefully performed so as not to involve the medullary centers.

16. List the advantages and disadvantages of intrathecal neurolysis.

Advantages: ease of performance (usually done as a one-time injection) and completeness and long duration of the block. Disadvantages: the possibility of spread to anterior motor nerve roots, thereby producing paralysis. The patient must remain in an unchanged position for at least 30 minutes after injection, and there is initial burning with injection of alcohol.

17. List the advantages and disadvantages of epidural neurolysis.

Advantages: positioning of the patient is not as critical; neurolysis can be carried out over a large number of dermatomes; permanent motor block is unlikely if phenol is used; and neurolysis can be carried out over a period of two to four days by repeated injections of phenol through an epidural catheter. Disadvantages: incompleteness and shorter duration of nerve blockade and the need for repeat injections over several days. A larger dose and volume of neurolytic solution are needed; hence, inadvertent intrathecal migration can be disastrous. Success rates with epidural neurolysis have not been adequately documented, although anecdotal reports of success range from 33 to 90%.

18. What is cryoanalgesia?

The application of extremely low temperatures using a cryosurgical probe achieves pain relief by blocking peripheral nerves or destroying the nerve endings with extreme cold. The cryoprobe works on the principle of the Joule-Thompson effect. It is composed of an inner tube, an outer tube, and a working tip. When high pressure gas is allowed to expand in the probe tip, there is a rapid fall in temperature. When nitrous oxide is used, for example, the cryoprobe tip cools to $-60°$ C.

19. By what mechanism does prolonged neural blockade occur after cryoprobe application?

Application of a cryoprobe produces a local icy lesion (cryolesion) at the nerve. After the nerve is frozen, axonal disintegration, wallerian degeneration, and disruption of the myelin sheath occur, although the integrity of the epineurium and perineurium is maintained. Thus, the conduction block produced by a cryolesion is a temporary effect, and regeneration of the nerve eventually occurs.

20. What influences the duration of the block after cryolesioning?

Duration of nerve blockade depends on the rate of axonal regrowth and the distance of the cryolesion from the end organ. Clinically, a peripheral cryolesion results in sensory blockade from weeks to months, typically one to two months. The closer the iceball is to the nerve and the larger the cryolesion, the better the chance for successful and prolonged blockade.

21. What is radiofrequency neurolysis?

This technique uses high-frequency waves to produce thermal coagulation of the nerves. A probe is inserted percutaneously, and electrical impulses are given until the patient feels paresthesias in the painful area, indicating that the correct nerve has been located. The patient is then sedated and the current increased to coagulate the nerve.

22. List the advantages and disadvantages of radiofrequency lesioning.

Advantages: an irreversible lesion is produced, resulting in permanent blockade or prolonged block, and small probes can be used. Disadvantages: the possibility of neuritis as with chemical ablation and the expense of the radiofrequency equipment compared with that of phenol or alcohol.

23. List the advantages and disadvantages of cryolesioning.

Advantages: a reversible lesion is produced, neuritis rarely occurs, and cost of equipment involved is less than that of radiofrequency neurolysis. Disadvantages: a transient nerve block is produced that may require repeat cryolesioning; a large cryoprobe is required, so the percutaneous procedure can be uncomfortable; and success of blockade depends greatly on the proximity of the iceball to the nerve.

24. Why do neuritis and neuroma occur occasionally after neurolysis?

Regeneration of peripheral nerve in particular sometimes results in neuritis or neuroma. It has been suggested that alcoholic neuritis is related to incomplete destruction of somatic nerves and that the incidence is less when a complete and prolonged block has been obtained. Nerve irritation is less common in cranial nerves than in other peripheral nerves. Some agents, such as alcohol, have more of a propensity to produce local irritation.

25. What is deafferentation pain?

Deafferentation pain is usually a burning pain that can be more uncomfortable than the original pain. Central nervous system maladaptation to deafferentation, as well as a local phenomenon, may account for this complication of neurolysis.

26. List the following neurolytic techniques in order of greatest to least incidence of neuritis: radiofrequency, phenol, cryoanalgesia, alcohol.

1. Alcohol
2. Phenol
3. Radiofrequency
4. Cryoanalgesia

27. What are indications for lumbar sympathetic neurolysis?

Lumbar sympatholysis has been shown to be useful in controlling pain associated with peripheral vascular disease; specifically, patients with pedal ischemic rest pain with a cool extremity and without gangrene are the ideal candidates. It is performed in patients who are not candidates for peripheral bypass procedures because of technical or medical reasons. This procedure is less often used for sympathetically mediated pain that responded very well to local anesthetic blockade but only for the duration of the local anesthetic. There are small series and case reports of good results in using sympatholysis for otherwise unresponsive, prolonged ischemia of the digits in Raynaud's disease, although long-term success is minimal.

28. How can lower abdominal or pelvic cancer pain be managed with neurolysis?

Plancarte and co-workers (1990) described a superior hypogastric plexus block at the anterolateral border of the first sacral vertebral body for alleviating pain from pelvic cancer. Intrathecal neurolysis can also be performed; however, bladder and bowel dysfunction occur in a high proportion of patients.

29. Describe the treatment for trigeminal neuralgia that is unresponsive to conventional medical management.

Neurolysis with radiofrequency lesioning, glycerol, phenol, or alcohol has been successfully used for the treatment of trigeminal neuralgia. In one series, radiofrequency retrogasserian rhizolysis has been reported to be successful in 95% of patients with a recurrence rate of 16% over four to twelve years. Glycerol rhizolysis is less uncomfortable for the patient, with good results reported lasting a median of two years. In one of the largest series using alcohol, 70% of patients had no recurrence of pain when followed for more than three years. Phenol was used with a similar long-term success rate. Neurosurgical microvascular decompression procedures have also been reported to be successful in 80 to 90% of patients.

30. What are the complications of trigeminal neurolysis?

Side effects, which are usually transient, include Horner's syndrome from block of the para-trigeminal sympathetic fibers. In addition, corneal anesthesia with consequent loss of corneal reflex and possibly paralytic keratitis, loss of sensation on the ipsilateral side of the face and half of the tongue, paresthesia, herpetic eruptions, and anesthesia dolorosa are reported complications of this procedure.

BIBLIOGRAPHY

1. Bonica JJ: Management of Pain, 2nd ed. Philadelphia, Lea & Febiger, 1990, pp 1980–2039.
2. Brown DL, Bulley CK, Quiel EC: Neurolytic celiac plexus block for pancreatic cancer pain. Anesth Analg 66:869–873, 1987.
3. Ferrer-Brechner T: Epidural and intrathecal phenol neurolysis for cancer pain. Anesthesiol Rev 8:14–19, 1981.
4. Holland AJC, Youssef M: A complication of subarachnoid phenol blockade. Anaesthesia 34:260–262, 1979.
5. Ischia S, Luzzani A, Ischia A, et al: A new approach to the neurolytic block of the coeliac plexus: The transaortic technique. Pain S4:T34, 1987.
6. Jain S, Foley K, Thomas J, et al: Factors influencing efficacy of epidural neurolysis therapy for intractable cancer pain. Pain S4:T34, 1987.
7. Korevaar WC, Kline MT, Donnelly CC: Thoracic epidural neurolysis using alcohol. Pain S4:T33, 1987.
8. Plancarte R, Amescua C, Patt RB, et al: Superior hypogastric plexus block for pelvic cancer pain. Anesthesiology 73:236, 1990.
9. Plancarte R, Velazquez R, Patt RB: Neurolytic blocks of the sympathetic axis. in Patty RB (ed): Cancer Pain. Philadelphia, JB Lippincott, 1993, pp 384–420.
10. Raj PP, Denson DD: Neurolytic agents. In Raj PP (ed): Clinical Practice of Regional Anesthesia. New York, Churchill Livingstone, 1991.
11. Siegfried J, Brogg G: Percutaneous thermocoagulation of the gasserian ganglion in the treatment of pain in advanced cancer. Adv Pain Res Ther 2:463–468, 1979.
12. Singler RC: An improved technique for alcohol neurolysis of the celiac plexus. Anesthesiology 56:137–141, 1982.
13. Stovner J, Endresen R: Intrathecal phenol for cancer pain. Acta Anaesth Scand 16:17–21, 1971.
14. Swerdlow M: Intrathecal neurolysis. Anaesthesia 33:733–287, 1978.
15. Waldman SD, Wilson WL, Kreps RD: Superior hypogastric block using a single needle and computed tomography guidances: Description of a modified technique. Reg Anesth 16:286–287, 1991.

36. SYMPATHETIC NEURAL BLOCKADE

Meir Chernofsky, M.D.

1. What distinguishes a sympathetic block from other neural blockade procedures?

The goal of sympathetic blockade is to preserve motor function and touch sensation while selectively blocking the sympathetic nerves. Because sympathetic fibers travel to almost all tissues in the body to innervate the vasculature, almost all nerve blocks involve sympathetic blockade. The separation of somatic and sympathetic function (differential blockade) is sometimes incomplete.

2. How can a differential sympathetic blockade be achieved?

There are three general ways to block sympathetic nerves while preserving somatic function. The first is to block sympathetic nerves with the same local anesthetic agents (in similar concentrations) used for somatic blockade, but to perform the blocks at anatomic locations where sympathetic nerves are separate and distinct from somatic nerves. The second approach is to perform the block at locations that combine somatic and sympathetic nerve fibers, but to use low concentrations of local anesthetic. As postsynaptic sympathetic nerves are small and unmyelinated, they are more sensitive than some larger or myelinated somatic fibers to dilute local anesthetic. This approach is useful for spinal and epidural blockade.

The third approach to sympathetic blockade is to use specific sympathetic antagonists. For example, the antihypertensive agent guanethidine can be injected into the vasculature of a limb, with a tourniquet applied and inflated to a pressure greater than the systolic arterial pressure. After a short period during which the agent has had a chance to distribute into local tissues, the tourniquet is deflated, and one has achieved a local selective lysis of sympathetic function. This technique is a variation of intravenous regional anesthesia, the Bier block. It is usually a poor choice if ischemia is the primary problem.

3. What is the general role of sympathetic blockade in pain management?

Sympathetic blocks may be helpful for four general types of clinical problems. In some body regions, afferent pain fibers travel with sympathetic nerves. For example, the fibers that conduct painful impulses from the pancreas are closely associated with the celiac plexus. Therefore, neural blockade of the celiac plexus is a convenient way to provide pancreatic analgesia. The primary target of such a procedure is the afferent fibers that travel with the sympathetic trunk, although a sympathetic role in the maintenance of such pain has not been ruled out.

Secondly, the sympathetic nervous system is believed to play a primary role in a certain class of painful syndromes. Directed blockade of the sympathetic fibers may be both diagnostic and therapeutic in cases of sympathetically maintained pain. However, even reflex sympathetic dystrophy (RSD), which was once believed to be the prime example of these syndromes, is now called CRPS-I (chronic regional pain syndrome), indicating our lack of knowledge of the pathophysiologic basis.

Thirdly, physicians skilled in neural blockade are occasionally asked to become involved in the treatment of ischemic syndromes of the limbs. The patient may or may not have pain, and the sympathetic nervous system is not implicated in the pathologic process. However, by inducing sympathetic neural blockade, the tonic baseline level of arterial vasoconstriction is reduced. Depending on the vascular pathology, blood flow to the ischemic area may be improved.

There is also a grab-bag of indications for sympathetic blockade that do not fit into one of the above categories. For example, stellate ganglion block, discussed below, may be useful in the diagnosis and treatment of certain cardiac dysrhythmias related to prolonged QT syndrome.

4. Without going into specific indications just yet, what are some of the common types of sympathetic blocks?

Blocks that take advantage of isolating the sympathetic fibers at sympathetic plexi or trunks include the so-called stellate ganglion block, the lumbar sympathetic block, the celiac plexus block, and the hypogastric plexus block. Techniques that exploit the potential of differential blockade by using low concentrations of local anesthetics include differential spinal and epidural blocks. Agents used in the Bier technique in the upper or lower extremity include reserpine, guanethidine, and the ganglionic agent, bretylium. Finally, as pointed out above, almost all somatic nerve blocks also block sympathetic nerves.

5. What is reflex sympathetic dystrophy (RSD)? What does it look like clinically? What is the role of the sympathetic nervous system?

RSD is a syndrome of pain and disability (altered sensory, motor, and sympathetic neural function) in a distal extremity. It is characterized by decreased function and signs of sympathetic overactivity. RSD is thought to be initiated by trauma. The degree of the initial trauma may vary from a major fracture with neurovascular injury to a trauma so minor that it is not recalled by the patient. In patients with major nerve injury, the syndrome is called CRPS-II (formerly causalgia). Various medical conditions, such as stroke and myocardial infarction, also may be the inciting factor for RSD.

RSD is a chronic, progressively evolving syndrome with different signs at different stages. Pain and decreased function are present at all stages. Initially, there may be signs of sympathetic overactivity, such as increased sweating in the distal limb, which is pale and cool to the touch. As the condition progresses, some of these signs become less obvious, and atrophy becomes more prominent. The extremity, more commonly the hand, becomes hypersensitive and tender and is guarded by the patient. In the late stages, there is radiologic evidence of bone-thinning (Sudeck's atrophy).

The clinical signs and the marked relief after sympathetic block in early cases points to sympathetic overactivity as an important factor in maintenance and perhaps initiation of the syndrome. However, this mechanism has recently been called into question.

Treatment of RSD becomes less satisfactory in the later stages of disease. When the condition is neglected, it may progress to a disability that dominates the life of the patient. Patients may become so desperate that they request amputation. Unfortunately, early surgical adventures with amputation in RSD demonstrated that a chronic pain syndrome remains even after the limb is gone. Therefore, early diagnosis, with a trial of therapy when possible, is important.

6. What is a stellate ganglion block? How is it performed?

There is a series of sympathetic ganglia on either side of the cervical vertebral column and on either side of the thoracic vertebrae. The stellate ganglion is less a consistent anatomic structure than a general area in which the inferior cervical ganglia and first thoracic ganglia are fused—or at least in close proximity.

Virtually the entire sympathetic nerve supply to the head and neck synapses in or near the stellate ganglion. A good portion of the sympathetic innervation to the ipsilateral upper extremity also synapses in the stellate ganglion, with the remainder synapsing in adjacent ganglia. A consistent blockade of the head, neck, and upper extremity sympathetic innervation may be achieved by applying a quantity of local anesthetic (5–12 ml) to the area of the stellate ganglion. When the proper quantity of local anesthetic is used, spread to adjacent ganglia is common, leading to reliable upper extremity sympathectomy.

The most common technique is an anterior neck approach. The patient is placed in the supine position, and the neck is extended as tolerated. After antiseptic preparation, a 3-cm needle (22–23 gauge) is introduced perpendicular to the skin (and perpendicular to the floor) at the level of the cricoid cartilage between the trachea and the anterior border of the sternocleidomastoid muscle. Retracting the sternocleidomastoid muscle laterally and palpating the anterior aspect of the C6 vertebrae with two fingers facilitates introduction of the needle and avoids puncture of the carotid artery. The needle is advanced until bone is encountered. If bone is not encountered at this location, the needle is withdrawn to the subcutaneous tissues and reintroduced in a slightly caudad or cephalad direction.

When bone is encountered, the needle is withdrawn about 0.5 cm. (If this step is not done, a higher incidence of somatic blockade of the upper extremity will result.) After careful aspiration testing is negative for blood or cerebrospinal fluid, 5–12 ml of local anesthetic is introduced in fractional doses and the needle is withdrawn. Because placement of the needle is inexact with regard to the targeted vertebral level, the author prefers to hedge his bet with the higher volume of local agent.

Many variations and other approaches are also possible. Any one of many anesthesia texts or neural blockade handbooks provides more detailed information about block technique and should be studied before a stellate ganglion block (or any of the other blocks discussed in this chapter) is attempted.

7. What are the contraindications to stellate ganglion block?

Most of the contraindications are a matter of common sense and are relative rather than absolute. Patients who are anticoagulated or taking high-dose aspirin are at increased risk for bleeding. A local infection over the proposed site of injection is a somewhat more absolute contraindication. Patients with bullous disease of the upper lobes of the lung are at greater risk for accidental pneumothorax and must be approached with more caution. Because one of the possible complications of stellate ganglion block is vocal cord paralysis, patients with contralateral vocal cord paralysis are at risk for severe airway abnormality if the ipsilateral cord becomes paralyzed. Patients who have abnormal anatomy because of prior surgery or injury present greater technical difficulty because of the differences in anatomic landmarks. Such patients are probably better approached with alternative techniques, such as intravenous regional sympatholysis.

8. What are the results, risks, and side effects of a stellate ganglion block?

Stellate ganglion block causes sympathetic blockade of the ipsilateral face and arm. Therefore, a successful block produces an ipsilateral Horner's syndrome (ptosis, miosis, and anhydrosis), flushing of the face, and increased temperature of the arm. These effects are normal and last for the duration of the blockade. Slightly blurred vision and a sense of fullness around the eye may result. Local trauma from the blockade or blockade of the recurrent laryngeal nerve may produce hoarseness. Neck tenderness is fairly common, but frank hematoma is less likely. In severe cases, hematoma may threaten the airway.

Inadvertent blockade of components of the brachial plexus may lead to upper extremity numbness and weakness or paralysis, both temporary in the vast majority of cases. If pain relief occurs in the presence of somatic blockade, the pain syndrome may have been due to a peripheral lesion, but a sympathetic origin cannot be inferred.

Passive ranging of the painful joints may be dangerous in the face of somatic blockade because pain, which may warn of extreme passive strain on a structure, is blocked.

Serious complications of stellate ganglion blockade include carotid puncture with hematoma and vertebral artery puncture. Introduction of even small amounts of local anesthetic into either of these arteries may lead to seizures (usually short-lived). Introduction of small amounts of local anesthetic into the cerebrospinal fluid may lead to high (or total) subarachnoid neural blockade with respiratory arrest, coma, hypotension, and sometimes cardiac arrest. A generalized toxic reaction to the local anesthetic load also may occur if too much local agent gains access to the circulation too fast. If the needle enters too deeply, a pneumothorax may occur. Late complications include the remote possibility of mediastinitis after puncture of the esophagus as well as the possibility of late airway compromise from hematoma or trauma.

9. How can the above complications be prevented or managed?

There is no foolproof way to avoid complications. Their incidence may be reduced by proper training and experience. However, the chance of permanent injury to the patient as a result of seizure, accidental spinal anesthesia, or pneumothorax can certainly be reduced to acceptable levels with proper preparation:

1. Perform the block only on fasting patients to avoid aspiration in case of loss of consciousness.

2. Perform the block only in a setting in which an anesthesiologist (or an emergency physician with excellent airway management skills) is immediately available to manage complications.

3. Start an intravenous lifeline in every patient before the block is attempted so that emergency drugs can be administered without delay.

4. Perform the block with monitoring of blood pressure, cardiac rate and rhythm, and oxygen saturation.

5. Administer supplemental oxygen to all patients, or have it immediately available in case of signs of trouble.

6. Have an emergency airway cart and emergency drugs available, and inspect these items frequently. They should not be under lock and key while a block is in progress.

7. Take all complaints from the patient seriously, and have a high index of suspicion for pneumothorax.

10. What is the role of the stellate ganglion block in treatment of RSD?

In cases of suspected upper extremity RSD, an initial block may be performed with a short-acting local anesthetic such as lidocaine 1%. This initial block is diagnostic; its purpose is to determine whether the block is technically feasible, whether it produces sympathetic blockade of the upper extremity, and whether this blockade results in (1) subjective pain relief, (2) any increase in functional ability of the hand, or (3) objective signs of improvement on examination and functional testing.

If the first block is successful either subjectively or objectively, a series of blocks may provide sufficient relief for appropriate physical therapy. After each block, a physical therapist works with the patient to achieve functional improvement. Behavioral therapy is an important adjunct to the therapy of RSD.

11. Which somatic nerve is most likely to be blocked unintentionally in attempting a stellate ganglion block?

With an anterior approach, the stellate ganglion is anterior to the trunks of the brachial plexus. The ganglion and plexus are separated by only a layer of fascia at this location. Therefore, all of the somatic nerves formed by the C5–T1 roots may inadvertently be blocked by diffusing anesthetics. If one performs the block slightly cephalad to the described location, the deep cervical plexus may be blocked, producing loss of sensation to the neck.

12. In what other ways can sympathetic block be induced at this level? Is a stellate ganglion block the best approach? If so, why?

There are other approaches to stellate or upper thoracic sympathetic chain blockade. The area, for example, may be approached posteriorly. Approaches other than the classic anterior approach do not have easy endpoints by palpation, and the use of radiographic guidance is strongly recommended.

Sympathetic blockade of the upper extremity also may be achieved by temporarily isolating the involved upper extremity with a tourniquet (inflated above venous pressure) and injecting a sympathetic blocking agent into a vein in the hand. The technique is similar to the Bier block, a popular method of achieving regional anesthesia of the hand. Problems with this approach include side effects of the sympathetic blocker, either because the tourniquet is accidentally deflated or because some shift of drug to the central compartment is inevitable, even with good technique. The side effects include hypotension, nausea, and dizziness.

Drugs that have been used for intravenous regional sympathetic blockade include reserpine, guanethidine, and bretylium.

The posterior approach to the sympathetic chain is practical if the anterior approach involves an anatomic problem. Intravenous regional sympathetic blockade can be used in patients in whom any nerve block is contraindicated—for example, in anticoagulated patients. The intravenous regional sympathetic block is also longer-lasting than a local anesthetic neural blockade. For uncomplicated patients with definite or possible RSD, the stellate ganglion block is the first-line technique.

13. Other than RSD, what are some commonly accepted indications for stellate ganglion block?

The pain of herpes and postherpetic neuralgia of the head and neck down to upper thoracic dermatomes may be managed by stellate block. Aggressive treatment of the pain associated with early herpes zoster may prevent or modify the development of postherpetic neuralgia. The so-called shoulder-hand syndrome, which is a continuum of problems, including painful decreased range of the upper extremity after stroke and other vascular episodes, may be controlled with stellate ganglion block. Physical therapy may be facilitated, just as with classic RSD.

The pain of Paget's disease, phantom limb pain, and other pain associated with upper extremity denervation of benign or malignant origin may respond to this block. Severe coronary ischemic pain may improve with stellate block, and the dysrhythmias associated with prolonged Q-T syndrome may be temporarily managed.

For ischemic problems of the upper extremity, including atherosclerosis and microemboli, perfusion may be improved with stellate ganglion blocks. The ischemic pain associated with scleroderma, isolated Raynaud's disease, and other vasospastic conditions also may respond.

14. How does the treatment of lower extremity RSD differ from treatment of upper extremity RSD? What major alternative to classic sympathetic block is more practical for lower extremity RSD than for upper extremity RSD?

In principle, lower extremity RSD is approached with the same type of algorithm as upper extremity RSD. The first-line block used is the lumbar sympathetic block, described below. The requirement for a multidisciplinary approach, including behavioral medicine and physical therapy, is identical to management of upper extremity RSD.

The introduction of very dilute concentrations of local anesthetics into the epidural space may bring about sympathetic blockade and analgesia without inducing sensory and motor blockade. The cervical epidural route is a viable alternative for the induction of upper extremity sympathetic blockade, and the lumbar epidural route is effective for lower extremity sympathetic blockade. However, a lumbar epidural is technically easier than a cervical epidural, with fewer potential complications.

A major advantage of the lumbar epidural route for the management of lower extremity RSD is that an epidural catheter can be inserted on an outpatient basis and left in place for several days. Therefore, repeat blockade to facilitate therapy on a more or less daily basis is easier to perform.

When the epidural route is used to achieve sympathetic blockade, pain relief is nonspecific, because the concentrations of local anesthetic may induce somatic analgesia in addition to sympathetic blockade. Diagnostically, one cannot conclude that the source of the pain is solely sympathetic if a somatic blockade is achieved.

The option of intravenous regional sympathetic blockade with a Bier technique is equally practical for the lower extremity. Considering the relatively larger volume of the venous capacitance in the lower extremity, a larger volume of medication must be used compared with the same block in the upper extremity.

15. How is a lumbar sympathetic block performed?

The lumbar sympathetic chain consists of presynaptic and postsynaptic sympathetic nerves and ganglia in close association with the lumbar vertebral bodies, lying anterolaterally on both sides. Therefore, the vertebral bodies themselves are the best landmark.

In one common approach, the patient is positioned prone, with a pillow under the abdomen. Precautions (including an intravenous line and appropriate monitoring) are established. The spinous processes of L3 are identified and marked. The entry point of the needle is 7–9 cm lateral to the midline at the L3 level.

After the area is prepared, a wheel of local anesthetic is raised. Then a stiletted needle at least 12 cm in length (21–22 gauge, preferably marked in centimeters) is introduced at the above point toward the midline, making an angle of 45° with the skin. The needle is advanced while the injectionist maintains verbal contact with the patient. At this point, there are three possible outcomes. If paraesthesias are encountered, one has probably encountered the lumbar plexus within the psoas muscle. In this case, one should withdraw the needle to the skin and redirect. The needle may be too far lateral and may have to be reintroduced 1–2 cm more medially. Alternatively, one may have used too shallow an angle. If bone is encountered at 3–5 cm depth (the second possible result), one has encountered a transverse process. One should withdraw to the skin and redirect the needle cephalad or caudal.

The desired endpoint is the encountering of bone at a depth of 8–11 cm. This bone is the vertebral body. At this point, the injectionist should note the insertion depth, withdraw to skin, and redirect at a *slightly* higher angle. This step is repeated until bone is either not encountered at a depth of 2 cm beyond the point of the original encounter or until one can easily walk off the bone and advance the needle by 1–2 cm. When the needle is in proper position, there should be little resistance to advancement or injection. After careful aspiration, a 3-cc test dose of local anesthetic is injected. If after several minutes there is no evidence of spinal block or systemic symptoms, 12–15 cc of local anesthetic is injected in 5-cc increments with repeated aspiration and verbal contact with the patient. The same agents used for stellate block are appropriate for lumbar block. Variations to this technique include more medial entry points and multiple needle techniques.

16. Which somatic nerve is most likely to be blocked unintentionally during an attempt at lumbar sympathetic blockade?

The most likely somatic nerve to be blocked is part of the lumbar plexus in the substance of the psoas. If this occurs and pain is relieved, one cannot automatically conclude that the pain is sympathetically mediated. Accidental epidural and spinal blockades are also possible.

17. What are the important complications of lumbar sympathetic blockade? How can they be managed or prevented?

The litany of problems possible with lumbar sympathetic block is somewhat similar to those for stellate ganglion block. The good news is that airway complications, mediastinal complications, and pleural trauma are out of the picture.

Common problems include discomfort from the introduction of the needle, hematoma, and persistent paresthesias (which usually resolve after days or weeks). Potentially serious complications involve the proximity of the target area to the epidural space, subarachnoid space, and either the aorta and vena cava (in the case of higher insertion or lower-lying bifurcation) or iliac vessels.

Accidental injection of 12–15 cc of local anesthetic into the epidural space should not be catastrophic. A normal epidural blockade results; the patient must be monitored for high block and major sympathetic blockade with hemodynamic instability.

Accidental injection of 3 cc of a test dose of local anesthetic into the subarachnoid space results in a spinal block, with implications similar to an epidural blockade. Introduction of much more than 3 cc results in a high or total spinal block with apnea, loss of consciousness, and profound hypotension with vascular collapse.

Similarly, accidental injection of 3–4 cc (for example, 60–80 mg of lidocaine or 5–10 mg of bupivacaine) of most local anesthetic mixtures directly into the vasculature results in mild toxic symptoms, whereas larger amounts may cause major toxic manifestations such as seizures and cardiac arrest.

Careful aspiration for blood or cerebrospinal fluid is mandatory for all blocks, as is incremental injection with careful observation of the patient. Unfortunately, these precautions do not prevent all such complications.

18. For what reasons may a sympathetic block not improve the signs and symptoms of RSD? How can one decide which of these factors is operative in a particular patient?

Assuming that the diagnosis of RSD is correct, a sympathetic block may fail to relieve symptoms if it was technically inadequate, if the condition is fairly advanced, or if there are confounding factors such as significant peripheral nerve damage. This last condition, called causalgia in the older literature, is now known as CRPS-II.

If a sympathetic block does not seem to be effective, objective measurement should be made to demonstrate a decrease in sympathetic activity in the involved limb. If a sympathectomy is not demonstrated, it is worthwhile to try again on another day, perhaps with a greater volume of local anesthetic or with a slightly different approach (more cephalad or caudad direction of the needle). If a block that produces no relief is shown to produce limb sympathectomy, we encourage the patient to undergo a second attempt. Most patients who have had a successful series of blocks state that some attempts were not as effective as others.

Sometimes the diagnosis of RSD is hard to pin down. If a series of two sympathetic blocks completely fails to relieve symptoms and if it was demonstrated that the blocks indeed achieved sympathectomy of the involved area, the pain is probably not sympathetically mediated. However, in the absence of another diagnosis, the type of multidisciplinary program used for RSD may still be the patient's best hope. Future blocks may be used simply to facilitate analgesia and range of motion.

19. Which objective measurements of effect of limb sympathetic blockade can be used in the clinical setting?

Early in the course of RSD, the vasculature innervated by the overactive sympathetic nerves should remain reactive, i.e., able to dilate if the sympathetic input is reversed. This is the rationale of sympathetic blockade. The most obvious measurements to confirm the efficacy of a block relate to temperature and blood flow.

The simplest and most widely used measurement is to place thermometer probes on the distal part of the involved extremity and on the contralateral healthy extremity. The most reassuring response is a lower baseline temperature on the involved side (compared with the healthy side), which rises 2° Kelvin within 20 minutes of neural blockade. The problem with this measurement is that it is neither specific nor sensitive. There may be no baseline difference between the two sides, and surface temperature may poorly reflect tissue temperature for many reasons.

If one is lucky, the veins of the distal extremity may become more prominent after blockade. This observation, however, is hardly quantitative or even objective.

In classic RSD, increased sympathetic activity leads to increased sweat production. A number of tests, some based on serial measurement with indicator papers, quantify a decrease in sweat production after a successful sympathetic block. Quantitative sudomotor axon reflex testing (QSART) is more specific but more difficult.

The psychogalvanic reflex is a change in the conductivity of skin secondary to sudden stimulation of the special sensory organs. It is thought to be mediated by vasomotor changes and is diminished after sympathetic blockade. This reflex can be measured by a simple oscilloscope, such as an electrocardiograph monitor.

Plethysmographic measurements of pulsatile blood flow should increase after a successful block. Thermography, an elegant way to demonstrate changes in sympathetic activity, is used by some pain clinics.

Extracting useful information from a diagnostic sympathetic block is far more complex than a single objective measurement. The full range of peripheral neuroanatomic and psychological considerations in chronic pain may influence what happens after a block.

21. What is the celiac plexus?

The celiac plexus is a series of ganglia surrounding the celiac artery, just anterior to the aorta. The sympathetic innervation of the abdominal viscera originates with other sympathetic nerves but does not synapse in the sympathetic chain. The sympathetic nerves exit the sympathetic chain as splanchnic nerves to synapse in a number of ganglia. Most of these are loosely associated in the celiac plexus. Most of the afferent nociceptive innervation of the visceral structures of the abdomen travel in close association with the celiac plexus. Therefore, by blocking the celiac plexus, one can interrupt nociception from the viscera and also affect any sympathetically mediated pain in this area.

22. How is celiac plexus block performed? What are the risks?

As with other sympathetic blocks, a number of approaches are possible. The most common is a posterior approach, which is similar in principle to the lumbar plexus block. The patient is placed prone with a pillow beneath the abdomen. Intravenous access is secured, and appropriate monitoring is established.

The needle used is a 21- or 22-gauge stiletted needle at least 12–15 cm in length, preferably with distances marked in centimeters. The entry point is 7–8 cm lateral to the midline. The exact starting point is just inferior to the end of the twelfth rib and lateral to the T12 spinous process. After local infiltration at the entry point, the needle is advanced toward the midline, making an angle of 45° with the horizontal in the cross-sectional plane. The vertebral body is sought at a depth of 10–12 cm. Bone encountered within 5–6 cm is probably the transverse process. In this case, the needle is withdrawn to subcutaneous tissue and directed superiorly or inferiorly. In view of the anatomy, superior direction is a better choice. If no bone is encountered by 13 cm or so, the needle is withdrawn to subcutaneous tissue and the angle with the horizontal is decreased slightly.

Ideally, bone should be encountered as described. When it is, one should attempt to redirect the needle anteriorly (higher angle) and walk off the vertebral body. A pop is then felt as the needle is advanced by 2 cm. At this point, aspiration tests are carried out and the block is activated.

With a smaller-gauge (e.g., more malleable) needle, one has less ability to walk off the vertebra and is more likely to need to withdraw and redirect. However, smaller needles may do less damage if they penetrate vital structures.

When one believes that the needle is correctly placed, a test dose is performed, as described above for the lumbar plexus block. If the test appears to be negative, the local anesthetic mixture is injected. Large volumes may be necessary because of the extent of the loosely defined anatomic structure; 15 ml is the minimum. The local agent may be bupivacaine 0.25–0.5%, with or without epinephrine 2–5 µg/ml. For follow-up blocks, a neurolytic mixture is often used.

The block may be performed with fluoroscopic or computed tomographic guidance. Guidance is necessary when the anatomy is distorted by disease or body habitus. Proper placement of the needle is suggested by a characteristic pattern of spread of a contrast bolus.

The risk and complications of celiac plexus block are similar to those of lumbar plexus blockade. The aorta, of course, is in close proximity to the celiac plexus. Aortic penetration should not be catastrophic, barring coagulopathy or severe atherosclerosis. However, one certainly does not want to inject therapeutic substances into the aorta. Frequent aspiration tests are the key.

23. What is the clinical problem in treating the pain of pancreatic carcinoma? What is the role of local anesthetic celiac plexus blockade? What other approaches may be helpful?

The pain from pancreatic carcinoma may arise from a number of sources: invasion and destruction of the pancreatic duct system; mass effect; invasion of neighboring structures, including nerves; and various degrees of intestinal obstruction. Although systemic narcotics are usually the first modality used, they may become ineffective or cause intolerable side effects.

Many nerve blocks target the pain of pancreatic carcinoma, including epidural blockade, subarachnoid blockade, and celiac plexus block. However, the celiac block is particularly attractive because it is effective and because neurolytic agents can be delivered to the celiac plexus with relatively low risk of somatic neurolysis. Subarachnoid and epidural block, when indicated for this type of pain, are used to deliver opioids, with or without very low doses of local anesthetic. Such therapy may not be completely effective for visceral pain, which is mediated by pathways quite different from somatic pain. Subarachnoid or epidural neurolytic block is less practical for this indication.

The other advantage of celiac plexus neurolytic block is that its usual duration of effect (weeks to months) coincides with the unfortunately short life span of the patient. If necessary, a second block can be made weeks or months after the first block. Although patients often have an expected life span of weeks to months after diagnosis, they are alert until the end. To free the patient of significant pain and to preserve the alert state are real services.

The role of local anesthetic celiac plexus blockade for this indication is diagnostic. If a block with bupivacaine 0.25–0.5% relieves the pain, a neurolytic block is likely to provide prolonged relief.

24. For what other painful conditions may celiac plexus blockade have a role? What is the potential problem with the use of this block to treat benign pain?

Celiac plexus blockade is potentially useful for any painful condition of the abdominal viscera, including malignancies and benign pain such as that associated with chronic pancreatitis. Local anesthetic celiac plexus blockade may be used as a diagnostic maneuver for painful abdominal conditions. A condition that arises from the viscera or involves sympathetically mediated pain may be relieved with a celiac block. Pain arising from musculoskeletal or neural structures should not be relieved.

The pain of chronic pancreatitis may be severe and disabling. As with almost all chronic pain syndromes, there is likely to be significant associated behavioral dysfunction. If a local anesthetic celiac plexus block is effective, celiac neurolytic block may be considered. The problems are twofold. First, the analgesic effect is often temporary, and it is not known how many times such a procedure may be safely repeated. Even so, a few weeks to months of relief can help to break the chronic pain cycle and allow other modalities to take effect.

The second problem is loss of a potential signal that something is wrong. Patients with benign chronic abdominal pain may be subject to intraabdominal catastrophes such as perforations and obstructions of the gastrointestinal tract. Obviously, time is of the essence in diagnosing and treating such problems. If the potential to feel visceral pain is lost, such conditions may progress until the patient's chances of survival are diminished. This is a particular problem if the cause of the pain is alcoholic pancreatitis. An alcoholic patient may be less reliable in noting and reporting other signs of a surgical emergency, such as vomiting and abdominal pain.

Celiac plexus blockade with local anesthetic has a potential but limited role in the management of surgical anesthesia and pain. The block may supplement neuraxial block and permit various procedures in the upper abdomen to be performed without general anesthesia. Celiac plexus blockade was used in some centers for cholecystectomy when open cholecystectomy was common.

25. When using a celiac plexus block, how does one decide which side to block?

The celiac plexus is not a lateralized structure, but it is a diffuse structure. For a diagnostic block, it is acceptable to block from one side. If the result is poor, a repeat block with bilateral needle placement may be attempted. For neurolytic block, bilateral needle placement is sometimes done to get the best spread without excessive volume of neurolytic agent. However, when the block is performed with radiographic assistance, even neurolytic block can be performed with one needle.

26. What is the clinical challenge in treating severe malignant pelvic pain? What is the role of sympathetic blockade?

Various cancers of the reproductive organs and lower gastrointestinal tract may cause severe pelvic pain. When oral analgesics fail to control the pain and one must resort to nerve blocks, the options are continuous spinal or epidural opioids, with or without local anesthetics, and various neuroablative procedures. All of these options yield excellent results for well-selected patients; however, they are quite invasive. In addition, neurodestructive procedures are not ideal; they occasionally result in somatic blockade, which can be distressing to a terminally ill patient who wants to maintain as much function as possible for as long as possible. The other side of the coin is that neurodestructive procedures are not as permanent as they sound. The life expectancy of some patients with malignant infiltration of the pelvis may be months and even years.

Of the many possible pathologies of pelvic pain, nerve invasion and destruction are prominent. When the pain is sympathetically mediated, a simple series of blocks can forestall the need for more invasive procedures.

27. How is a hypogastric plexus block performed? What are the risks?

The hypogastric plexus is a series of nerves that lie anterior to the lower lumbar vertebrae and then branch out to a number of minor plexi in the pelvis. This plexus system contains mainly sympathetic postganglionic nerves and afferent fibers.

Although the details of this block are beyond the scope of this chapter, the various components of the hypogastric plexus can be blocked with the patient in the prone position. Fluoroscopic assistance is usually required because hypogastric plexus block does not have a palpable endpoint. The basic approach is not unlike that used for the lumbar sympathetic block; hypogastric plexus block is performed lateral to L5 vertebrae. The needle is directed caudad, and the goal is placement anterior to the lumbosacral junction. Proper needle placement yields a consistent picture on fluoroscopy and can be confirmed by injection of contrast, which shows a characteristic pattern of spread.

28. Almost all of the indications for sympathetic blockade are chronic problems. Why, then, do we perform local anesthetic sympathetic blocks, which wear off within several hours of the procedure?

Local anesthetic sympathetic neural blockade is performed to make a diagnosis, to interrupt a cycle of pain, or to facilitate other interventions. When one is planning the management of a poorly defined, nonspecific chronic pain problem, the management plan may be altered based on response to a sympathetic block. For example, if atypical food pain of relatively recent onset responds to a lumbar sympathetic local anesthetic blockade and if one can demonstrate that no incidental somatic blockade resulted, it is acceptable to proceed with an accepted protocol for RSD. As mentioned above, this is most often a multidisciplinary protocol involving a series of blocks, physical therapy, behavioral therapy, and perhaps intravenous sympatholytic injections. Systemic medications may include nonsteroidal antiinflammatory drugs and antidepressants. If, in the same patient, a lumbar sympathetic block produces good evidence of sympatholytic effect but no relief, further management is planned in other directions.

The most common use of repeated blocks is to facilitate physical therapy. This is the classic way of managing RSD, but it is also appropriate for many other painful conditions. During the effective period of the block, stretching and range-of-motion exercises can be accomplished with less discomfort. Teamwork is essential in coordinating the block with therapy. Beyond the obvious challenge of making sure that the therapy appointment is scheduled within the effective period of the block, a mutual understanding of the diagnosis is essential. Furthermore, the author insists that a fully certified physical or occupational therapist is involved in the exercise. Depending on the diagnosis, therapy carried out by an inexperienced individual may push the patient too hard and do more harm than good.

Neural blockade with local anesthetics almost never cures a pain problem by itself. If the block is to serve its purpose as an adjunct to the multidisciplinary care plan, the patient's expectations for the block must be realistic. If patients expect a block to be curative and then feel that they are referred for behavioral therapy when it is not, a certain loss of hope and trust is inevitable.

BIBLIOGRAPHY

1. Bell S, Cole R, Robert-Thomason IC: Coeliac plexus block for control of pain in chronic pancreatitis. BMJ 281:1604, 1980.
2. Bonica JJ: Causalgia and other reflex sympathetic dystrophies. In Bonica JJ (ed): The Management of Pain, 2nd ed. Philadelphia, Lea & Febiger, 1990, pp 220–243.
3. Bridenbaugh PO, Cousins MJ: Neural Blockade in Clinical Anesthesia and the Management of Pain. Philadelphia, J.B. Lippincott, 1988.
4. Brown DL, Bulley TK, Uiel EL: Neurolytic celiac plexus block for pancreatic cancer pain. Anesth Analg 66:869–873, 1987.
5. Carron H, Litwiller R: Stellate ganglion block. Anesth Analg 54:567–570, 1975.
6. Glynn CJ, Basedow RW, Walsh JA: Pain relief following postganglionic sympathetic blockade with IV guanethidine. Br J Anaesth 53:1297–1302, 1981.
7. Moore DC, Bush WH, Burnett LL: Celiac plexus blockade: A roentgenographic, anatomic study of technique and spread of solution in patients and corpses. Anesth Analg 60:369–379, 1981.
8. Plancarte R, et al: Hypogastric plexus block: Retroperitoneal approach. Anesthesiology 71:A739, 1989.
9. Roberts WJ: A hypothesis on the physiological basis for causalgia and related pains. Pain 24:297–311, 1986.
10. Yanagida H, Kemi C, Suwa K: The effects of stellate ganglion block on the idiopathic prolongation of the Q-T interval with cardiac arrhythmia (the Romano-Ward syndrome). Anesth Analg 55:782–787, 1976.

37. INTRASPINAL OPIOIDS

Mark D. Canning, M.D., Zahid H. Bajwa, M.D.,
and Carol A. Warfield, M.D.

1. What is meant by intraspinal opioid?

This term refers to the use of opioid medications administered in close proximity to the spinal cord. This is in contrast to systemic administration (oral, intramuscular, intravenous); the primary site of action for systemic opioids has been shown to be supraspinal receptors in the brain, whereas intraspinal opioids act primarily on the spinal cord.

2. How are intraspinal opioids given?

Intraspinal opioids may be injected into the epidural space (outside the dura mater) or into the intrathecal space (subarachnoid or spinal). Either method may be single-shot or continuous. With single-shot administration, the spinal or epidural needle is withdrawn following injection. For continuous administration, a small catheter is placed, and the drug is given via the catheter. Drugs may then be administered by intermittent bolus or via a continuous infusion device.

3. How long have intraspinal opioids been in use?

In 1855, the Wood needle allowed for the first parenteral administration of morphine. However, it was not until 1979 that Wang, Nauss, and Thomas reported the first human study demonstrating the safe, effective intrathecal application of morphine. Behar and associates reported epidural applications soon after.

4. What is the rationale for using intraspinal opioids?

Nociceptive input (i.e., a painful stimulus) travels to the spinal cord via primary afferents, A-delta and C fibers. These fibers synapse with second-order neurons located in the dorsal horn of the spinal cord. From there, nociceptive input is transmitted to supraspinal centers in the brain via ascending tracts.

Melzack and Walls' gate control theory proposed that interneurons in the dorsal horn act to modulate nociceptive input. They postulated that gates could be opened and closed by stimulation and inhibition via interneurons in the spinal cord. These interneurons were later determined to be located in the substantia gelatinosa. Spinal opioids exert their primary effects in the substantia gelatinosa (lamina II) of the dorsal horn.

5. What evidence is there for opioid action in the substantia gelatinosa?

Iontophoretic and micro injection data have demonstrated the substantia gelatinosa as the primary site of action for intraspinal opioids. These early studies have been confirmed by radiolabeled studies. The mechanism in the substantia gelatinosa is presynaptic inhibition of neurotransmitter release, although postsynaptic effects probably have a role.

6. How do opioids reach the substantia gelatinosa?

Once administered, subarachnoid opioids reach the spinal cord via two mechanisms: (1) direct spread from the cerebrospinal fluid (CSF) and (2) vascular absorption from the CSF, which is then delivered to the spinal cord. For epidural routes, entrance into the CSF is via direct spread through the dural cuff and then transfer to the cord by the two mechanisms noted above. In addition, vascular absorption from the epidural space with subsequent delivery to the cord also occurs.

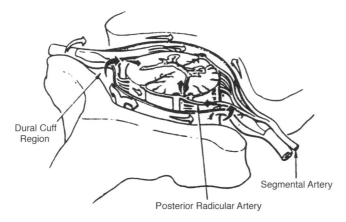

Dural Cuff
Region

Segmental Artery

Posterior Radicular Artery

Cross-section depicting opioid spread in epidural space (white arrows) and in spinal cord and CSF (black arrows). (From Cousins M, Bridenbaugh P (eds): Neural Blockade in Clinical Anesthesia and Management of Pain. Philadelphia, J.B. Lippincott, 1988, with permission.)

7. Which specific properties of the opioid molecule play a role in reaching the dorsal horn?

Several pharmacokinetic properties determine the degree to which intraspinal opioids reach the dorsal horn: lipid solubility, molecular weight and shape, surface area exposed (i.e., "spread"), and route of administration (epidural vs. subarachnoid). The most important of these appears to be molecular weight.

8. Are all opioids created equal?

No. The most useful property for classifying intraspinal opioids is lipid solubility. Opioids can be divided into two classes: lipophilic (lipid-soluble) vs. hydrophilic (lipid-insoluble). Fentanyl, sufentanil, and meperidine are lipophilic drugs. Morphine and hydromorphone are hydrophilic. The octanol water coefficient is the standard for grading and comparing lipophilicity.

Relative Octanol: Water Coefficients (Compared to Morphine)

OPIOID	O:W
Morphine	1
Hydromorphone	4
Meperidine	40
Fentanyl	400
Sufentanil	1600

9. What pharmacodynamic role does lipophilicity play?

Increased lipid solubility decreases the time required for transfer of drug across lipid barriers (blood vessels, cell membranes). Clinically, this translates to more rapid-onset, shorter duration of action after spinal administration, higher equianalgesic doses, and higher incidence of systemic side effects.

10. Why are higher equianalgesic doses required for lipophilic drugs?

Because of the highly vascular and adipose-filled nature of the epidural space, a significant amount of lipophilic drug will be absorbed by both blood and fat. This serves to reduce the amount of drug "available" to reach the dorsal horn.

11. What factors determine duration of action of spinal opioids?

Termination of action is accomplished after the opioid diffuses away from the receptor and returns to the CSF or is carried away from the spinal cord by venous return. Affinity for the receptor and lipophilicity determine the duration of action. To date, the role for intraspinal metabolism is unclear.

12. What are the common side effects?

Classically, intraspinal opioid side effects are similar to those observed with systemic administration: respiratory depression, urinary retention, pruritus, and nausea and vomiting. Tolerance and physical dependence may also occur.

13. Which is the most common side effect?

Pruritus has been shown to occur quite commonly; however, according to studies by Reiz and Westburg and by Bromage, Camporesi, and Chestnut, the incidence is highly variable: 15 to 100%. The exact mechanism is unknown, but probably does not involve histamine release. Pruritus responds to low dose naloxone (5µg/kg/hr) without decreasing analgesic effectiveness.

14. How common is urinary retention?

The incidence of urinary retention is 10 to 50% and does not differ from that of systemically administered narcotics, although the onset and severity may differ (see Stenseth and Breirik and Gustafsson et al). Reducing the administered dose does not decrease the incidence. The mechanism is inhibition of the volume-evoked micturition reflex. Urinary retention does respond to low dose naloxone.

15. Is nausea more likely with the spinal route than with systemic administration?

The incidence for intraspinal-related nausea is probably 17 to 34% and may be reduced with lipophilic drugs, epidural administration (vs. intrathecal), and continuous therapy (vs. single shot). The mechanism is opioid receptor stimulation at the chemoreceptor trigger zone. Antiemetics are the first-line therapy for nausea.

16. Is opioid withdrawal a potential problem?

Patients physically dependent on systemic narcotics may achieve pain relief from intraspinal opioids or local anesthetics. If systemic opioids are stopped abruptly, there is risk of withdrawal because the amount of intraspinal opioid reaching supraspinal centers may not be enough to prevent withdrawal.

17. What is the incidence of respiratory depression?

Respiratory depression is most commonly associated with intrathecal morphine and the narcotic-naive patient. The incidence is less than 1% with the epidural route and slightly higher for intrathecal opioids. Intraspinal opioids have not been shown to have higher incidence than systemic opioids.

18. What is the time course of respiratory depression?

Respiratory depression is generally classified as early or late. Early respiratory depression generally occurs within 1 to 2 hours postinjection. Late respiratory depression peaks at six hours but can occur up to 12 hours postinjection. Each type has a different mechanism and thus differing onsets.

Early respiratory depression occurs as a result of vascular absorption and is primarily seen after epidural administration. Overdoses of opioid (e.g., accidental spinal injection, dosage error) in the subarachnoid space can result in early respiratory depression via a nonvascular mechanism, but these are rare. Because lipophilic drugs (fentanyl, meperidine) are readily absorbed in the highly vascular epidural space and because higher doses are administered, they are much more likely to produce early respiratory depression.

Late respiratory depression occurs as a result of rostral migration of drug in the CSF. Ultimately, the opioid reaches the floor of the fourth ventricle. The drug can then be absorbed into the medulla and affect the respiratory center. Clearly, hydrophilic drugs (hydromorphone, morphine) are at highest risk for this type of migration because of greater "spread" and relatively higher CSF concentrations. Lipophilic drugs generally do not develop great enough CSF concentrations or significant rostral spread because they are rapidly absorbed.

19. How does vascular absorption occur?

Via two mechanisms. Epidural veins are responsible for the most significant amount of absorption and deliver the drug, via the azygous vein, to the systemic circulation. Once the drug reaches the systemic circulation, its effects, side effects, and metabolism resemble a systemically administered opioid.

Absorption via the basivertebral venous plexus provides an alternative route of blood-borne redistribution. However, the basivertebral route bypasses the azygous return and delivers the drug cephalad to the brain. Hence, it is felt that even small concentrations of drug carried via this system might have more deleterious effects, either alone or in combination with systemically redistributed drug.

20. Is bolus administration superior to continuous infusion?

The bolus administration and continuous infusion methods each have advantages and disadvantages. Bolus administration of opioid is advantageous in that a sophisticated infusion device is not required. Practically, only hydrophilic agents can be used because of their longer duration of action. However, increased side effects, including respiratory depression, can result. In addition, local anesthetic cannot be combined with the regimen; the dose-sparing, synergistic combination of local anesthetic and opioid is becoming increasingly more popular.

Continuous infusion offers the advantage of use with local anesthetic and decreased risk of side effects. Ideally, the infusion also offers steady levels of opioid (and analgesia). Finally, the likelihood for contamination (due to the closed system) is also reduced when compared with the bolus technique.

Continuous vs. Bolus: Relative Advantages of Epidural Administration Techniques

	ADVANTAGES	DISADVANTAGES
Continuous Infusions	Can use shorter-acting opioids, which are more titratable	Requires sophisticated infusion device
	Consistent analgesia (less peaks and troughs)	Higher cost
	Decreased risk for contamination	
	Device eliminates need for physician to periodically inject catheter	
	May be combined with local anesthetic solutions	
	Reduced incidence of side effects	
Intermittent Bolus	Does not require sophisticated infusion device	Cannot be combined with local anesthetic
	Simplicity of periodic injection	Difficult to titrate dose
	Inexpensive	Higher incidence of rostral spread and side effects
		Increased risk for contamination
		Requires staff to periodically inject catheter

21. Which route is preferred: intrathecal or epidural?

Epidural is the preferred route in postoperative pain management therapies, primarily because the risk of a spinal headache is greatly reduced. In chronic and cancer pain therapies, the increased risks associated with intrathecal administration (including respiratory depression and chronic CSF leak) and the greater likelihood of meningitis should the catheter become infected lead many clinicians to opt for the epidural route. However, there are two important reasons to use an intrathecal catheter in the chronic/cancer pain setting:

1. A high opioid requirement is more easily met by the intrathecal route, since spinal dosing is generally 1/10th that of equianalgesic epidural dosing.

2. Catheter-tip fibrosis, which leads to ineffective analgesia and is a common epidural catheter complication, does not occur when the intrathecal route is chosen.

22. When are intraspinal techniques contraindicated?

Allergy to intraspinal opioids and systemic infection are absolute contraindications. Coagulation disorders are only relative contraindications to intrathecal and epidural techniques; however, the risk of an expanding hematoma causing spinal cord compression is a real risk. Most centers have established guidelines for acceptable aberrant coagulation parameters.

23. In terms of pain relief, what advantages do intraspinal opioids have?

In the acute situation, intraspinal administration presents a high concentration of opioids directly to the dorsal horn and will modulate nociceptive input in the dorsal horn. Somatic input is largely reduced when adequate doses are given. Visceral input, however, is only partially blocked; for this reason, intraspinal opioids are often combined with local anesthetics. This combination serves to block all nociceptive input, both visceral and somatic.

24. Do these advantages apply to the chronic pain patient?

In addition to the advantages noted above, intraspinal opioids allow for pain control in patients tolerant to systemic opioids and those unable to take these medications systemically (e.g., because of nausea and vomiting secondary to oral morphine).

25. When are intraspinal opioids used for acute pain?

The most common indications include perioperative pain management, peripartum pain management, and acute pain secondary to trauma.

26. Are intraspinal opioids alone effective for acute pain?

Intraspinal opioids are effective in relieving somatic pain, but not completely effective in relieving visceral pain. Many centers use morphine alone for acute pain relief; however, the majority use combinations of opioids and local anesthetics. Yaksh has demonstrated the synergistic effect of using local anesthetics with lower doses of opioids.

27. Are intraspinal opioids useful for labor and delivery?

Intrathecal and epidural opioids have been used for both labor and delivery. Epidural opioid administration has become the method of choice for laboring parturients. When combined with local anesthetic, excellent analgesia results. The risk of spinal headache in young patients has steered many away from the use of intrathecal opioids, but with smaller, well-designed needles, this is no longer a common complication.

28. Are there other acute settings where intraspinal opioids may be of use?

Trauma patients in whom systemic opioids may be detrimental (e.g., ventilatory depression with severe obstructive lung disease or multiple rib fractures) may benefit from neuraxial blockade of nociceptive stimuli.

29. Are intraspinal opioids useful for chronic pain?

When conventional pain therapies fail or reduce the quality of life, intraspinal opioids may be indicated. In general, this occurs when patients have pain responsive to oral or parenteral opioids but suffer from intolerable side effects with systemic opioids.

Cancer pain is the most common indication. Noncancer pain syndromes, such as reflex sympathetic dystrophy, ischemic extremity pain, or postherpetic neuralgia, are more likely to respond to the intraspinal administration of local anesthetic, rather than an opioid.

Continuous administration of opioid via an indwelling catheter can provide long-lasting pain relief with little systemic effects. Choices for administration include patient-controlled, bolus, or infusion techniques. Catheters may be injected via an externalized port, percutaneous reservoir, or implanted pump.

BIBLIOGRAPHY

1. Behar M, Magora F, Olshwang D, et al: Epidural morphine in treatment of pain. Lancet 1:527, 1979.
2. Bromage P, Camporesi E, Chestnut D: Epidural narcotics for postoperative analgesia. Anesth Analg Curr Res 59:473, 1980.
3. Brownridge P: Epidural and intrathecal opiates for postoperative pain relief. Anesthesiology 38:74, 1983.
4. Chaney MA: Side effects of intrathecal and epidural opioids. Can J Anaesth 42:893, 1995.
5. Cousins M, Cherry D, Gourlay G: Acute and chronic pain: Use of spinal opioids. In Cousins M, Bridenbaugh P (eds): Neural Blockade in Clinical Anesthesia and Management of Pain. Philadelphia, JB Lippincott, 1988.
6. Gustafsson L, Schildt B, Jacobsen K: Adverse effects of extradural and intrathecal opiates: A report of a nationwide survey in Sweden. Br J Anaesth 54:479, 1982.
7. Melzack R, Wall P: Pain mechanisms: A new theory. Science 150:971, 1965.
8. Nehme A: Intraspinal opioid analgesia. In Warfield C (ed): Principles and Practice of Pain Management. New York, McGraw-Hill, 1993.
9. Penning J, Yaksh T: Interaction of intrathecal morphine with bupivacaine and lidocaine in the rat. Anesthesiology 77:1186, 1992.
10. Reiz S, Westburg M: Side effects of epidural morphine. Lancet 2:203, 1980.
11. Stenseth O, Breirik H: Epidural morphine for postoperative pain: Experience with 1085 patients. Acta Anaesth Scand 29:148, 1985.
12. Wang J, Nauss L, Thomas J: Pain relief by intrathecally applied morphine in man. Anesthesiology 50:149, 1979.

38. NEUROSTIMULATORY AND NEUROABLATIVE PROCEDURES

Jason E. Silvers, B.S., and James N. Campbell, M.D.

1. What is spinal cord stimulation?

Spinal cord stimulation (SCS) provides electrical stimulation over the dorsal columns of the spinal cord through the placement of epidural electrodes. Although the mechanism by which SCS relieves pain remains unclear, SCS results in significant pain relief for an appropriately selected group of patients.

2. What are the criteria for choosing patients who may benefit from spinal cord stimulation for treatment of pain?

1. The patient should have a clear diagnosis for which the procedure is indicated.

2. Standard therapies to treat pain have been exhausted or are unacceptable to the patient.

3. When feasible, temporary relief of the patient's pain symptoms should be demonstrated by a trial of stimulation.

4. The pain should be distributed such that spinal stimulation can stimulate the sensory fibers that serve the painful area and create paresthesias. It is difficult to stimulate the sensory fibers that serve the spinal column, and thus spinal axis pain usually does not respond to spinal cord stimulation. In spinal cord injury, the sensory fibers that would ordinarily serve the painful area may be severed. The underlying substrate for stimulation (the dorsal columns) is thus missing. Not surprisingly, spinal cord stimulation does not relieve pain in such patients.

3. Give examples of conditions which may, and of those which usually do not, respond to spinal cord stimulation.

May respond:
    Radicular pain from failed back surgery
    Ischemic pain from peripheral vascular disease
    Pain from peripheral nerve injury
    Phantom limb pain or stump pain
    Complex regional pain syndrome (reflex sympathetic dystrophy, causalgia)
Usually do not respond:
    Postherpetic neuralgia
    Pain from spinal cord injury
    Axial pain in failed back syndrome

4. Why is spinal cord stimulation for failed back surgery syndrome more applicable to radicular neuropathic pain than to axial low back pain?

It is easier to generate paresthesias in radicular distributions than in the midline of the lower back. Radicular paresthesias are elicited at almost all electrode positions, whereas achieving stimulation overlap of the lower back is technically difficult and may require complex electrode placement and extensive psychophysical testing.

5. What are implantable pumps for intrathecal drug delivery?

Implantable pumps consist of reservoirs, placed subcutaneously, which connect via a catheter into the intrathecal space. Implantable pumps allow physicians to administer opiate analgesics directly into the cerebrospinal fluid. The pumps are programmable so that neurosurgeons can adjust dosages and delivery rates. More questions on this technique are given in the chapter on spinal anesthesia.

6. What are the dose advantages of spinal epidural and subarachnoid opiate delivery versus systemic administration?

Spinal epidural opiate delivery has a dose advantage over systemic administration of one order of magnitude. On a milligram basis, epidural opioids are ten times more potent than systemically administered opioids. Subarachnoid delivery has a two order of magnitude (100×) dose advantage. Of note, visceral pain responds best to intraspinal opiate delivery, while head and neck pain respond best to intracerebroventricular delivery.

7. How can externalized catheters be used to treat pain symptoms?

Externalized catheters are placed percutaneously and connect directly into the intrathecal space. Neurosurgeons can administer medications directly from the outside into the cerebrospinal fluid. However, externalized catheters are associated with high infection rates and therefore must be changed frequently.

8. Name several advantages and disadvantages of battery-powered, programmable, implantable pump designs and passive implantable pump designs.

	Battery-powered	*Passive*
Advantages	Allow for noninvasive adjustments of dosages and infusion rates; can deliver complex rate profiles (e.g., bolus administration)	Low start-up costs; no life-limiting components (i.e., no battery)
Disadvantages	Limited by battery longevity and high start-up costs	Lacks flexibility, nonprogrammable

9. What is the most common indication for opiate delivery via implantable pumps?

The ability to administer opiates directly into the cerebrospinal fluid has been one of the most important advances for the treatment of regional and widespread cancer pain. Opiate receptors are present on the central terminals of the sensory fibers that innervate the painful area and thus can be directly activated in this way. Direct delivery to the spinal cord also has the advantage over systemic administration in that there may be fewer associated symptomatic side effects due to the smaller doses necessary for adequate pain relief. *Implantable pumps should be used only in patients in whom oral delivery of opiates has failed whether because of unacceptable side effects or lack of efficacy.*

10. What is a cordotomy and what are the desired results?

A cordotomy surgically destroys the spinothalamic tract. The spinothalamic tract, located in the anterolateral part of the spinal cord, carries nociceptive information from the contralateral side of the body to the brain. Pain relief occurs a few spinal segments below the level of the lesion, but on the side of the body *opposite* the side of the cordotomy.

11. How does an open cordotomy compare with a percutaneous cordotomy?

Open cordotomy requires a small laminectomy and incision in the spinothalamic tract, while percutaneous cordotomy uses radiofrequency lesions to destroy this portion of the cord. A percutaneous cordotomy is done with local anesthesia and, prior to producing the destructive lesion, stimulation can be done to assure that the painful area will be covered by the cordotomy. Percutaneous cordotomy is usually performed at the C1–2 level, allowing for a high body level of pain relief. Although results from open cordotomy are favorable, percutaneous cordotomy is less invasive and results are comparable.

12. What are the potential risks of a bilateral cordotomy performed at upper cervical levels?

Respiratory depression—this may take the form of "Ondine's curse" or sleep apnea
Neurogenic bladder

Horner's syndrome—usually transient, from injury to the sympathetic fibers in the cervical
    cord
Transient hypotension
Bowel and bladder incontinence—usually transient

13. How do rhizotomy and dorsal root ganglionectomy procedures treat pain symptoms?

Both of these procedures are destructive techniques aimed at interrupting transmission of nociceptive impulses from the periphery to the spinal cord, before these impulses reach the cord. A
rhizotomy destroys the dorsal roots (carrying afferent sensory fibers, including "pain" fibers, or
nociceptors) proximal to the dorsal root ganglion. A dorsal root ganglionectomy removes the
dorsal root ganglion, which contains the cell bodies of the afferent sensory fibers, including nociceptors. However, rhizotomies, dorsal root ganglionectomies, and combined procedures most
often do not confer long-term benefit.

14. How do rhizotomy and cordotomy differ in treating specific cancer lesions?

Rhizotomies affect only the areas served by the specific root that is cut (dermatomes), while
cordotomies affect the entire side of the body from the level of the lesion down. Therefore, rhizotomies are considered only in very localized pain syndromes, and cordotomies can be used for
more widespread pain.

15. What is thought to be the anatomic basis for trigeminal neuralgia?

One proposed structural basis for trigeminal neuralgia is vascular compromise of the trigeminal nerve. Trigeminal neuralgia may also result from multiple sclerosis, collagen vascular disease, and other structural diseases that compress the trigeminal nerve near the brainstem. A
broader discussion is available in the chapter on trigeminal neuralgia (tic douloureux), along with
questions on medical management.

16. Name three percutaneous ablative techniques used to treat trigeminal neuralgia and the side effects associated with these procedures.

1. Radiofrequency retrogasserian rhizolysis attempts to produce graded anesthesia in the affected division of the trigeminal nerve. The procedure is based on the thermocoagulation of specific roots.
2. Retrogasserian glycerol rhizolysis involves glycerol injection into the trigeminal cistern.
The osmotic agent produces a "chemical neurolysis."
3. Balloon microcompression involves inflation of a Fogarty-type of balloon near the
gasserian ganglion.
Side effects: Loss of sensation is usually moderate or not noticeable, particularly with glycerol injection. In severe cases, corneal anesthesia may lead to loss of vision. A different type of
pain may emerge in the area rendered anesthetic (sometimes referred to as anesthesia dolorosa).
The mechanisms of pain production in injured nerves are discussed in the chapter on neuropathic
pain.

17. What is a neuroma?

Neuromas represent unsuccessful attempts at nerve regeneration. When axons are severed
(axotomy), the proximal part of the axon may grow out, attempting to regain continuity with the
distal part. Neuromas form after axotomy if nerve regeneration is unsuccessful. A neuroma consists of densely packed clusters of regenerative sprouts which form after nerve fibers are severed.
Neuromas may produce spontaneous pain. They are also particularly sensitive to mechanical
pressure and to circulating catecholamines.

18. Describe the surgical treatment options for a neuroma.

Simple excision of a neuroma rarely provides adequate pain relief. As along as a severed
nerve fiber has a viable cell body and regeneration of that fiber does not occur, a neuroma will

form. Surgical therapy should be directed at relocating the neuroma to a different site, away from scar tissue and mobile structures such as tendons and joints. The new site should also be protected from external stimuli. One option is to embed the neuroma into deep muscle. Another surgical option involves repairing the nerve with a graft to prevent the neuroma from reforming.

19. Which neurons in the spinal cord do DREZ lesions target?

The DREZ operation produces discrete lesions in the dorsal root entry zone of the spinal cord, particularly in Rexed layers I, II and V. These layers contain the secondary sensory neurons, which carry nociceptive input from the periphery to the brain through the spinothalamic tract.

20. What is the principle behind the DREZ operation?

The DREZ operation is a very useful procedure for pain problems that arise from lesions of the sensory roots near their entry into the spinal cord. DREZ lesions attempt to destroy neurons in the superficial layers of the spinal cord. Avulsion injuries of the brachial plexus, where the sensory roots are literally torn from the spinal cord, are ideal cases for treatment with the DREZ operation. In these syndromes, it is postulated that a hyperactive or hypersensitive pool of neurons in the dorsal horn is responsible for maintaining the pain syndrome.

21. What is sympathetically maintained pain (SMP)?

In some patients with neuropathic pain, abnormal activity in the sympathetic nervous system is presumed to maintain the pain. SMP most likely results from the emergence of abnormal sensitivity of peripheral nerve pain fibers (nociceptors) to norepinephrine. The release of norepinephrine from the sympathetic nervous system activates nociceptors and thus produces pain.

22. How can sympathetically maintained pain be diagnosed?

One of the major stumbling blocks in treating SMP has been diagnosis. SMP must be considered in any patient suffering with severe facial or extremity pain. Also, almost all patients with SMP have cooling hyperalgesia (pain to a mild cooling stimulus). A sympathetic block will relieve pain in every patient suffering from SMP. However, there are false positives associated with sympathetic blocks, and placebo effects may be difficult to detect. If a technically well-done sympathetic block fails to relieve the patient's pain symptoms, the patient does not have SMP. Phentolamine infusion, and possibly topical clonidine, may also be used to test for SMP.

BIBLIOGRAPHY

1. Campbell JN: Diagnosis and treatment of pain associated with nerve injury. In Benzel EC (ed): Practical Approaches to Peripheral Nerve Surgery. Park Ridge, IL, AANS Publications Committee, 1992.
2. Coffey RF: Neurosurgical management of intractable pain. In Youmans JR (ed): Neurological Surgery. 4th ed. Philadelphia, W.B. Saunders Co., 1996.
3. Loesser JD: Dorsal rhizotomy for the relief of chronic pain. J Neurosurg 36:745–754, 1972.
4. Nashold BS, Nashold JRB: The DREZ operation. In Tindall GT, Cooper PR, Barrow DL (eds): The Practice of Neurosurgery. Baltimore, Williams & Wilkins, 1996.
5. North RB: Spinal cord stimulation for chronic intractable pain. In Devinsky O, Beric A, Dogali M (eds): Electrical and Magnetic Stimulation of the Brain and Spinal Cord. New York, Raven Press, 1993.
6. North RB, Kidd DH, Campbell JN, et al: Dorsal root ganglionectomy for failed back syndrome: A five-year follow-up study. J Neurosurg 74:236–242, 1991.
7. Onofrio BM, Yakash TL: Long-term pain relief produced by intrathecal morphine infusion in 53 patients. J Neurosurg 72:200–209, 1990.
8. Raja SN, Treede RD, Davis KD, Campbell JN: Systemic alpha-adrenergic blockade with phentolamine: A diagnostic test for sympathetically maintained pain. Anesthesiology 74:691–698, 1991.

39. PSYCHOLOGICAL CONSTRUCTS AND TREATMENT INTERVENTIONS

Dennis Thornton, Ph.D.

1. List three possible psychological mechanisms for pain.

The first purely psychological mechanism is the concept of somatization. Psychic distress and conflict are converted into somatic complaints in an unconscious attempt to reduce intrapsychic tension. A second mechanism is psychosomatic: underlying muscle tension results in regional discomfort. While this may be difficult to prove by examination, the fact that relaxation techniques and the use of anxiolytic drugs provide relief lends credence to the theory. The third mechanism represents the rare occurrence of somatic delusions or hallucinatory pain. These phenomena may occur in schizophrenia or in cases of severe depressive illness.

2. Do all pain patients display these types of dynamic issues?

No. There are a variety of pathways in which individuals can come to display pain behaviors. Histories of being raised in dysfunctional homes with abuse, alcoholism, or mental illness are common in chronic pain patients. The resulting harsh superego is reflected in alcohol and drug abuse, self-sabotaging behaviors, marital discord, suicide attempts, and workaholism. An injured worker may experience not only the loss of employment but also an absence of personal gratification and a diminished sense of self, leaving him vulnerable to re-emergence of anger, depression, and other negative emotions repressed from childhood. Such dynamic factors then negatively influence the patient's ability to invest in, and benefit from, psychological interventions.

3. What is the relevance of psychoanalytic theory to understanding the experience of pain?

Psychoanalytic theory divides the psyche into three functions: the id: unconscious source of primitive sexual, dependency, and aggressive impulses; the superego: subconsciously interjects societal mores, setting standards to live by; the ego: representing a sense of self, mediates between realities of the moment and psychic needs and conflicts. Psychoanalytic writings discuss how pain frustrates the satisfaction of dependency and sexual needs as well as appropriate dissipation of aggressive feelings. The blocked expression of these needs leads to inner turmoil. Chronic pain, when sanctioned as a bona fide physical problem, allows for unconscious gratification of ambivalent dependency needs. Underlying anger may be expressed indirectly, in the form of passive-aggressive behaviors, where the patient holds family members and treating practitioner alike as hostages to endless complaints and demands for attention. The experiences of pain satisfy the superego's need to suffer and atone.

4. From a psychoanalytic perspective, how can the experience of pain be employed as a defense mechanism?

Pain can be viewed as an ego defense mechanism in that the focus on somatic sensations deflects attention from intrapsychic conflicts and anxieties. The experience of physical pain is unconsciously perceived as more acceptable than the emotional pain. Szasz coined the term "l'homme douloureux" to signify the dynamic by which the patient represses his fears of loss and rejection and the tension from these conflicts is displaced onto the body. The ensuing chronic pain behavior then serves as a form of interpersonal communication. Individuals frustrated and angry over their inability to alter their life situation in turn baffle health care professionals who attempt to treat the physical complaints, which are symbols of the underlying emotional pain.

5. List the core dynamic features associated with the patient prone to psychogenic pain.

The concept of the pain prone patient was originated by George Engel, a psychoanalytically oriented psychiatrist, who observed particular personality characteristics in patients reporting chronic somatic symptoms, predominantly pain. These characteristics included:

1. Overriding guilt, with pain serving as a means of atonement.
2. A background of poor parenting, neglect, abuse and/or illness.
3. A history of defeat, stemming from masochistic character structure.
4. A strong but frustrated aggressive drive.
5. Pain serving to replace an object loss.
6. A sadomasochistic sexual development.
7. Pain that has symbolic meaning, usually identification.
8. A psychiatric disorder, including conversion hysteria, depression, hypochondriasis, and paranoid schizophrenia.

Engel employed the term psychogenic to denote that the pain experienced was initiated, maintained, or enhanced by memories, thoughts, or unconscious processes. The process of displacement of psychic pain onto the soma is interpreted as a defense against anxiety or as a compromise solution to unconscious conflicts.

6. What is meant when pain patients are described as experiencing some form of "gain" from their pain experience?

The construct of gain is described in three basic forms, all of which are means by which pain behaviors are reinforced. The process of gain is described as primary, secondary, or tertiary.

7. What is primary gain?

Avoidance of a psychic conflict by converting it to a physical ailment. This conversion process is usually interpreted as a defense against anxiety or as a compromise solution of unconscious conflicts. While the underlying conflict is kept out of consciousness, the conflict remains unresolved and there is a continued buildup of psychic tension always ready for discharge. The anxious individual then discharges the pent-up energy by responding to ordinary or mildly painful stimuli in an exaggerated way.

8. How is the term secondary gain applied?

It applies to factors that reinforce the display of pain-related behaviors. The reinforcing factors alluded to are most commonly litigation and disability payments. However, demonstration of caring and concern is also a factor. Under these circumstances, there is a perceived incentive for the patient to persist in the complaint of pain. If the pain is resolved, the plaintiff's case will be weakened, or the love may be lost. Similarly, the injured worker who is partially improved may be pressured to return to work. Feeling in a weakened state, not ready to resume full responsibilities, it becomes easier to retreat into pain rather than face the threat of attempting to return to functioning and failing.

9. How is tertiary gain different from primary and secondary gain?

Where constructs of primary and secondary gain apply to the individual, tertiary gain is external to the patient and involves family members or significant others who benefit from directly or indirectly reinforcing pain behaviors. The gain may be that interpersonal or family problems are suppressed as long as the patient remains ill, for example, the parent who feels inadequate and successfully avoids having to work and interact with the world by having to care for an ill child. By continuing to report that the child is symptomatic, the parent has a face-saving excuse for remaining dysfunctional. Similarly, the angry spouse may undermine the patient's efforts toward regaining independence because a new balance has been achieved with the advent of chronic pain and disability.

10. Name some characteristics often associated with chronic pain syndromes.

a. Preoccupation with pain.
b. Strong and ambivalent dependency needs.

    c. Characterologic masochism (meeting other people's needs at one's own expense).
    d. Inability to take care of self-needs.
    e. Passivity.
    f. Lack of insight to deal appropriately with anger and hostility.
    g. Use of pain as a symbolic means of communication.

11. How did the term pain-prone disorder originate?

It was coined by Blumer and Heilbronn in an attempt to account for psychodynamic factors that they felt significantly influenced the presentation of somatic symptoms. Chronic pain was viewed as a variant of depression, even though patients might not see themselves as depressed, but suffering from physical ailments. In this light the depressive symptoms were masked. The authors proposed that this psychobiologic disorder was based on the following criteria:
    a. Characteristic premorbid traits.
    b. Specific psychodynamic features.
    c. Family history and other possible psychobiologic markers.

12. Explain the concept of masked depression.

Depressed patients commonly complain of various somatic complaints. Many patients who present with chronic pain syndromes also report a panoply of neurovegatative symptoms, such as sleep and appetite disturbances, decreased libido, fatigue, irritability, withdrawal from and general lack of interest in normal activities, deterioration in relationships, and fixation on somatic sensations. However, these same patients rarely acknowledge true dysphoria, insisting that they are not depressed, or if sadness is acknowledged, it is ascribed directly and solely to pain or some other organic problem. In this respect, the underlying depression is unlikely to be addressed adequately because the patient is resistant to the notion that psychological factors play an etiologic role in the symptoms. Further, focusing on the pain symptoms may protect the patient from more severe depressive symptoms.

13. How has classic learning theory been applied to the field of chronic pain?

Psychologist B.F. Skinner, the father of operant conditioning, identified two classes of responses that can be displayed by an organism: respondents and operants. Respondents are essentially reflexive in nature and are under the control of the antecedent stimulus, like Pavlov's dog being trained to salivate at the sound of the tone preceding the presentation of food. In contrast, operants involve actions potentially subject to voluntary control. Here the magnitude of the response depends on the nature and duration of the antecedent stimulus. In this sense, the behavior is under the control of the environmental consequences (reinforcements) and is, therefore, time-limited. If the behavior (e.g., moaning) is positively reinforced (by attention from others), it will increase in relation to the amount of reinforcement received and the meaning of that consequence (attention) to the person. On the other hand, if the behavior is not reinforced (others ignore the moaning), the behavior will gradually extinguish. This learning theory model has been presented as an alternative to the medical model to explain how individuals evolve into chronic pain patients: their pain-related behaviors are reinforced by those around them.

14. According to learning theory, what are the three principal pathways by which chronic pain syndromes develop?

Operantly acquired pain behaviors are maintained through three basic pathways:
    1. Direct and positive reinforcement of pain behavior.
    2. Indirect but positive reinforcement of pain behavior by avoidance of adverse consequences.
    3. Failure of well behavior to receive positive reinforcement.
These three categories are not mutually exclusive.

15. Give an example of direct and positive reinforcement of pain behaviors.

Continued rest can become a major positive reinforcer of pain behavior. If certain movements result in pain, the person is less likely to perform such behaviors and will instead rest in bed. Initially, this may decrease the level of discomfort (direct positive reinforcement). However, as the overall activity level decreases, so does the pain tolerance. This results in longer and longer rest periods and a downward spiraling in general functioning. Rest, as a pain contingent reinforcer, becomes self-perpetuating.

The use of analgesic medications used on an as needed basis can also foster pain behaviors. In both acute and chronic pain circumstances, patients may feel forced to learn the drill quickly. "If the doctors will not keep me comfortable, I will have to complain and act in pain in order to get relief." In many inpatient programs, the cycle of drug-related pain behaviors is disrupted through detoxification.

16. Can others, aside from health professionals, reinforce pain behaviors?

Monetary rewards play a significant role in the maintenance of pain behaviors in a substantial proportion of chronic pain patients. Another example of how others impact the display of pain behaviors was demonstrated in a study that examined how chronic pain patients, participating in an inpatient pain program, acted in the presence of their spouses in comparison to how they acted in the presence of the staff. The spouses were classified as either solicitous or nonsolicitous, with the former group described as responding to patients' pain behaviors in a manner that would reinforce the display of such behavior. As expected, patients with solicitous spouses displayed pain-related behaviors more frequently in the presence of their spouses than when interacting with neutral staff, who did not reinforce these behaviors. Patients with nonsolicitous spouses did not show an increase in frequency of pain-related behaviors in the presence of their mates.

17. Provide an example of indirect reinforcement (avoidance learning) of pain behaviors.

Much of our everyday behavior results from avoidance learning. We act to minimize or avoid behaviors and/or circumstances that may lead to adverse or punishing consequences. Pain may allow a person to avoid the unpleasant job, the test for which he was unprepared, or the argument with his spouse. Behaviors that are successful in avoiding the undesired circumstances are reinforced. Once established, these behavior patterns are extremely resistant to change. This pattern is offered as a major explanation for why so many injured workers fail to return to work once they are out of work for any prolonged period of time.

18. Comment on the way in which failure to reinforce well behaviors can take place and continue the pain cycle.

There is a clear overlap between the failure to reinforce well behaviors and the direct and indirect reinforcement of pain behaviors. The wife who actively encourages her husband to spend another day in bed resting his back before considering returning to work is both discouraging well behavior (return to work) and directly reinforcing a pain behavior (resting), which may or may not be coupled with the husband's own desire to avoid work. Similarly, the husband who rushes in to assist his wife with physical chores because of her sore hand is discouraging her attempts to resume normal responsibilities. A more appropriate response would be to offer assistance and respond only upon the spouse's cuing that help is needed.

19. What is social learning theory?

Social learning theory is a psychological construct that proposes that behavior is not merely a result of inherited or acquired psychological conditions and environmental forces. Rather, individuals develop in a more complex manner by interacting in a meaningful way with their environment, with both actions and environment impacting each other. New experiences reshape views of the past and vice versa.

20. How does social learning therapy apply to the understanding of chronic pain?

It is accepted that family members and other culturally important figures serve as models for both desirable and undesirable behaviors. Children are particularly open to the effects of modeling adults. Studies of children with recurrent abdominal pain were shown to be over five times as likely to have relatives (parents or siblings) who had similar symptoms in the study period than children who did not report recurrent abdominal pain. Fear of dental procedures has been demonstrated to be transmitted from fearful parents to their young offspring. Adults who scored high on a scale for hypochondriasis, dependency, and use of health services recounted that when they were ill as children, their own parents were very likely to call the doctor. There is a relatively high incidence of relatives with similar or other chronic illness reported by adults with chronic pain syndromes.

21. What is cognitive behavior therapy?

Cognitive behavior therapy is a theoretical approach that acknowledges the importance of both cognitions and behaviors in the acquisition and maintenance of behavioral patterns. Cognitive behavior treatments have been applied to a wide range of psychological disorders, including depression and anxiety, as well as pain.

22. What is implied by a cognitive-behavioral treatment approach to pain management?

A cognitive-behavioral approach focuses on and promotes adaptive changes in the thoughts, feelings, beliefs, and behaviors of pain patients. Emphasis is placed on enlisting the patient as an active participant in the treatment program. This is often a unique experience, since many patients are maintained in a passive role when receiving unidimensional, medically oriented treatments, e.g., surgery and/or medications. Being offered the opportunity to become a collaborator in their treatment helps pain patients attain a greater perception of self-control as well as coping skills that can mitigate suffering. A cognitive-behavioral approach is generally active, structured, and time-limited, in contrast to more psychoanalytically oriented psychotherapy where the patient talks and the therapist listens. The patient is engaged in a dialogue regarding the personal effects of pain, learns concrete coping strategies, and works to establish steps to achieve mutually identified goals. Treatment also calls for the patient to assume personal responsibility in the form of self-monitoring, practicing relaxation and other techniques, and eventually conducting "personal experiments" to challenge and modify maladaptive beliefs, cognitions, and behaviors identified as promoting continued pain behaviors.

23. What are the basic tenets of a cognitive-behavioral perspective?

Five basic statements can be made regarding the underlying structure of a cognitive-behavioral perspective:

1. Individuals are active processors of information and not just passive reactors.
2. Thoughts (e.g., appraisals, expectancies, beliefs) can elicit and influence mood, affect psychological processes, have social consequences, and can also serve as an impetus for behavior; conversely, mood, physiology, environmental factors, and behavior can influence the nature and content of thought processes.
3. Behavior is reciprocally determined by both the individual and environmental factors.
4. Individuals can learn more adaptive ways of thinking, feeling, and behaving.
5. Individuals should be active collaborative agents in changing their maladaptive thoughts, feelings, and behavior.

24. What are the primary objectives of cognitive-behavioral treatment programs as applied to the rehabilitation of patients with chronic pain?

The main emphasis is on functioning, as opposed to simple reduction of pain. Other goals involve reduction in the patient's reliance on analgesic medication, decreased use of the health care system, and eventual resumption of responsibilities, e.g., functioning at home and/or return to employment.

With the above as central objectives for pain management, cognitive-behavioral principles are applied as an integral component of the interdisciplinary treatment approach. Cognitive-behavioral strategies are designed to assist the patient to achieve the following goals:

1. Reduce the patient's sense of suffering and being overwhelmed by pain.
2. Instruct the patient in the acquisition and implementation of effective coping strategies to promote more adaptive adjustment to pain.

3. Promote a fundamental shift in self-perception from a stance of passive helplessness to being proactive toward rehabilitation, fostering a sense of self-efficacy.
4. Assist the patient in recognizing the interplay between psychosocial factors, especially thoughts, feelings, and the experience of pain.
5. Provide instruction for and model the use of cognitive-behavioral techniques to reduce distress.
6. Enhance patient skill level to help anticipate setbacks, and devise plans to reduce their probability and successfully deal with those that occur.
7. Promote an active role in daily activities enhancing the patient's self-confidence and willingness to divest himself of pain-related behaviors.

TREATMENT APPROACHES

25. How effective have psychoanalysis and psychodynamic psychotherapy been in the treatment of individuals with chronic pain syndromes?

While psychodynamic principles have contributed significantly to understanding the psychological problems that can foster pain behaviors, insight-oriented psychotherapy alone has not been shown to be a very effective treatment approach. Because many pain patients are so focused on somatic symptoms and believe them to be evidence of underlying organic disease, there is little motivation to attain insights into the psychological underpinnings of their problem. In those instances where individuals have been motivated and treatment has been successful, it has been time-consuming and costly. For these reasons, intensive traditional psychotherapy tends not to be the treatment of choice for this patient population. When employed in conjunction with cognitive-behavioral or other treatments designed to alter maladaptive behaviors, the addition of insight can promote positive change.

26. Name four principal behavior therapy techniques used in treating chronic pain patients.

1. Graded activation program: Patients are taught to gradually increase their level of physical activity.
2. Social reinforcement: Significant others are enlisted as participants in the treatment program and alter their responses to the patient's behaviors to discourage the display of pain-related behaviors and reward the display of well behaviors.
3. Time-contingent use of medications: Analgesic medications are provided on the basis of time rather than the report of pain or display of pain behaviors.
4. Self-control techniques: The patient is taught self-regulatory skills to diminish the experience of pain and focus on well behaviors.

27. When should a graded activation program be started?

Diaries are helpful and can be tailored to specific needs. Information includes "up time" (time spent in active endeavors where the patient is resting, sitting, sleeping, etc.); pain intensity rating; use of medication; socialization (time spent alone or with others); as well as mood, thoughts, feelings, or self-cognitions. Diaries are best used when they are maintained for at least seven consecutive days and are reviewed with the clinician while still current.

28. What are some of the potential benefits derived from the use of a diary?

Diaries have been shown to be a reasonable reflection of the patient's experience of pain, helping the clinician gauge perceived pain intensity. Pain normally fluctuates over time, and patterns can be surmised and influential factors identified. Medications and their effectiveness can be readily assessed. Diaries can assess the efficacy of the specific interventions. Monitoring their behavior increases patients' awareness of factors influencing their pain. Since the maintenance of a diary requires some effort and must be completed by the patient, it serves as an excellent means of assessing patients' cognitive organization. It also addresses their level of motivation to engage themselves actively in rehabilitative efforts.

29. Describe how the concept of time-contingent use of medications is generally employed.

The primary objective of this strategy is to break the association between the display of pain behavior and the reduction of pain by analgesic medication. By providing medications on a fixed schedule, the pain behaviors are no longer reinforced, but appropriate relief can be provided. Time-contingent dosing can also be used to eliminate analgesic medication in an inpatient program.

First, a diary is employed to assess the baseline consumption of medication. Second, the total intake is divided into even doses and then provided at set intervals in the form of a "pain cocktail." The medication is combined with a liquid, e.g., orange juice, to mask the exact amount of drug provided. Over time, the amount of medication is reduced to zero, but the pain cocktail still provided. Data have shown that patients receiving medication on a time-contingent basis reported less pain both during and after detoxification compared to those receiving medication on an as needed basis.

30. What are some of the formalized relaxation techniques?

Relaxation techniques can be grouped according to the basic approach employed. The specifics of each technique can be altered to suit the needs of the individual and are not mutually exclusive, that is, elements of one technique can be combined with other techniques.

Breathing relaxation: Adapts principles and exercises of classic yoga. Breathing is usually an automatic function, without conscious control. When conscious attention is focused on breathing, attention is removed from areas of tension. The focus is on the promotion of altered breathing, primarily abdominal or diaphragmatic breathing. This approach is extremely flexible and adaptive and often serves as the base technique to be learned.

Progressive relaxation: Created to assist individuals in becoming more aware of muscle tension and relaxation through a process of tensing, then relaxing specific muscle groups in sequence. The structured procedure requires about 20 minutes to complete.

Autogenic relaxation: Uses a series of self-statements to promote a state of inner calm and muscle relaxation. For example, "My mind is quiet," "My arms and legs feel quiet, heavy, comfortable and relaxed," etc. These self-statements are generally pleasant and soothing, making this approach quite popular.

Guided imagery: This approach encourages the use of imagination to create pleasant scenes and experiences to promote a sense of well-being. Popular themes are the creation of a private place where the individual can go to contemplate, reflect on issues, and experience a decrease in pain. Taking an imaginary trip to the beach is commonly employed. The more sensory modalities engaged, the more profound the effect.

Meditation: Borrowed from Eastern teachings, the process of meditation is founded in the principle of uncritically focusing on one thing at a time. This may be a word, such as a mantra or a short phase, meaningful to the meditator. Staring at a flame, flower, or other object can also act as an anchor. It is important to note that the act of meditation is not simply focusing on one object to the exclusion of everything else. The mind is always drifting, and the meditator accepts this and strives toward maintaining an inner harmonious focus.

31. What is the role of self-help groups for treating chronic pain patients?

Self-help organizations have grown in popularity and organizations exist locally and nationally for a wide variety of medical conditions, including chronic pain. Participation can be beneficial for pain sufferers. First and foremost, it provides a sense that "I am not alone." This is significant since many patients with chronic pain report that their suffering is unseen by others and may be questioned, and they experience a profound sense of isolation. Discovering that others have the same condition, have comparable experiences with the health care system, and harbor similar emotions can provide a sense of relief and belonging. Some of the groups are oriented toward teaching one another a variety of self-management techniques and reinforcing their use.

32. Are there potential drawbacks to patients participating in self-help pain organizations?

On the whole, the experience is positive. However, the quality of any local group is determined more by the individual leaders and members than by the sponsoring organization. This is true for all self-help groups. Group leaders are almost exclusively chronic pain sufferers themselves. While this level of responsibility may assist some in their rehabilitation, a few may unconsciously seek to cloak themselves in pseudoprofessional, caretaker roles as a means of diverting their energies from their own recovery. Others may use such organizations as an alternative to the traditional health care system and to chastise it for failing to help them. Patients should be encouraged to inquire about self-help organizations and use them as an adjunct to mainstream interventions.

33. Is group therapy also applicable to treating chronic pain patients?

Group therapy has been applied successfully in treating patients with chronic pain. Cognitive-behavioral techniques often comprise the mainstay of skills training. Groups tend to be psychoeducationally oriented, teaching patients about pain, the use of medication, self-management techniques, and providing instructions for relaxation procedures, appropriate exercise, and methods to enhance self-esteem. Follow-up data indicate that patients frequently report a decrease in depressive symptoms and a reduction in pain, and they use fewer drugs. They were also more active.

34. Should all chronic pain patients receive marital or family therapies as an adjunct to medical and physical interventions?

Marital and/or family therapies, like all interventions, do not work for everyone. Couples therapy employed with headache sufferers revealed that those couples who completed therapy did benefit from treatment as opposed to those who dropped out, as assessed by the applied outcome measures. Of note is that dropout couples reported marital discord of greater severity and duration than the completers. Therefore, recommendations for marital therapy should be made on a selective basis.

35. What information about self-help is available to patients?

There are two national self-help organizations for patients with chronic benign pain syndromes. The primary focus of these groups is to provide patients and concerned family members with relevant information related to chronic pain conditions. The American Chronic Pain Association is specifically geared to the lay public and self-help. A fundamental premise is that further medical interventions are not likely to provide additional relief. Therefore, it is incumbent upon the individual to learn new ways of dealing with his pain in order to lead to productive life. Guidelines are provided for conducting self-help groups. The National Chronic Pain Outreach Association presents itself as a clearing house for both patients and professionals. It publishes a quarterly magazine about new treatments, maintains a listing of self-help groups and pain specialists, and offers self-help kits for those who want to initiate a self-help group of their own.

American Chronic Pain Association
P.O. Box 850
Rocklin, California 95677
(916) 632-0922

National Chronic Pain Outreach Association
7979 Old Georgetown Road, Suite 100
Bethesda, Maryland 20814-2429
(301) 652-4948

There are additional self-help organizations for headache sufferers. The American Council for Headache Education (ACHE) is directly affiliated with the professional organization, the American Association for the Study of Headache (AASH). The National Headache Foundation is an independent charitable organization that provides patient-related information. There are also self-help groups around the country for specific pain syndromes. Local directories can provide information about self-help clearing houses where information about support groups of all sorts can be obtained.

ACHE
875 King's Highway, Suite 200
West Deptford, NJ 08096

National Headache Foundation
52525 North Western Avenue
Chicago, IL 60625

36. Are there professional organizations for which information about pain syndromes as well as services can be obtained?

In the United States, there are two organizations that deal specifically with pain syndrome: (1) the American Pain Society (APS), which is the national affiliate of the International Association for the Study of Pain (IASP). These organizations are interdisciplinary and academically oriented. The APS holds annual scientific meetings to keep professionals abreast of both clinical and research advances. (2) The American Academy of Pain Management is a smaller organization with a medical orientation. It, too, holds annual meetings to inform and instruct clinicians in the application of pain management techniques.

American Pain Society
4700 W. Lake Avenue
Blenview, IL 60025-1485
(708) 375-4715

37. What other organizations are available to both professionals and the lay public to obtain information about the quality of services provided?

The Commission for Accreditation of Rehabilitation Facilities (CARF) is an independent organization that accredits various rehabilitation facilities, e.g., those for spinal cord injury, head trauma, and general rehabilitation, and pain centers. CARF emphasizes a multidisciplinary, rehabilitation orientation, where patients play an active role in their rehabilitation. Stringent criteria are applied to those facilities applying for accreditation. Those facilities that have achieved CARF accreditation have demonstrated themselves to be centers of excellence.

Commission for Accreditation of Rehabilitation Facilities
101 North Wilmont Road, Suite 500
Tucson, AZ 85711
(602) 748-1212

BIBLIOGRAPHY

1. Arnoff GM, Rutrick D: Psychodynamics and psychotherapy of the chronic pain syndrome. In Arnoff GM (ed): Evaluation and Treatment of Chronic Pain, 2nd ed. Baltimore, Williams & Wilkins, 1992.
2. Arnoff GM: Psychological aspects of nonmalignant chronic pain: A new nosology. 1992.
3. Bandura A: Behavior therapy and the models of man. Am Psychol 29:859–869, 1974.
4. Block AR, Kremer EF, Gaylor M: Behavioral treatment of chronic pain: The spouse as a discriminative cue for pain behavior. Pain 9:243–252, 1980.
5. Bouckoms A, Hackett TP: The pain patient: Evaluation and treatment. In Cassem NH (ed): Massachusetts General Hospital Handbook of General Hospital Psychiatry, 3rd ed. St. Louis, Mosby, 1991.
6. Craig KD: Special modeling influences: Pain in context. In Sternbach RA (ed): The Psychology of Pain, 2nd ed. New York, Raven Press, 1986.
7. Davis M, Eshelman ER, McKay M: The Relaxation and Stress Reduction Workbook, 4th ed. New Harbinger Publications, 1995.
8. Fordyce WE: Behavioral Methods for Chronic Pain and Illness. St. Louis, Mosby, 1976.
9. Mersky H: Psychiatry and pain. In Sternbach RA (ed): The Psychology of Pain, 2nd ed. New York, Raven Press, 1986, pp 97–120.
10. Rosen G, Kvale A, Husebo S: Group therapy of patients with chronic pain. Tidskr-Nor-laegeforen 110:3602–3604, 1990.
11. Roy R: Couple therapy and chronic headaches: A preliminary outcome study. Headache 29(7):455–457, 1989.
12. Sanders SH: Component analysis of a behavioral treatment program for chronic low back pain. Behav Ther 14:697–705, 1983.
13. Sholevar GP, Perkel R: Family systems intervention and physical illness. Gen Hosp Psychiatry 12(6):363–372, 1990.
14. Szasz TS: Pain and Pleasure: A Study of Body Feelings. New York, Basic Books, 1968.

40. PHYSIATRIC MODALITIES IN PAIN MANAGEMENT

Mark A. Thomas, M.D., and Brian Kahan, D.O.

1. What are the electrotherapy modalities used in the treatment of pain?

Transcutaneous electrical nerve stimulation (TENS), percutaneous electrical nerve stimulation, interferential current therapy, high-voltage/high-volt galvanic stimulation (HVS), low-voltage stimulation, pulsed electromagnetic therapy, and cranial electric stimulation have all been reported as useful in treating pain from a variety of causes. The choice of modality should be based on chronicity of symptoms, pathology, goal of treatment, and patient's tolerance. Of the modalities noted, the most widely applied (and practical) are TENS in its various forms and HVS.

2. What is the presumed mechanism of action for transcutaneous electrical nerve stimulation (TENS) in the treatment of pain?

TENS is thought to act by preferential stimulation of peripheral somatosensory fibers, which conduct more rapidly than nociceptive fibers. This results in a stimulation of inhibitory interneurons in the second lamina of the posterior horn (substantia gelatinosa) that effectively blocks nociception at the spinal cord level. This is the gate theory as proposed by Melzack and Wall (1965). (See Chapter 00.) TENS will provide placebo analgesia in about 10 to 25% of patients treated. It has also been suggested that TENS may stimulate the central endogenous pain control systems, although this has not been verified.

3. What are the indications for the application of TENS in the treatment of pain?

TENS has been used in virtually all types of both acute and chronic pain. Reported success rates vary significantly in published series, with a bottom end of about 10 to 30% effectiveness, depending on the population studied.

There is good evidence that over 50% of patients respond positively to TENS applications for the following diagnoses: myofascial facial pain, pain due to peripheral neuropathy, menstrual or uterine pain, ischemic pain (including angina), and pain due to degenerative joint disease. Responses may be temporary.

4. How is TENS applied, and what are the best parameters to provide analgesia?

TENS may be applied over a peripheral nerve, in a dermatomal distribution, or to a contralateral or residual extremity. In general, electrodes are placed caudal or cephalad to the painful site rather than alongside it. Frequency and amplitude can be varied to achieve maximum efficacy.

In studies investigating the analgesic effect of TENS, patient response was better for lower treatment frequencies (4 Hz for ischemic pain; 2 Hz for chronic low back pain).

5. What are the contraindications to the use of TENS?

Contraindications include a pacemaker or other implanted electronic device, metal prosthesis, or implant at the site of application. About 1.5% of patients will have cutaneous reaction to the gel or electrodes. Diagnoses for which TENS has not been found to be more effective than placebo include anorectal pain, pain due to central or autonomic nervous system pathology, or pain from psychiatric illness or psychosocial distress.

6. What are the indications and contraindications for the use of high-volt stimulation (HVS) in the treatment of pain?

HVS is used for analgesia and for relaxation of muscle spasm. It is helpful for treating pain due to musculoskeletal pathology. This type of electrotherapy has not been as well studied as

TENS, although a similar mechanism of action is thought to be involved. Contraindications include a pacemaker or other implanted device, such as a metal prosthesis or hardware.

7. How does HVS work in the treatment of painful conditions?

Direct muscle stimulation results in tetanic contraction; when this cannot be sustained, the muscle relaxes because of fatigue. This reduces nociceptive input and local edema and improves local circulation. Activation of central pain modulation and a strong placebo response cannot be discounted.

8. What are the side effects that may result from the use of HVS?

Muscle aching or soreness may result from sustained contractions and fatigue. The stimulus may be painful and poorly tolerated.

9. What is actinotherapy?

Actinotherapy is a therapeutic use of projected light sources.

10. Which therapeutic light modalities are used in treating the patient with pain?

For primary analgesia, recent literature suggests that low-energy laser therapy may be beneficial. In specific instances, ultraviolet or infrared light may be useful for reducing pain by the treatment of pain-producing pathology.

11. How does laser treatment work, and how is it applied?

Low-energy laser is applied directly to the painful area or to related trigger points or acupuncture points. Although some efficacy has been demonstrated in sizable patient series, the mechanism is unclear. Low-energy laser has been shown to postpone posttraumatic neural degeneration and to produce analgesia.

12. What are the benefits of therapeutic heat?

1. Increase extensibility of collagen tissues.
2. Decrease joint stiffness.
3. Relieve pain.
4. Release muscle spasms.
5. Resolve inflammatory infiltrates, edema, and exudates.
6. Increase blood flow.

13. What factors are instrumental in deciding which heat modality to apply?

1. Size of area to be treated.
2. Amount of penetration needed.
3. Degree of safety for the specific disease or injury.
4. Ease of application.
5. Availability of source.
6. Individual preference.

14. What are the contraindications to heat therapy?

1. Anesthetized area.
2. Obtunded patient.
3. Vascular disease.
4. Hemorrhagic diathesis.
5. Malignancies.
6. Acute trauma.

15. What are the indications for superficial heat modalities?

Since these modalities have their greatest effect at the skin surface, they are generally indicated for patients who have mild musculoskeletal complaints.

16. Describe the temperature distribution, application, and indications for superficial modalities.

Modality	Temperature Distribution	Application	Indication(s)
Hydrocollator	Skin surface, conduction	Wrap in six layers of cloth before applying, 165–170° F 20 to 30 minutes	Arthritis, bursitis, contusions, edema, local infections, spasms, synovitis, sprains, strains
Paraffin	Skin surface, conduction	Dip method or immersion method 125–130° 20 to 30 minutes	Conditions of hands and feet, scleroderma, arthritis, bursitis, joint stiffness, contractures, scar tissue, Sudeck's atrophy, tenosynovitis
Fluidotherapy	Skin surface, convection	Immersion of extremity into machine for 20 to 30 minutes with active ROM 102–118°F	Same as paraffin, sickle cell, desensitization, RA
Hydrotherapy	Skin surface, convection	Immersion less than 105° F	Arthritides of multiple joints, stiffness, wound care, debridement
Radiant	Subcutaneous, convection	Near infrared (700–1400 mu) Far infrared (1400–40,000 mu) 18 inches away from skin	Large areas, muscle spasms, myofibritis, same as paraffin
Cold	Subcutaneous	Direct	Acute sprains, strains, inflammation except RA, spasticity, analgesia

17. Describe the temperature distribution, application, indications, and contraindications for the use of deep heating modalities.

Modality	Temperature Distribution	Application	Indications	Contraindications
Short-wave diathermy	2 to 3 cm below skin surface, muscle	10 to 100 megacycles	Heating of superficial muscles, PID, PVD proximal to occlusion	Metal implants, IUDs, pacemakers, pregnancy, viscous areas
Microwave	Penetrates into muscles and tissues	900 to 2456 megacycles	Heating of deep musculature	Same as short wave, brain, bony prominences
Ultrasound	Absorption depends on tissue protein content with bone having greatest absorption; increased absorption at junctions of heterogeneous tissues	0.8–2.5 W/cm², stroking. underwater, pulsed, and multiple field methods	Neuromuscular disease, musculoskeletal diseases, hyperemia, contractures, RSD, neuromas	Viscous areas, pregnant uterus, metal implants with cement, recent fractures, cancer patients

18. What types of therapeutic exercises are used in the treatment of pain?
1. Range of motion.
2. Stretching.
3. Strengthening.
4. Endurance techniques.

19. What are the psychological effects of exercise?
Exercise and physical activity have been shown to improve mood, quality of life, and intellectual function. Folkins and Sime suggest that the mental health benefits of exercise include:

(1) increased perception of control and mastery throughout improvement in fitness; (2) improved self-monitoring ability in a biofeedback paradigm; (3) achievement of a meditative state that relates to improved mental health; and to (4) distraction from anxiety.

It is believed that this positive impact on mental health is due to increased catecholamine circulation, increased endorphin level, increased distraction away from symptom sequences, and increased body temperature, which contributes to decreased muscle tension, elevated mood, decreased anxiety, and improved sleep patterns.

20. What are the benefits of range of motion (ROM)?

ROM has been shown to be highly effective in patients with pain. It acts not only to maintain functional ability and to prevent contractures but also to desensitize the patient, prevent edema, and prevent spasms.

21. What types of range of motion should be used?

ROM can be applied either actively (AROM), active-assisted (AAROM), or passively (PROM). PROM implies that all the effort comes from the therapist and none from the patient. AROM implies that all the motion is provided by the patient. AAROM is a combination of both, where the patient actively moves the joint through its range and then a therapist applies a static force to provide a stretch.

22. List the indications and contraindications of the three types of range of motion.

Type	Indications	Contraindications
PROM	Performed when a patient can't move a joint actively or a patient is anxious about moving the joint and there are no contraindications to motion of the joint	Unstable joints, insensate areas, connective tissue disease, acute flare of RA
AAROM	Spasms, re-education of the efferent side, utilization of the afferent side of a motor pattern, contractures	Insensate joint, infection, acute attack of RA
AROM	Improve strength, flexibility, endurance, patient confidence	Ligamentous damage, insensate joint, fractures, acute attack of RA

23. What is the rationale for stretching a painful area?

Stretching attempts to improve the elastic component of the muscle, thus returning it to its normal resting length. This can be done directly by a static stretch causing the muscle to lengthen, or indirectly by adding an isometric contraction with the stretch to activate the Golgi tendon organs that cause reciprocal inhibition and relaxation of the muscles.

24. How can stretching be applied?

1. Lateral—the force is applied at a right angle to the long axis.
2. Longitudinal—the force is applied in the direction of the long axis.
3. Traction—separation of the origin and insertion.

25. What are the different strengthening methods used?

1. Isometric
2. Isotonic
3. Isokinetic

26. How do these methods differ?

Isometric exercise is performed by exerting against an immovable object or by holding an object in a static position. This exercise helps to prevent muscle atrophy during the acute pain phase or when other exercises are contraindicated.

Isotonic exercise involves movement of a constant weight or load through a specified range of motion. This exercise can build strength and endurance.

Isokinetic exercise involves movement performed at a constant rate with a variable force throughout a specified range of motion. The advantage of this exercise is that it stresses the muscle being used throughout the entire range.

27. How does endurance training help the pain patient?

Endurance training concentrates on improving the patient's cardiovascular status through aerobic exercises. Aerobic exercise provides the physiologic benefits discussed earlier. Furthermore, general conditioning has been shown to lessen the impact of chronic back pain.

28. List some of the types of traction available and their advantages.
1. Sustained traction—more effective in separating joint surfaces.
2. Intermittent mechanical traction—more effective in mobilizing joint surfaces.
3. Manual traction—better tolerated by patients.

29. List some of the indications for spinal traction.
1. Nerve root impingement secondary to osteophyte encroachment.
2. Herniated nucleus pulposus with disc protrusion.
3. Compression fractures after the subacute phase.
4. Degenerative joint disease.
5. Grade I spondylolisthesis.
6. Hypomobile joints.
7. Muscle spasms.
8. Joint pain.

These are the most common clinical situations in which traction is used. However, there are few well-controlled studies to demonstrate the efficacy of traction in back pain.

30. List the contraindications to traction.

All traction is contraindicated when there is structural disease secondary to infection, malignancy, gross instability, or severe osteoporosis. Cervical traction is contraindicated in patients with rheumatoid arthritis and vertebral-basilar insufficiency.

31. How is cervical traction applied?

Cervical traction can be applied manually or mechanically. Manual traction is applied by a therapist's hand. The advantages are that the load and angle of pull can vary and the patient may be able to relax more efficiently. The disadvantages are that the technique is subjective, since the load applied cannot be quantified. This technique is tiring. Mechanical traction can be applied through various types of devices. The angle of pull should be varied, depending on the area where the desired effect is needed. With the cervical spine in neutral, the greatest effect is at the occipito-atlantal joint. The addition of 5° of flexion will allow one to progress distally down the cervical spine to a maximum of 35°, which affects C7–T1.

Duration of traction should be increased gradually, in increments of 3 minutes, to a maximum of 20. The maximum force that can be applied is 25–30 pounds. This will vary, depending on the size of the patient.

32. Describe the technique for applying lumbar traction.

As with cervical traction, lumbar traction can be applied manually or mechanically. Manual traction may include the aid of a therapist or may be assisted by gravity. Mechanical traction uses a friction-free couch with pelvic and thoracic harnesses. It is useful in (1) scoliosis secondary to unilateral muscle spasm; (2) unilateral facet joint hypomobility; and (3) protective lumbar scoliosis. Treatment time should not exceed 20 minutes. Prolonged lumbar traction may increase semispinalis activity and spasm. The tractal force is usually 50% of the patient's body weight.

33. How is manipulative therapy thought to relieve pain?

Clinical studies on manipulation have been hard to control, and as a result, practitioners have had difficulty accepting it as an effective mode of treatment. Controlled studies by various clinicians have suggested that manipulation relieves pain by (1) changing the patient's pain threshold; (2) changes in posterior joint function; (3) reduction of disc protrusion; (4) increased range of motion; and (5) improved circulation.

34. List the contraindications for manipulative therapy.

1. Severe degenerative joint disease.
2. Vertebral basilar insufficiency.
3. Down's syndrome
4. Spina bifida.
5. Osteoporosis
6. Dwarfism

35. How is massage therapy thought to relieve pain?

1. Prevents formation of adhesions.
2. Decreases blood pressure.
3. Increases lymphatic flow.
4. Increases blood flow.
5. Provides relaxation.
6. Loosens scar tissue.

It should also be kept in mind that any hands-on technique tends to reinforce a patient's confidence.

36. Name three different techniques of massage.

1. Ischemic compression (acupressure).
2. Deep friction massage.
3. Rolfing.

37. Describe how deep friction massage is thought to benefit a patient.

Cyriax was the first to describe deep friction massage. His method delivers deep massage transversely across tissue fibers over a very small area. The purpose is to relieve pain, free adhesions, break up scar tissue, and restore mobility. It is believed to relieve pain by causing traumatic hyperemia, stimulating mechanoreceptors, and increasing tissue perfusion.

38. What is a trigger point?

According to Travell, a trigger point is a focus of hyperirritability in a tissue that, when compressed, is locally tender and, if sufficiently hypersensitive, gives rise to referred pain and tenderness either distally or proximally to the site of origin.

39. Describe the concept behind ischemic compression (acupressure).

Ischemic compression was made popular by Travell and Simons for the treatment of trigger and tender points. The technique involves sustained pressure over the painful area for a period of about 90 seconds. It is believed that the ischemic pressure causes a reactive traumatic hyperemia that inactivates the trigger or tender point.

40. Describe the concept of myofascial release.

Myofascial release is based on soft-tissue mobilization. Its premise is that fascial immobility causes dysfunction throughout the musculoskeletal system. Normally fascia is very mobile, but reorganization occurs in response to immobilization, injury, and scarring.

When using this technique, the practitioner applies gentle pressure or stretch until a point of resistance is obtained. The stretch is then maintained until a release is felt, usually manifested by increased range of motion at the particular site.

41. Describe the concept of muscle-energy techniques for myofascial pain.

Muscle energy is a manual technique that involves the voluntary contraction of a patient's muscle in a precisely controlled direction, at varying levels of intensity, against a distinctly executed counterforce applied by the operator. It can be used to lengthen a shortened, contracted, or spastic muscle. It may also reduce localized edema and mobilize an articulation with restricted mobility.

42. What is the concept of muscle energy, and how is it applied?

Muscle energy techniques take advantage of the relaxation that follows a prolonged muscle contraction.

The direct muscle-energy technique requires that the patient's affected area be stretched until a pathologic barrier is felt. Muscle contraction is used with the direction of force toward the restriction. This force is held for 5 to 7 seconds; then the patient is instructed to relax while the examiner maintains the patient's current position. The examiner then repositions the affected area until the pathologic barrier is felt, and the process is repeated.

The indirect muscle-energy technique is similar to the direct technique with regard to setup, but the direction of force applied is opposite to the pathologic barrier.

Each technique is usually repeated three times or until there is improvement in the pathologic barrier. The amount of force applied should not cause the patient to strain. At the end of treatment, the affected area is moved passively to its neutral position.

43. What functional signs should be elicited in patients complaining of pain?

In examining the patient in pain, some of the most useful information is found through observation. In general, try to observe the patient when he or she is not aware of your presence. Concentrate on how he or she walks, gets out of a chair, gets on to the examining table, and takes off garments. These observations can point out areas of pain and restricted range of motion.

One should also examine how the patient gets dressed and leaves your office. Patients tend to be more relaxed after the doctor's visit is over. Observation at this time might detect subtle findings that weren't present during the initial evaluation because the patient was more guarded.

44. What are the fundamentals of the spinal exam?

The spine consists of cervical, thoracic, lumbar, and sacral areas. Each area should be examined individually and collectively. The spinal column should be examined in at least two situations:

1. A dynamic situation, where the spinal column is being loaded (i.e., standing, sitting, or forward bending).

2. A static situation, where the spine is unloaded (i.e., supine, prone, or lateral recumbent).

The examiner should look at the spine from the anterior, posterior, and lateral aspect. One should check that normal curvature (cervical lordosis, thoracic kyphosis, lumbar lordosis) is maintained and note any asymmetry or unleveling (e.g., shoulder or sacral). From the lateral aspect, one should note whether there is any *increased* kyphosis or lordosis. This can be done by either hanging a plumb line from the office ceiling or drawing an imaginary line posterior to the external auditory meatus to the lateral malleolus. The line should bisect the humeral head and greater trochanter and travel slightly posterior to the knee to the lateral malleolus.

45. Describe examination of the extremities.

Examination of the extremities should consist of having the patient perform active range of motion, followed by the examiner's performing passive range of motion for each joint to be tested. Limits of range and areas throughout the range that cause pain should be recorded.

46. How do braces and splints work?

Orthotics (braces) and splints act to support or re-orient moving body parts, generally joints or tendons. They may be useful in treating painful conditions that result from pathologic movement, weight bearing, or muscular overuse. The mnemonic is **CALF**: correct/control; align; limit; facilitate:

- Correct alignment or direction of movement.
- Control/guide direction, amplitude, and rate of movement.
- Align body segments into a more stable or less painful configuration.
- Limit/stop motion at pre-set point.
- Facilitate a specific motion.

47. What are the indications for using a brace to treat pain?

Braces are used when movement produces pain. The most common painful conditions in which bracing is useful to alleviate or reduce pain include spondylo- or retrolisthesis, low back pain, degenerative joint disease, tendinitis or epicondylitis, ligament sprain (all joints), muscle tear, and fracture.

BIBLIOGRAPHY

1. Bradsford J: Physical Agents. In DeLisa JA, Gans BM (eds): Rehabilitation Medicine: Principles and Practice, 2nd ed. Philadelphia, JB Lippincott, 1993.
2. Geiringer S: Traction manipulation and massage. In DeLisa JA, Gans BM (eds): Rehabilitation Medicine: Principles and Practice, 2nd ed. Philadelphia, JB Lippincott, 1993.
3. Duncombe A: Modalities of physical treatment. Phys Med Rehabil StateArt Rev 5(3):493–521, 1991.
4. Jhee WH: Exercise and rest. Phys Med Rehabil State Art Rev 5(3):527–537, 1991.
5. DeLateur B: Strength and local muscle endurance. Phys Med Rehabil Clin North Am 5(2):269–295, 1994.

IX. Organizational Issues

41. PAIN CLINICS

Nelson Hendler, M.D., M.S.

1. What is a multidisciplinary pain treatment center?

A multidisciplinary pain treatment center is made up of various medical disciplines as well as ancillary personnel to assist with the diagnosis and management of patients with chronic and persistent pain. Centers can be organized in either an outpatient or inpatient setting; they may be free-standing or hospital-based. They are usually characterized as **multidisciplinary chronic pain treatment centers** (those using numerous clinicians and a broad spectrum of modalities to treat any number of syndromes), **monomodality centers** (using only a single type of treatment, such as nerve blocks, biofeedback, or hypnosis, etc.), and **syndrome-specific clinics** (treating only one disorder). In a truly multidisciplinary center, both the diagnostic component and the treatment component should be multidisciplinary.

2. How should a multidisciplinary pain treatment center be organized?

The central element of organizing a multidisciplinary chronic pain treatment center is to establish a common philosophy among the various physicians and other health care personnel involved. These philosophical concerns deal with (a) the use of certain pharmacologic agents, (b) the interpretation of various diagnostic studies, (c) attitudes toward the role of psychiatry, physical therapy, and adjunctive treatments, and (d) the goal of the chronic pain treatment center—i.e., rehabilitation, reduction of pain, and restoration of function.

3. What are the essential elements of a multidisciplinary pain treatment center?

A well-run multidisciplinary pain treatment center requires that a single health care provider function as the leader of the team. This person should assume responsibility for coordinating all of the medical efforts, laboratory studies, ancillary therapies, and medications and should be available during all hours that the pain treatment center is open to provide continuity of care. Members of the team may be from any and all disciplines. The most common cadre is an admixture of anesthesiologists, neurologists, psychiatrists, psychologists, physiatrists, neurosurgeons, orthopedic surgeons, and nurses. In centers treating orofacial pain, dentists are indispensable. Social workers and non-medical personnel round out the team. The exact composition of the team is less important than the philosophy of working as a team toward the functional rehabilitation of patients in pain. Essentially any health care provider with expertise in pain management can be the team leader for a specific patient, though it is usually more practical for the leader to be a physician.

4. What is the role of a psychiatrist in a multidisciplinary chronic pain treatment center?

The psychiatrist should have a good working knowledge of psychopharmacology and assume the responsibilities for regulating medications, ranging from the use of antidepressants to the employment of opioid and sedative/hypnotic drugs, if needed. He or she should be knowledgeable about drug interactions or withdrawal from opioids and benzodiazepines, as well as appropriate alternatives for these medications. The psychiatrist should either run or supervise group psychotherapy sessions and biofeedback, as well as family counselling sessions.

5. What is the role of an anesthesiologist in a multidisciplinary pain treatment center?

An anesthesiologist can be an invaluable member of the multidisciplinary team. As noted in the chapters on temporary blockade, permanent blockade, sympathetic blockade, or spinal anesthesia, they have the capability of providing both diagnostic and therapeutic blocks. They may also provide greater insight into drug interactions and novel means of drug delivery. Additionally, an anesthesiologist working in conjunction with the neurosurgeon and the orthopedic surgeon of the team can provide a continuity of care, ranging from diagnostics through the anesthesia needed for surgery.

6. What is the role of the neurosurgeon?

The neurosurgeon can provide diagnostic and surgical skills not available from other specialties. As described in the chapter on neurosurgical techniques, they can provide both stimulatory and ablative procedures for pain relief.

7. What is the role of the psychologist?

The psychologist can provide skills usually not offered by a psychiatrist in the area of administration and interpretation of psychological testing and neuropsychological testing, and assessment of cognitive functioning. Working alone or in conjunction with the psychiatrist, they provide group therapy, supportive psychotherapy, family counseling, and individual counseling. Additionally, the psychologist can coordinate the activities of the social workers and help to deal with the multiple social issues usually associated with chronic pain. Many psychologists have special training in cognitive/behavioral techniques and biofeedback. These modalities are described in greater detail in the chapter on psychological therapies.

8. What is the role of a physiatrist?

A physiatrist can provide valuable input in the area of rehabilitation, both occupational and vocational. He or she may supervise the occupational therapist and vocational rehabilitation specialist. The physiatrist can manage the physical therapist and select appropriate physical testing and rehabilitation efforts, such as muscle strengthening and muscle retraining. A physiatrist is also of great assistance in postoperative care and rehabilitation. Specific physiatric interventions are covered in the corresponding chapter by Thomas.

9. Who should lead a multidisciplinary pain treatment center?

The answer to this is rather complex. The experience of many chronic pain treatment centers indicates that care is facilitated by a physician leading a multidisciplinary chronic pain treatment center. A physician can prescribe and regulate medications, coordinate medical testing, and serve as a medical coordinator among the various consultants. This role would be very difficult for a Ph.D. who may be knowledgeable in these areas, but unfortunately would not have the legal ability to prescribe medications and medical diagnostic studies. However, if the Ph.D. or other provider works in conjunction with a licensed physician, this problem can be minimized. The type of physician again becomes an interesting issue. The personal characteristics of the physician as well as the medical knowledge are of paramount importance; the specialty training becomes a secondary issue. The physician in charge should be able to work well with the other members of the team and should be empathetic in understanding patients with chronic pain. Therefore, a compassionate neurologist, a psychiatrist with a knowledge of medicine, or a neurosurgeon or orthopedic surgeon who is willing to make time to take a careful history and listen to patients, would be ideal selections. Therefore, the characteristics would include

Organizational skills
People skills
Knowledge of pharmacology and psychopharmacology
Knowledge of medical testing
Knowledge of surgical procedures

Willingness to provide continuity of care on a daily basis

Knowledge of insurance issues and sociologic issues

Willingness to provide administrative details, such as report writing, testimony, etc.

10. Which is better: an inpatient or an outpatient chronic pain treatment center?

This question actually begs other questions rather than providing answers. Both settings have advantages and disadvantages. An outpatient chronic pain treatment center reduces costs for the insurance carrier and for the patient and probably is appropriate for the vast majority of chronic pain patients. Most chronic pain patients do not need residential treatment unless they are severely depressed or unable to manage their medications. The inpatient setting may facilitate drug withdrawal and provide testing and consultations that are not readily available in the patient's home area. In the last case, a hospital-based inpatient chronic pain treatment center or a free-standing residential unit may be ideal.

11. After entering a pain treatment program, how rapidly must opioid analgesics be discontinued?

The question has been a subject of debate in recent years. In the 1960s and 70s, the "common wisdom" was to withdraw all chronic pain patients who did not have cancer from all opioid drugs. However, many patients with pain of non-cancer origin can be maintained on stable doses. Addiction is rare in patients treated appropriately. On the other hand, increased regulatory activity on the part of the Drug Enforcement Agency forces a physician to document the need for opioids and the rationale for the prescription. While opioids are not devoid of side effects, they may be less disturbing than the side effects found with other drugs used in treating chronic pain. As with any drugs, the balance between benefits and side effects must be weighted for each patient. Therefore, drug withdrawal is not always indicated.

12. What psychological tests should be done on admission to a pain treatment center?

At a minimum, assessment of the patient's psychological state should include:

An inventory to determine the severity of the depression.

Suicide Risk Test to determine the potential for suicide, which, interestingly, does not always correspond with the severity of the depression.

The SCL 90 to assess the patient's psychological states, which vary from week to week.

A Personality Inventory to determine the patient's personality traits; this is different than the patient's psychological state, which is measured by the SCL 90. However, it must be strongly emphasized that the Millon and the Minnesota Multiphasic Personality Inventory (MMPI) cannot be used to assess the validity of the complaint of pain.

The Mensana Clinic Back Pain Test. While not used at all centers, has been shown to correlate with the presence or absence of demonstrable organic pathology.

13. How do you spot a malingerer within a chronic pain treatment center?

True malingering is unusual. It represents the conscious effort to deceive, not a psychiatric illness. One of the hallmarks of a malingerer is the refusal to participate in diagnostic studies. Obviously, if the patient is malingering, he or she may be concerned that studies will reveal the absence of organic pathology. Most chronic pain patients emphatically state that they will do anything to get rid of their pain. A patient who is unwilling to participate in testing or treatment becomes suspect. The major exception to this rule is a patient who strongly objects to surgical intervention. It would be perfectly reasonable not to do additional diagnostic studies in search of a surgical lesion in an individual who has already stated their unwillingness to participate in surgery. An unwillingness to have surgery is a realistic concern, and the need for diagnostic studies in this individual may then become a medical/legal issue; that is, when the patient needs to prove that there is an organic basis for the complaint even though he or she will not go on for surgery. That raises the ethical issue of providing testing with potential morbidity to a patient who may not act upon the results of that testing.

14. What percentage of patients at a chronic pain treatment center are "fakers"?

The incidence of malingering, which is a conscious attempt to deceive, is very small, as is the incidence of hysterical conversion reaction, which is an unconscious attempt to protect against a distressful psychological event. Physicians involved in diagnosing and treating patients within the chronic pain treatment center should treat all patients as though they have organic pathology.

15. How are chronic pain treatment centers certified?

The Committee on Accreditation of Rehabilitation Facilities (CARF) has a certification program for both inpatient and outpatient chronic pain treatment centers, as well as monomodality and multidisciplinary chronic pain treatment centers. While CARF accreditation is no guarantee of quality of the chronic pain treatment center, certification does, at least, indicate an effort on the part of the chronic pain treatment center to reach certain minimum standards. The American Academy of Pain Management also offers certification for chronic pain treatment centers.

16. How do multidisciplinary pain treatment centers differ from other types?

Multidisciplinary chronic pain treatment centers offer a full range of treatment and diagnostic evaluations, unlike monomodality centers, which focus on a single technique, or disease-specific centers that deal with only a single entity. Examples of disease-specific centers include headache clinics, cancer pain treatment centers, back pain clinics, facial pain clinics, pelvic pain clinics, and a host of others that focus on a single complaint of disease entity. Monomodality clinics may offer only acupuncture, physical therapy, relaxation training, biofeedback, chiropractic care, or psychiatric services. No single modality will treat all types of pain, but there is a tendency in monomodality clinics to try to treat more types of pain than can be effectively treated by their single modality. Also, there is a tendency to bias diagnoses toward the type of medical problem that is amenable to the type of treatment that the monomodality clinic offers. "When all you have is a hammer, everything looks like a nail."

17. What is the cost of the multidisciplinary pain treatment center?

Costs can vary from center to center, depending on the approach used. They can be as low as a single, outpatient consultation fee or as high as full hospital per diem rate.

18. What is the ideal result of multidisciplinary pain treatment center clinic evaluations?

The ideal result would be to establish an accurate diagnosis and treatment plan that is appropriate for the diagnosis. The treatment plan may be carried out within the center or referred back to physicians in the patient's area.

19. Which multidisciplinary pain treatment center is the best?

The answer to the question is best determined by the results that one wants to obtain. If the diagnosis is in doubt, a multidisciplinary pain diagnostic and treatment center that would determine the appropriate diagnosis is the best approach. If the diagnosis is already firmly established, a center with particular expertise in that area may be indicated. Under these circumstances, a disease-specific clinic may be ideal.

20. How should a pain center be chosen?

Ideally, by comparing published outcome data. Unfortunately, they are not readily available. Lacking that criterion, local or national reputation and representation in peer-reviewed journals should be sought.

21. Where can I get a list of multidisciplinary pain treatment centers?

The International Association for the Study of Pain, the American Pain Society, the American Academy of Pain Medicine, the American Academy of Pain Management, and CARF should be able to provide any interested physician with a list of the multidisciplinary chronic pain treatment centers.

22. What are the pitfalls in interpreting outcome studies?

This is probably the most important question of this chapter. Outcome study results can be distorted and biased by both patient selection and reporting practices. Patient selection is a critical determining factor in assessing the accuracy of a published outcome study. If patients are preselected by their ability to complete a rigorous program, the success rate will be skewed to the higher end. If "all presenters" are taken, the rate may be low. Another bias that occurs in patient selection is age of the injury. Insurance companies report that if an injured worker has been out of work for two years or more, the return-to-work rate is less than one percent. However, they also report that if an injured worker has been out of work for less than one year, the return-to-work rate is 85%. Reporting practices depend on "the definition of success." There are different criteria required for different groups. Some of the criteria commonly used are return to work (not valid in many elderly), decreased pain intensity (often of little value if there is no functional improvement), decreased drug intake (not valid if medications produce better function), or increased functional ability.

BIBLIOGRAPHY

1. Hendler N, Talo S: Role of the pain clinic. In Foley KM, Payne RM (eds): Current Therapy of Pain. Philadelphia, B.C. Decker, 1989, pp 22–23.
2. Hendler N: Validating the complaint of chronic back pain: The Mensana Clinic approach. Clin Neurosurg 35:385–397, 1989.
3. Pilowsky I, Katsikitis M: A classification of illness behaviour in pain clinic patients. Pain 57(1):91–94, 1994.
4. Sheehan J, Ryan M, McKay J, et al: Pain clinic attenders: An audit. Irish Med J 87(2):52–53, 1994.
5. Sullivan MD: Psychosomatic clinic or pain clinic. Which is more viable? Gen Hosp Psychiatry 15(6):375–380, 1993.
6. Sullivan MD, Loeser JD: The diagnosis of disability. Treating and rating disability in a pain clinic. Arch Intern Med 152(9):1829–1835, 1992.
7. Talo S, Hendler N, Brodie J: Effects of active and completed litigation on treatment results: Workers compensation patients compared with other litigation patients. J Occup Med 31(3):265–269, 1989.
8. Weir R, Browne GB, Tunks E, et al: A profile of users of specialty pain clinic services: Predictors of use and cost estimates. J Clin Epidemiol 45(12):1399–1415, 1992.

42. REGULATORY ISSUES

Ellen Cooper, M.S.

1. Do patients with painful medical conditions generally receive adequate treatment for pain?

No. Both acute pain and chronic pain due to cancer are generally undertreated. This is particularly true of treatment with opioid drugs. Surveys of patients in the postoperative period demonstrate that up to 75% suffer pain of moderate or severe intensity. Because virtually all postoperative pain can be controlled with proper medication, an alarmingly high number of patients suffer from unnecessary pain. Similarly, in patients with advanced cancer, simple drug regimens can provide relief for more than 70%; however, 70% of patients with advanced cancer still report significant pain. On a global scale, the statistics are even more alarming. More than 3½ million people suffer from cancer pain, but only a small fraction receive adequate treatment. This is particularly striking in view of the fact that pain can be controlled with appropriate drug regimens in approximately 90% of these patients.

2. What factors stand in the way of adequate pain treatment?

Barriers to good analgesic therapy exist on the professional, societal, and governmental levels. From a professional point of view, physicians and nurses often have the misconception that the prescription of opioid medications will lead inexorably to tolerance, dependence, and addiction. Even physicians who understand that this is not true tend to underprescribe medications, possibly because of fear of other side effects. Furthermore, the fear of regulation by outside agencies also tends to impede a physician's prescribing practices. Many physicians do not understand government regulations on opioid prescribing. Their fears are often unjustified. Certain government regulations, however, do limit prescribing practices. For example, in states that require a triplicate prescription for opioid medications, opioid prescribing decreases by about 50%. Patients also have many misconceptions about opioids. Their fear that the opioids represent a "last-ditch effort" makes them reluctant to take these drugs early in their disease. They also may be afraid of addiction, other side effects, or societal stigma that goes along with taking opioid medications.

3. Are patients with medical illness and no history of substance abuse at significant risk of addiction if opioids are administered?

Studies in patients with cancer have demonstrated that the main reason for escalating drug intake is progression of disease rather than aberrant behavior. This same pattern has been demonstrated in patients with pain due to nonmalignant disease. Although tolerance and physical dependence may occur, addiction is a rather rare phenomenon in patients treated appropriately with opioid medications for their pain.

4. What is pseudoaddiction?

Pseudoaddiction is a term most often used in reference to patients with cancer who demonstrate behaviors similar to those of addicts. Examples may include drug-seeking behavior, exaggerated complaints and symptoms, premature running out of medications, and family concerns about prescriptions. Such behaviors are usually the result of gross undertreatment of pain. Patients feel the need to exaggerate symptoms to obtain adequate medications. Adequate pain relief eliminates the abnormal behavior. This behavior can also be considered in patients with chronic pain.

5. Define addiction, physical dependence, and tolerance.

Addictive disease refers to a condition that inclines a person toward the use of a substance or substances in an uncontrolled, compulsive, and potentially harmful manner. The active state of addiction is characterized by preoccupation with obtaining or using a substance, loss of control over use of the substance, and continued use despite adverse consequences.

Physical dependence refers to the development of a withdrawal syndrome after abrupt cessation of a drug or on administration of an antagonist. Physical dependence is an expected consequence of prolonged use of a dependency-producing substance and may be accompanied by tolerance to pharmacologic effects of the substance.

Tolerance is present when increasing doses of a substance are required to sustain effects.

6. What are the differences among opiates, opioids, and narcotics?

Opioid is a generic term used to refer to codeine, morphine, and other natural and synthetic drugs whose effects are mediated by specific receptors in the central and peripheral nervous systems. The original term, opiate, was taken to mean any derivative of *Papaver somniferum*, the poppy plant that produces opium. Opioid also includes the endogenous opioids, such as endorphins and enkephalins. The term narcotic was initially used to denote a drug capable of producing sleep (narcosis). It was mainly applied to the opioids. However, narcotic has now become more of a legal term, used in reference to all substances covered by the 1961 Single Convention on Narcotic Drugs, including opiates as well as synthetic substances such as meperidine and fentanyl. The term covers not only the opioids but also cocaine and many other drugs of abuse.

7. What is the historical background that led the federal government to become involved in monitoring opioids?

Twentieth century governments recognized the dangers of abuse and trafficking of opioids, including opium, morphine, and heroin. Concerns, particularly about the opium trade in China and the Philippines, prompted governments throughout the world to join together and set controls on the ever-increasing diversion of illegal substances.

Studies of addicts in the 1950s and 1960s seemed to show that many addicts had their first exposure to opioids from prescriptions during a painful illness. This finding was incorrectly extrapolated to suggest that medical treatment was a common cause of addiction.

8. Which federal legislation regulates the prescribing practices of opioid analgesics?

The Harrison Narcotic Act of 1914 is the hallmark legislation that marked the federal government's interest in the prescribing and controlling of opioids. In 1961, the International Narcotics Control Board (INCB) was established to receive reports from governments about the movement of opioids and to ensure that supply and demand for opioids were in balance, hoping to prevent undersupply for legitimate purposes. All governments involved are required to furnish the INCB with statistics on an annual basis. In 1971, the Federal Comprehensive Drug Abuse Prevention and Control Act repealed all previous laws and took over the control of prescription drugs. Opioids and drugs with potential for abuse were placed into five schedules.

Hill summarized the source of the government's authority to regulate as follows:

> Government regulations on controlled substances are authorized by two legislative sources: a) Health Care Practice Acts (HPAs) including medical, nursing, pharmacy, dental, etc., which set standards of practice for the use of controlled substances and all other aspects of professional practice, and b) Controlled Substances Acts (CSA) which mandate how such substances are to be handled when used for medical purposes. States exert influence on health care practice through enactment of HPAs and the evaluation of practitioners' practices, based on standards set forth in them. Federal influence is primarily through CSAs.

9. What are the schedules into which all opioids and drugs with potential for abuse are classified?

Schedule I—Drugs with high abuse potential and no accepted medical use.

Schedule II—Drugs with a high potential for abuse and severe liability to produce psychic or physical dependence. Schedule II controlled substances consist of certain opioid drugs and drugs containing amphetamines or methamphetamines as the single active ingredient or in combination. Examples are opium, morphine, codeine, hydromorphone, methadone, cocaine, and oxycodone. Most drugs that are effective in the management of pain due to cancer fall into this category.

Schedule III—Drugs with a potential for abuse that is less than for that of drugs in schedules I and II. Examples are drugs containing limited quantities of certain opioids and certain nonopioid drugs.

Schedule IV—Drugs with a low potential for abuse that leads only to limited physical dependence or psychological dependence relative to drugs in schedule III. Examples are chlordiazepoxide and diazepam.

Schedule V—Drugs with a potential for abuse that is less than that of drugs in schedule IV and consist of preparations containing moderate quantities of certain opioid drugs. Examples include antidiarrheal medications.

This schedule does not necessarily make sense in terms of prescribing practices. In New York and many other states, triplicate prescriptions are required for schedule II and schedule IV drugs but not for a number of drugs in schedule III. The schedule is statute, but prescribing practices are regulations. Legislatively, it is much easier to change a regulation than it is to change a statute. In the late 1970s, when benzodiazepines were abused heavily, their schedule could not be changed, but the regulation requiring a triplicate prescription was changed.

10. How does the federal government define an addict?

Federal law defines an addict as "any individual who habitually uses any narcotic drug so as to endanger the public morals, health, safety, or welfare, or who is so far addicted to the use of narcotic drugs as to have lost the power of self-control with reference to his addiction." This definition is somewhat vague, but publications by the Drug Enforcement Administration (DEA) have made it clear that the agency's function is not to hinder physicians from use of opioid analgesics for providing pain relief.

According to the medical definition of addiction, the patient must have a preoccupation with securing the drug, spend a great deal of time either using the drug or recovering from its effects, and continue to use the drug despite harmful effects.

11. What is the role of the Drug Enforcement Administration?

The DEA is the federal agency responsible for enforcing national drug laws. It is responsible for registering manufacturers, distributors, and practitioners who handle opioid drugs. The DEA works closely with the Food and Drug Administration and the National Institute on Drug Abuse, which determines annual quotas for amounts of the various opioids that can be manufactured and distributed.

12. What have been the benefits, if any, of the federal drug control laws?

Before the establishment of the international drug control system, legitimate manufacturers were the primary source of abused opioid drugs, including heroin. After 1925, legitimate production of opioids has rarely been a source of drugs in the illicit traffic. Because the federal definition of addict is generally vague, it has not particularly limited prescribing practices. The goal of the federal laws has been to ensure that a therapeutic drug is available to patients when it is needed; laws do not restrict the size of prescriptions or set limits on refills. Many state laws, however, limit prescriptions to a one-month supply and may even limit the number of doses.

13. What have been some of the disadvantages of the federal drug control system?

By essentially waging a "war on drugs," the government has restricted medical access to essential medications. The drugs often necessary for managing pain in cancer and other medical illnesses are also the commonly abused drugs. This unfortunate coincidence has negatively influenced the effective treatment of pain worldwide. Regulation of drugs communicates that they are dangerous and reinforces fears. Legitimate manufacturers are concerned about production, physicians are reluctant to prescribe them, and patients are reluctant to take them for fear of being labeled "addicts." Forcing physicians to register with the federal government to prescribe opioid medications has significantly curtailed their use.

14. How have state laws affected prescribing practices?

Although most state controlled substance laws are patterned after the Federal Uniform Controlled Substances Act, there are many important differences. Many state laws do not recognize the essential medical uses of controlled substances or the importance of ensuring availability within the state. Many state laws do not have provisions allowing opioid treatment of intractable pain. Unlike the federal definition of addict, the New York State Controlled Substance Law defines addict as "a person who habitually uses a narcotic drug and who by reason of such use is dependent thereon." In addition, such "addicts" must be reported to the commissioner of public health. According to the above definition, all patients in New York who depend on class II narcotics have to be reported as addicts.

There is a great deal of confusion among physicians about what the laws really state. Nearly one-fourth of physicians polled in one study felt that it was probably a violation of federal or state laws to prescribe opioids for chronic nonmalignant pain. One-half of the physicians surveyed thought that prescription was illegal for patients with a history of opioid abuse. In point of fact, the law considers prescription of opioids illegal only if it is done to maintain an addiction. Methadone maintenance can be prescribed only through a methadone maintenance program.

15. Have state laws affected prescribing practices and availability of controlled substances?

In the United States, multiple-copy prescription programs exist in at least ten states (California, Texas, Michigan, Illinois, New York, Rhode Island, Indiana, Idaho, Hawaii, and Washington). They have resulted in statewide reductions of more than 50% in the number of prescriptions written for opioids. Physicians must purchase registered and numbered books of prescriptions from the state. Each prescription has three copies: one goes to the pharmacist, one to the office chart, and one to the state. Many state laws limit the amount of medication that can be dispensed at one time, increasing costs and number of patient visits to a physician. In addition, because there are so many layers of laws, confusion sometimes abounds and physicians become more reluctant to prescribe class II narcotics, frequently substituting less effective class III or nonopioid medications.

16. What is the INCB?

The International Narcotics Control Board (INCB), a Vienna-based arm of the United Nations International Drug Control Program, monitors the implementation of the Single Convention on Narcotic Drugs, an international treaty. The INCB recommends steps that governments and health professionals should take to address this problem.

17. What do governments perceive as the major impediments to the medical use of opioids?

In a survey of 65 governments performed by the INCB, concern about addiction was the most frequently stated impediment, appearing in 72% of statements. The next most frequently stated issue was insufficient training of health care practitioners. Sixty-five percent of the governments surveyed reported that they had national policies to improve the use of opioids.

18. Are legal restrictions on opioid prescriptions prevalent throughout the world?

The following is a direct quotation from a cancer pain release:

WHO has observed that physicians and pharmacists may become reluctant to prescribe or stock opioid analgesics due to strict requirements and fear of punishment. In the survey, many governments reported they required special government issued prescription forms and other special permissions. The maximum sentence for a physician who fails to comply with prescriber requirements is 22 years in prison; the maximum fine afforded is up to one million dollars. Some governments reported having mandatory minimum penalties as high as ten years in prison for such offenses. Forty-three percent of the governments required health professionals to report patients who receive opioid prescriptions.

None of the regulations in the United States are as stringent as this statement indicates. The majority of the legislation is aimed at avoiding diversion of drugs rather than regulating appropriate prescribing practices.

19. What are the educational issues surrounding lack of appropriate prescribing practices?

Standard physician education falls short of appropriately preparing physicians for necessary training in pain management. Even physicians who understand the pharmacokinetics and pharmacodynamics of analgesic medications tend to underprescribe them. State cancer pain initiatives are addressing the issues of education of health care providers and interaction with regulatory agencies.

BIBLIOGRAPHY

1. Clark HW, Sees KL: Opioids, chronic pain, and the law. J Pain Symptom Manage.
2. Cleeland CS, Cleeland LM, Dar R, Rinehart LL: Factors influencing physician management of cancer pain. Cancer 58:796–800, 1986.
3. Cleeland CS, Rotond A, Brechner T, et al: A model for the treatment of cancer pain. J Pain Symptom Manage 1:209–215, 1986.
4. Foley KM: The treatment of cancer pain. N Engl J Med 313:84–95, 1985.
5. Hill CS: Government regulation influences on opioid prescribing and their impact on the treatment of pain of nonmalignant origin. J Pain Symptom Manage 11(5):287–298, 1996.
6. International Opium Convention of 1925, League of Nations Treaties Series, vol. 81:317: Convention of 1931 for Limiting the Manufacture and Regulating the Distribution of Narcotic Drugs. League of Nations Treaty Series 139:301, 1931.
7. Max MB: Pain relief and the control of drug abuse: Conflicting or complementary goals? In Hill CS Jr, Fields WS (eds): Advances in Pain Research and Therapy, vol. 11. New York, Raven Press, 1989.
8. Porter J, Jick H: Addiction rare in patients treated with narcotics. N Engl J Med 302:123, 1980.
9. United States Code 802 (17): J Pain Symptom Manage 8(5):304, 1993.

INDEX

Page numbers in **boldface type** indicate complete chapters.